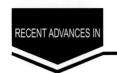

RECENT ADVANCES IN

Histopathology

CW00569503

Contents of *Recent Advances in Histopathology 16*

Edited by Peter P Anthony and Roderick N. M. MacSween

ISBN 0 443 04981 5
ISSN 0143 6953

You can place your order by contacting your local medical bookseller or Customer Services, Churchill Livingstone, Robert Stevenson House, 1–3 Baxter's Place, Leith Walk, Edinburgh EH1 3AF, UK. Tel: +44 (0)131 535 1021; Fax: +44 (0)131 535 1022

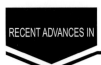

RECENT ADVANCES IN

Histopathology

Edited by

Peter P. Anthony MBBS FRCPath

Consultant Pathologist and Professor of Clinical Histopathology, Royal Devon and Exeter Healthcare NHS Trust and Postgraduate Medical School, University of Exeter, Exeter, UK

Roderick N. M. MacSween BSc MD FRCP(Glasg) FRCP(Edin) PRCPath FRSE FIBiol

Professor of Pathology, University of Glasgow; Honorary Consultant in Pathology, Western Infirmary, Glasgow, UK

David G. Lowe MD FRCS FRCPath FIBiol

Reader in Histopathology, St Bartholomew's and Royal London Hospital School of Medicine and Dentistry, Queen Mary and Westfield College, University of London, London, UK

NUMBER SEVENTEEN

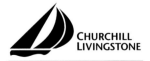

CHURCHILL LIVINGSTONE

EDINBURGH LONDON MADRID MELBOURNE NEW YORK SAN FRANCISCO AND TOKYO 1997

CHURCHILL LIVINGSTONE
Medical Division of Pearson Professional Limited
Distributed in the United States of America by Churchill
Livingstone Inc., 650 Avenue of the Americas, New York,
N.Y. 10011, and by associated companies, branches and rep-
resentatives throughout the world.

© Pearson Professional Limited 1997

First published 1997

ISBN 0 443 05766 4
ISSN 0143 6953

British Library Cataloguing in Publication Data
A catalogue record for this book is available from the British
Library.

Library of Congress Cataloging in Publication Data
A catalog record for this book is available from the Library of
Congress.

Medical knowledge is constantly changing. As new information becomes available, changes in treatment, procedures,
equipment and the use of drugs become necessary. The
editors and the publishers have, as far as it is possible, taken
care to ensure that the information given in this text is accurate and up to date. However, readers are strongly advised to
confirm that the information, especially with regard to drug
usage, complies with current legislation and standards of
practice.

Typeset by B. A. & G. M. Haddock, Scotland, UK
Printed in Singapore

Preface

The terms histopathology, anatomic pathology and cellular pathology are commonly applied to our discipline world-wide, with a degree of unease on our part and confusion on the part of others. It is, indeed, difficult to explain to a lay person what it is exactly that we do. Perhaps we should call ourselves clinical laboratory diagnosticians or some such. Whilst it is true that this is what we do most of the time, a glance at any textbook on the subject will reveal that there is much more to it than that. It is impossible to practise, teach or research in our discipline without both an understanding of basic science and a working knowledge of bedside clinical medicine in order to achieve the desired result. Whatever, the less than wholly satisfactory term we apply to ourselves may be a weakness, but what it reflects is our main strength. The current volume of Recent Advances demonstrates, again, the wide range of our repertoire. Take apoptosis, genes and their products, molecular biology, immunocytochemistry, breast cancer risk, criteria for benign versus malignant, microinvasion, difficulties in recognizing individual tumours, their natural history and response to treatment, endometriosis, renal disease, it is not all here, but each topic is dependent on fitting science, morphology and clinical practice together and, for the sake of completeness, a bit of epidemiology and the law are included as well. Once again, we are grateful to all our contributors for their excellent chapters on a variety of advances, problems and difficulties and we hope that the readers will find these of interest and useful. With this volume, two of us are leaving the series after 8 volumes and nearly 20 years. We have thoroughly enjoyed our collaboration and have derived enormous satisfaction from the knowledge that each number has been well received and appreciated. We have been efficiently supported by Churchill Livingstone and our thanks are due to them. David Lowe will carry on with James Underwood as co-editor. We wish them all possible success.

Peter Anthony
Roddy MacSween
David Lowe
1997

Contributors

T. J. Anderson PhD FRCPath FRSE
Reader in Pathology, The University of Edinburgh Medical School, Edinburgh, UK

R. M. Browne BSc PhD DDS FDSRCS
Professor of Oral Pathology, School of Dentistry, University of Birmingham, UK

C. H. Buckley MD FRCPath
Reader in Reproductive Pathology, St Mary's Hospital, University of Manchester, UK

B. Corrin MD FRCPath
Professor of Thoracic Pathology, Royal Brompton Hospital, London, UK

H. Fox MD FRCPath FRCOG
Emeritus Professor of Reproductive Pathology, St Mary's Hospital, University of Manchester, UK

A. J. Howie MD MRCPath
Senior Lecturer in Pathology, University of Birmingham Medical School, Birmingham, UK

J. Keeling FRCPath
Consultant Paediatric Pathologist, Royal Hospital for Sick Children, Edinburgh, UK

B. H. Knight CBE MD MRCP FRCPath DMJ
Professor of Forensic Pathology, University of Wales College of Medicine, Cardiff, UK

D. G. Lowe MD FRCS FRCPath FIBiol
Reader in Histopathology, St Bartholomew's and Royal London Hospital School of Medicine and Dentistry, Queen Mary and Westfield College, University of London, UK

D. G. MacDonald PhD FRCPath FDSRCPS(G)
Professor of Oral Pathology, University of Glasgow Dental School, Glasgow, UK

A. G. Nicholson BA, MRCPath
Consultant in Histopathology, Royal Brompton Hospital, London, UK

D. L. Page MD
Professor of Pathology and Director of Anatomic Pathology, Vanderbilt University
School of Medicine, Nashville, Tennessee, USA

R. H. W. Simpson BSc MMed FRCPath
Consultant Histopathologist, Royal Devon & Exeter Hospital, and Senior Lecturer
in Pathology, University of Exeter, UK

N. M. Smith BMedSci MRCPath
Consultant Paediatric Pathologist, Royal Hospital for Sick Children, Edinburgh, UK

T. J. Stephenson MA MD MHSM MRCPath
Consultant Histopathologist, Royal Hallamshire Hospital, Sheffield, UK

D. Tarin BSc DM FRCPath
Nuffield Reader in Pathology, Nuffield Department of Pathology and Bacteriology,
John Radcliffe Hospital, University of Oxford, Oxford, UK

A. H. Wyllie FRCPath FRCPE PhD FRSE FRS
Professor of Experimental Pathology, Head of Department of Pathology, The
University of Edinburgh Medical School, Edinburgh, UK

Contents

1

Apoptosis

A. H. Wyllie

Apoptosis is a coordinated and apparently internally programmed process that mediates the death of cells in a variety of biologically significant situations. Amongst these are the sculpting of tissues during development, atrophy in response to withdrawal of endocrine and other stimuli, selection of specific immunologically competent sub-populations in both T- and B-cell lineages during antigen stimulation and cytotoxic T-cell killing. Identical changes are observed in normal and tumour tissues exposed to low or moderate doses of chemotherapeutic agents or to ionising radiation. This chapter describes the structural changes that occur in apoptosis, their biochemical basis, the genes involved in their regulation and the pathology associated with some disorders in their regulation.

STRUCTURAL AND BIOCHEMICAL CHANGES IN APOPTOSIS

The characteristic morphological changes have been reviewed repeatedly (Kerr et al 1992, Wyllie et al 1988) and include dramatic shrinkage of cell volume accompanied by dilatation of the endoplasmic reticulum and convolution of the plasma membrane. The cell breaks up into membrane-bound near-spherical bodies containing structurally normal but compacted organelles. The nucleus, however, undergoes profound, initially discontinuous, chromatin condensation around the nuclear periphery. The nucleolus falls apart, its fibrillar centre lying bare of transcription complexes at the edge of the condensed chromatin. In those residual areas of the nuclear membrane not immediately underlined by condensed chromatin, nuclear pores appear to aggregate, but the nuclear lamina itself undergoes focal dissolution. These structural changes, completed with explosive rapidity, can be captured in histological and electron microscopic preparations, but are seen to advantage when apoptosis occurs *in vitro* under observation by time-lapse videomicroscopy. The ultimate fate of apoptotic cells in tissues varies. Some are swiftly phagocytosed. Others lose contact with their neighbours and basement membrane and so float into adjacent spaces. There is no acute inflammatory reaction. Because of this, and the speed with which apoptotic cells are removed, major cell losses can be effected within tissues with minimal disturbance of overall tissue structure.

1

Elements of apoptosis had been recognised before 1972, when the term was first used, but had been designated by a variety of names, often used exclusively in particular circumstances, so concealing the generality of the process (e.g. Councilman bodies in viral hepatitis, Civatte bodies in the epidermis, tingible bodies in macrophages of reactive lymph nodes). The changes of apoptosis contrast with those of *necrosis*, the disruption of cells observed in acute, high-dose toxicological exposure or severe hypoxia. Here, the injured cells swell and their plasma membranes rupture to release proinflammatory material from the cell interior into the extracellular space. The term apoptosis was originally introduced to emphasise the difference between the two modes of death and to suggest that the stereotyped morphology results from a common underlying mechanism. Spectacular biochemical and molecular biological evidence is now available to support this hypothesis.

Many of the biochemical processes responsible for these structural changes are understood. Several cytoskeletal proteins and the nuclear lamins undergo site-specific proteolysis. Activation of transglutaminase results in protein-protein cross-linking. Nuclease activation cleaves first large (50–300kb), then small (oligonucleosomal) fragments of chromatin. On the cell membrane, phosphatidylserine appears on the outer as well as the inner surface, and previously hidden residues, including charged amino sugars, become exposed on the cell surface, features which, amongst others, appear responsible for the recognition of apoptotic cells by their neighbours. No satisfactory explanation is yet available for the rapid cell shrinkage. Mitochondrial membrane potential alters some time before the structural changes begin.

Some of these features have been exploited to devise means for identifying and counting apoptotic cells in cultures and tissues. Chromatin condensation is still a satisfactory criterion, visualised either in tissue sections or in cell suspensions by staining with haematoxylin, Feulgen or acridine orange. The flat, ground-glass quality of the chromatin is unmistakable. The rapid reduction in cell volume, unaccompanied by breakdown of the selective permeability of the cell membrane, can be monitored by flow cytometry, often in association with some loss of DNA signal (to form the so-called hypodiploid peak). The multiple broken ends of nuclear DNA have been detected by various *in situ* end-labelling techniques, whilst those cells in which oligonucleosomal fragments are cleaved generate 'chromatin ladders' on DNA gel electrophoresis. A brilliant newcomer is Annexin V which selectively binds phosphatidylserine and therefore marks apoptotic cell membranes. Unfortunately Annexin V is helpful only when it can be applied selectively to the cell exterior (e.g. in cells in suspension, or by perfusion of tissues). Since normal cells have phosphatidylserine on the inner surface of the cell membrane, all cells are decorated indiscriminantly in tissue sections.

A GENETIC PATHWAY OF CELL DEATH

Observations made in the nematode *Caenorhabditis elegans* laid the foundations for understanding the genetic organisation of the control of cell death (Hengartner 1996). Because the development of this organism follows an invariate pattern, it is possible to define, in time and position, all 131 cell deaths that occur during development from egg to adult worm which contains around 1000 cells in all if germ cells are excluded. Structurally, these unquestionably 'programmed' deaths share many features with mammalian apoptosis, including cytoplasmic condensation and susceptibility to phagocytosis. The nematodes can be exposed to chemical mutagens to induce mutations randomly in the germline. Abnormal cell-death phenotypes (e.g. absence of expected deaths or presence of supernumerary deaths) can then be found in the resulting organisms, and the genes responsible can be identified by a combination of conventional and molecular genetic approaches. In this way, distinct genes or sets of genes have been shown to determine cellular susceptibility to death, the initiation or forestalling of the death event, and the recognition, phagocytosis and destruction of the dying cell. Amongst the most comprehensively studied nematode genes involved in this pathway are *ced3*, which initiates death (Yuan et al 1993), and *ced9* which inhibits it (Hengartner & Horvitz 1994). Strikingly, each of these genes is the homologue of a family of mammalian genes engaged in similar functions in apoptosis. It seems probable, however, that most of the other nematode death genes will have similar structural and functional homologues in mammals.

The effector pathway

Ced3 is a member of a family of cysteine proteases that exhibit preference for cleavage adjacent to Asp residues (Takahashi & Earnshaw 1996, Whyte 1996). It appears to be the only member of the family present in *C elegans*, but mammalian cells contain about 10 distinct members, of which the earliest to be purified was the interleukin-1β converting enzyme (ICE). There is some evidence that different members of this protease family are preferentially expressed in different cell types, but it is also certain that several proteases within a single cell can cooperate in a catalytic cascade. Partial redundancy may exist between the activities of different proteases. Four pieces of evidence show that these proteases drive the effector process of apoptosis. First, when added to suitably prepared nuclei from non-dying cells *in vitro*, the proteases swiftly induce in them all the characteristic structural changes that are seen in the nuclei of authentic apoptotic cells. Second, although present in most cells in inactive form, the proteases can be recovered in an activated state from cells about to enter apoptosis. Sometimes the level of transcription of the proteases also increases after injury. Third, apoptosis can be prevented by inhibitors of the cysteine proteases, some of them oligopeptides custom-designed to block the enzyme active site, others naturally occurring. Finally, animals in which the proteases (e.g. ICE) have been deleted in the germline by genetic manipulation show deficiency in induction of apoptosis by at least some stimuli.

Full understanding of the effector process of apoptosis will require complete definition of the substrates of these proteases. Curiously, interleukin-1β itself, being an extracellular cytokine, is unlikely to be a major player in the activation of apoptosis, but several other interesting intracellular proteins have cleavage sites specific for the ICE-family proteases. Thus, the cytoskeletal proteins fodrin and actin are cleaved by ICE-family proteases, as are lamins A, B and C, and major components of the peripheral nuclear 'cage'. These substrate associations probably underlie the changes in cell shape and attachment, and the dissolution of the nuclear lamina described above. There is still some uncertainty over the precise identity of the nucleases that cleave chromatin DNA, hence it is not yet possible to define how they may be activated through the protease cascade, but inhibitors of the ICE-family proteases do inhibit the chromatin cleavage of apoptosis. Further, the nuclear protein poly ADP-ribose polymerase – a high-abundance nuclear protein that contributes to recognition and repair of DNA double-strand breaks – is consistently cleaved and inactivated early in apoptosis by the ICE-family protease CPP32, perhaps preventing wasteful, and ultimately abortive, DNA repair reactions.

Bcl-2 related proteins

Ced9 shares 25% sequence homology with the proto-oncogene *bcl-2*, which can substitute for it functionally in *C. elegans* cells (Hengartner & Horvitz 1994). Again, *ced9* is the only known member of its family in the nematode, but *bcl-2* is a member of a large family of homo- and heterodimerising proteins, some of which are survival-supporting, like *bcl-2* itself and *bcl-xL*, whilst others are death promoting (e.g. *bax, bad* and *bcl-xS*) (Nuñez & Clarke 1994, Farrow & Brown 1996, White 1996). *Bcl-xL* and *bcl-xS* are the products of alternative splicing of the same transcript. Still further proteins, structurally more distantly related, interact with members of the *bcl-2* family and modify their activity. Amongst these are bag, a protein that enhances the survival function of *bcl-2* and *bik* (*nip4*). Hence, in mammalian cells, this family of proteins represents a level of control over the initiation of apoptosis that is capable of responding to multiple regulatory signals. *Bcl-2* has a C-terminal membrane anchor, and is largely found in association with the outer leaflet of the mitochondrial membrane, the cytosolic face of the plasma membrane, and the nuclear membrane. Perhaps surprisingly, the basis of its survival function is still not clear. It was suggested that it might protect against the injurious effects of oxygen radicals, but this cannot be its only mode of action, since *bcl-2* still protects cells from apoptosis in conditions in which oxygen radical generation is undetectable (Jacobson & Raff 1995). Very recent protein structural evidence suggests that *bcl-2* and *bcl-xL* may behave as pore-forming proteins, perhaps regulating transport of critical signalling molecules across mitochondrial and ER membranes.

Activation events

Most cells appear to be endowed with at least some members of the ICE family of proteases. The initiation of apoptosis must, therefore, be critically dependent upon the initial activation of the proteolytic cascade and the set-point of the intracellular balance between lethal and survival factors, such as proteins of the bcl-2 family and probably others. The existence of this type of ready-to-fire endogenous self-deletion mechanism would explain the uniform manifestations of apoptosis in many different situations, as described at the outset, but it also requires that an enormous variety of stimuli, physiological and pathological, must be able to access and ultimately activate the common effector pathway. It is already clear that several widely different signalling systems play this role.

Cytokines play an important part in the signalling of cell death. CD95/apo-1/fas is a transmembrane receptor of the CD40/TNF receptor family expressed in hepatocytes, enterocytes and some lymphocytes (Peter et al 1996). Historically, it was the first receptor associated with apoptosis to be discovered (Trauth 1989), and *fas* signalling is now known to be one of the key events in CTL killing (Krammer et al 1994). On binding the *fas* ligand – a cytokine of the tumour necrosis factor (TNF) family – CD95/apo-1/fas trimerises and initiates a chain of protein-protein interactions, first between its own cytosolic domain and a cytosolic protein called FADD (for 'protein containing fas activated death domain'), and then between FADD and a newly-discovered ICE-family protease, FLICE (for FADD-like ICE), so triggering the ICE-family protease cascade (Boldin et al 1996, Muzio et al 1996). This remarkable, direct, non-transcriptional coupling between activation of a cytokine-receptor by its ligand and the effector proteases may explain the rapidity of fas-induced killing.

TNF and its receptor may be coupled to a rather similar system, through a binding protein called TRADD (TNF receptor activated death domain protein), but the TNF receptor also signals by a separate pathway, involving a different region of its cytosolic domain, and requiring activation of the transcriptional regulator NFkB. Fluctuation of the prevailing levels (both upwards and downwards) of many other cytokines can also initiate apoptosis in the appropriate circumstances.

Ceramide is a signal for activation of apoptosis that is released from membrane lipids on digestion by sphingomyelinases. Sphingomyelinase is activated within seconds of plasma membrane damage, for example by ionising radiation (Haimovitz-Friedman et al 1994), and hence ceramide affords a means of coupling this type of cell injury to apoptosis. Fibroblasts from patients with Nieman-Pick disease, an inherited human disorder caused by constitutive loss of acid sphingomyelinase activity, show relative resistance to apoptosis in response to ionising radiation, indicating the importance of ceramide generation in signalling injury in, at least, this cell type. Interestingly, ceramide production is negatively regulated by protein kinase C, suggesting that cells with high protein kinase C activity might be preferentially protected against some types of injury. The role of ceramide signalling in apoptosis is yet to be completely clarified, but it seems probable that it modulates the balance of signals in the injured cell, *e.g.* between the MAP (mitogen activated protein) and JUN kinase pathways (Xia et al 1995). Sphingomyelinase activation and ceramide production have been shown to be one result of activation of *CD95/fas* and the TNF receptor. The significance of this is not clear, but it does offer an example of how signalling for apoptosis by one pathway (*e.g.* cytokine receptors) can tap into another, such as ceramide production, which under other circumstances (*e.g.* ionising radiation exposure) may itself be one of the lead events. Branching and converging mechanisms of this type go far towards explaining the stereotyped sequence of structural changes that accompany apoptosis: regardless of the initiating stimulus, the effector events eventually include a closely similar set of molecular interactions.

Finally, **cell killing by cytotoxic T-cells** exemplifies a rather different activation event (Greenberg 1996). Part of the killing mechanism depends upon signalling from *fas* ligand (present on the T-cell membrane) to *fas* on the target cell. Since cytotoxic T cells express both *fas* and *fas* ligand, this may provide a mechanism for internal regulation of their population. However, such a mechanism would not have the general quality required of a cytotoxic T-cell response, since not all potential target cells express *fas*. Cytotoxic T-cells also possess granules that release a variety of effector proteins, amongst them perforin, which permeabilizes the target cell membrane and granzyme B, which penetrates the target cell and is activated by perforin attack. Granzyme B is not a cysteine protease, although it shares the property of effecting cleavage after Asp residues, but it has the capacity to activate ICE and CPP32, and thus can trigger the effector events dependent on the cysteine protease cascade in the target cell.

ONCOGENE AND ONCOSUPPRESSOR GENE CHANGES

Many proto-oncogenes and oncosuppressor genes influence cell susceptibility to apoptosis.

C-myc is an immediate-early growth response gene, activated within minutes of mitogen stimulation. Its continued expression is required for re-initiation of consecutive cell cycles. In contrast, experimentally engineered expression of *c-myc*, in the absence of growth factor stimulation (e.g. in fibroblasts deprived of IGF-1), leads to apoptosis (Harrington et al 1994). All the domains of *c-myc* that are necessary for its mitogenic action are also obligatory for stimulation of apoptosis, and the growth factor-starved, *c-myc*

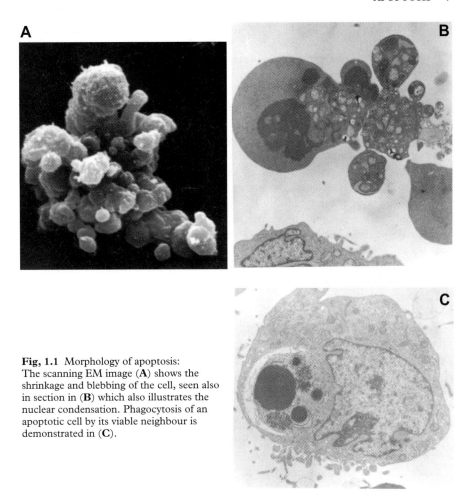

Fig, 1.1 Morphology of apoptosis:
The scanning EM image (**A**) shows the
shrinkage and blebbing of the cell, seen also
in section in (**B**) which also illustrates the
nuclear condensation. Phagocytosis of an
apoptotic cell by its viable neighbour is
demonstrated in (**C**).

stimulated cells show evidence of entry into S-phase prior to death, leading to
the view that the induction of apoptosis and replication by *c-myc* are somehow
two sides of a single process, the eventual outcome (successfully completed
rounds of cell replication or death by apoptosis) being determined by local
growth factor availability. Were a regulatory system like this to exist in tissues,
it could provide an interesting means of restricting cell proliferation to those
topologically defined areas in which the appropriate growth factors were available, and deleting potentially proliferating cells from areas where such factors
become scarce.

The association of susceptibility to apoptosis with stimuli for entry to the
cell cycle is not restricted to *c-myc*. Germline knockout of the oncosuppressor
gene ***rb-1*** produces populations of neurons in the developing CNS that cannot
leave the cell cycle and enter G_0: such cells are particularly susceptible to apoptosis (Clarke et al 1992). Similarly, cultured fibroblasts normally respond to

DNA injury by leaving the cell cycle and entering G_0, a process for which *rb-1* is essential. Such fibroblasts respond to DNA injury by apoptosis if their exit to G_0 is blocked by expression of the adenovirus E1a protein, or by the papillomavirus HPV16 E7 protein, which inactivates *rb-1* (Slebos et al 1994). Very similar results derive from fibroblasts engineered to express the transcription factor **E2F-1**, normally sequestered by active *rb-1* (Skowronski et al 1996).

The role of the proto-oncogene **bcl-2** and its family members in protecting cells from apoptosis has been discussed above. Several other proto-oncogenes have similar functions (although the mechanisms involved are still somewhat obscure), amongst them the protein tyrosine kinases *src* (Arends et al 1993, Liu et al 1995, Skowronski et al 1996), **abl** (Chapman et al 1994) and oncogenes of the *ras* family (Arends et al 1993, Wu & Levine 1994). The literature on ras proteins contains some apparent contradictions, however, perhaps because ras proteins are also involved in the signalling pathways that lead to death (Skowronski et al 1996).

p53 **and interferon response factor (IRF)-1** are oncosuppressor genes that signal DNA injury. Transcription of IRF-1 is also induced by viral infection. Both oncosuppressors can induce apoptosis in the appropriate circumstances (Clarke et al 1993, Lowe et al 1993, Tanaka et al 1996). Induction of apoptosis by *p53* is observed most consistently in cells committed to the cell cycle. Thus, there is a complex inter-relationship between *p53* changes, apoptosis, and the expression of genes (such as *rb-1*) that remove cells from cycle (Fig 1). The effects of *p53* and IRF-1 also appear to be interdependent. Perhaps most importantly, expression of either *p53* or IRF-1 may be coupled either to the initiation of apoptosis or to cell cycle arrest. The factors determining which of these very different end-points is chosen are not well defined: some are clearly cell type specific; others may relate to local concentrations of growth factors; still others depend on the nature of the injury stimulus.

Despite its major importance in triggering apoptosis in damaged cycling cells, *p53* appears to play a minor role in the apoptosis of normal development or in response to physiological regulatory stimuli in postnatal life. Thus, the majority of *p53* null mice are developmentally normal, and the apoptosis response of their thymocytes to glucocorticoids, or their prostatic epithelium to oestrogens, is intact.

APOPTOSIS AND THE PATHOGENESIS OF DISEASE

The preceding paragraphs have outlined the regulatory machinery that controls apoptosis. In the following paragraph examples of circumstances are discussed in which deviant regulation of apoptosis is responsible for the manifestations of disease.

Shigella dysentery

Shigella flexneri invades the lamina propia of the large bowel, gains access to the lymphoid tissue there, and is phagocytosed by macrophages. For non-virulent strains this can be the end of the story, but virulent strains possess plasmids encoding genes that permit escape from the phagosome into the cytosol, and then activation of the host cell's ICE-family proteases. The result is, therefore, apoptosis of the host macrophage and release into the lamina propia of activated ICE. Much of the pathogenesis of shigella dysentery is explained by this mechanism, which permits the organism to evade digestion, kill the protective mucosal macrophages (Zychlinsky et al 1994) and, through the pro-inflammatory cytokine IL-1, set up a florid inflammation.

Acquired immunodeficiency syndrome (AIDS)

The pathogenesis of AIDS is intimately associated with apoptosis. Peripheral blood lymphocytes of HIV-positive individuals tend to respond to mitogenic stimuli by apoptosis. The mechanism may relate to the effect of gp120 (an HIV protein which is released into the circulation) in stimulating expression of *fas*. Further, both gp120 and the viral tat protein increase cellular expression of *fas* ligand. *Fas*-armed cells are at increased risk of initiating apoptosis. Moreover, the cells deleted in this way are, preferentially, the CD4+ T-cells that would normally be responsible for generating or re-awakening immunological memory and so establishing immunity to intercurrent, opportunistic infections (Dhein et al 1995, Debatin 1996). Over the course of the disease, these CD4+ T-cells are progressively depleted, with corresponding failure in immune response to infections of this type. Eventually, the disease progresses to the familiar pattern of greatly depleted circulating CD4+ T-cells and repeated infection by low-virulence organisms.

Autoimmune disorders

The *lpr* and *gld* mouse strains carry constitutional loss-of-function mutations in, respectively, *fas* and its ligand (Wu et al 1993). The mice have huge lymph nodes with remarkably little cell proliferation, but also reduced apoptosis and a tendency for the development of an autoimmune disease similar to systemic lupus erythematosus (SLE). The implication is strong that, through failure of signalling via *fas*, auto-reactive T-cell clones have not been deleted. Similar genetic defects in *fas* or *fas* ligand are rare in human SLE, but patients with autoimmune disorders often possess soluble forms of *fas* and *fas* ligand in their circulation. It seems plausible that these soluble but ineffective molecules compete with their cell-bound homologues, and so diminish authentic *fas* signalling.

Degenerative diseases, stroke and other conditions

There is great temptation to attribute to apoptosis the loss of neurons in various CNS degenerations, e.g. Alzheimer's disease, Parkinson's disease and chronic infective dementias. Almost invariably, however, the identification of the mode of cell loss in these protracted human conditions is retrospective and speculative. One outstanding exception is the inherited condition of spinal muscular atrophy. Here there is an inherited defect of a gene implicated, for independent reasons, as an endogenous apoptosis inhibitor. Apoptosis inhibitors are also currently being explored as potentially beneficial therapeutic agents in the immediate aftermath of stroke and myocardial infarction, in the hope of arresting the death of hypoxic cells in the vicinity of the infarct.

Viral infection and persistence

Viruses, particularly DNA viruses, require a mechanism that protects their genome from the consequences of host cell apoptosis. Successful viral infection implies that the cell makes available to the virus its own replication machinery. However, as described earlier, powerful mechanisms exist to activate apoptosis when replicative cells are confronted with double-strand breaks (potential recombination sites) or with viral infection. Indeed, the core strategy of apoptosis – protease and nuclease activation, cell death and efficient phagocytosis and destruction of the deleted cells – seems ideally designed to abort viral infection. It is therefore significant that the genomes of many successful viruses – despite their relatively small size – code for proteins that block apoptosis by one route or another. Examples (Shen & Shenk 1995) include the adenovirus E1B55K and 19K proteins which, respectively, bind to *p53* or functionally imitate *bcl-2* through binding its natural inhibitors bik (nip4) and other related proteins; HPV16 E6, which inactivates *p53*; EBV BHRF-1, a *bcl-2* analogue; EBV LMP-1 which binds and putatively inactivates signalling molecules in the TNFR2 and CD40 receptor pathways; baculovirus *p35* and cow pox virus crmA, inhibitors of cysteine proteases, and baculovirus IAPs (inhibitor of apoptosis proteins), whose point of action in blocking apoptosis is not yet fully defined (Clem et al 1996), but which is homologous to the gene that is deficient in spinal muscular atrophy.

Carcinogenesis

The question therefore arises whether abrogation of apoptosis is a general mechanism in carcinogenesis (Lowe et al 1994, Wyllie et al 1994). Many non-viral carcinogenic agents also work through survival and replication of cells bearing mutations. In at least a proportion of cases, these mutations arise through double-strand breaks (e.g. after ionizing radiation) or single-strand breaks introduced in the process of modifying DNA altered by the production of photoproducts (e.g. after UV light) or bulky adducts (as following exposure to many chemical carcinogens). Although mechanisms exist to repair all these lesions, there is at least the theoretical possibility that the damaged DNA may be a sufficient stimulus for the initiation of apoptosis.

Would failure in apoptosis, therefore, permit clonal outgrowth of cells with inappropriate recombination events, facilitated by double-strand breaks, or other forms of DNA modification resulting from inappropriate repair? Worse still, might cancer therapeutic agents, which also introduce DNA damage, have the effect of accelerating the acquisition of new aggressive mutations in certain tumours where mechanisms of apoptosis are deficient? These questions are still not resolved, but there are several points to be made.

First, there is interesting circumstantial evidence that the silencing of *p53* leads to the production of tumours in cell populations in which there is a high level of apoptosis through deficiency in *rb*. Thus, in tissues of genetically modified animals bearing tissue-specific inactivation of *rb* there is a high level of apoptosis, but simultaneous inactivation of *p53* in these tissues renders them prone to carcinogenesis (Howes et al 1994, Pan & Griep 1994, Saenz-Robles et al 1994). Similarly, human diploid fibroblasts lacking functional *rb* die or produce clonogenic survivors at low frequency on exposure to a metabolic growth signal (the drug N-phosphonoacetyl-L-aspartate, PALA), whereas those lacking both *rb* and *p53* show ten-fold greater survival, including many cells with aneuploid genomes including intrachromosomal amplification (White et al 1994), features often found in the genome of malignant tumours. Similarly, in a skin carcinogenesis model in which chemicals were applied directly to the skin of mice, so producing both benign and malignant tumours, the animals without *p53* showed accelerated development of carcinomas relative to wild type mice. However, these observations fall short of the demonstration that blockade of apoptosis leads directly to the appearance of cells with a high mutation incidence – an observation critical to the hypothesis under test. Indeed, in the murine skin carcinogenesis model the results show that, although more malignant tumours were engendered in the *p53*-deficient animals through exposure to the carcinogen, the total number of tumours was reduced. It is difficult to explain this result if the only effect of the *p53* deficiency were to rescue from death cells damaged by the carcinogen. In another animal model, blockade of apoptosis in the lymphoid system through constitutive expression of *bcl-2* produced lymphomas of low-grade malignancy, whilst concurrent blockade of *p53*, in the absence of exposure to carcinogens, produced much more aggressive tumours (Strasser et al 1994). This result would not be predicted if the only role of *p53* deficiency were to permit survival of cells committed to death as a result of incidental DNA damage, since this is precisely the effect predicted for *bcl-2* expression, which shows a different phenotype. Critical experiments are therefore required to demonstrate the survival of mutated cells in *p53*-deficient tissues. Unexpectedly, the probability that such cells survive and proliferate proves to be related to cell type.

There is now good evidence that in the lymphoid lineage exposure to ionizing radiation in the absence of *p53* permits the survival of substantially increased numbers of mutated cells, whereas exposure to similar doses of ionizing radiation in the presence of *p53* permits the survival of an immeasurably small proportion of the population (Griffiths et al 1996). Mutation incidence in pre-B cells derived from the bone marrow of *p53* null animals, measured by the production of *hprt*-deficient colonies *in vitro*, was at least 10-fold higher than in the unirradiated controls. Moreover, analysis of the *hprt* locus in the mutated colonies revealed a high proportion of major rearrangements of the gene, the type of lesion predicted following deletion and recombination events, the DNA lesions that might otherwise have been detected and have triggered apoptosis in the presence of *p53*. These observations are, of course, entirely compatible with the high incidence of lymphoid tumours in *p53* null animals in general.

However, *p53* null animals exposed to ionizing radiation show high levels of apoptosis in many other tissues in which tumours are recorded rarely or not at all, such as the gastrointestinal tract or the liver (Clarke et al 1994). Similar mutation incidence measurements from the gastrointestinal tract reveal that presence or absence of *p53* has very little effect on mutation at doses up to 400 rads, although higher doses are indeed accompanied by many-fold enhanced mutation incidence. These data can be explained on the basis that *p53* is not the only mechanism coupling radiation damage to cell death in the gastrointestinal tract. Although the *p53* null animal experiences intense apoptosis in the basal region of the gastrointestinal crypt within 2–6 hours of exposure to radiation, none of which appears in the wild-type animal, there is a second phase of apoptosis affecting crypt cells 24–48 hours later, and this occurs regardless of the *p53* genotype. Interestingly, this second, *p53*-independent phase of apoptosis is not present in lymphoid populations.

These data thus emphasize that the role of *p53* in coupling DNA damage to apoptosis may vary from tissue to tissue, and this may have a significant bearing on the importance of *p53* in permitting mutagenic events associated with cancer. This role in coupling a cellular stress to death may also affect tumour progression (i.e. the evolution of more aggressive properties). Thus, there is evidence that *p53* is induced in hypoxia. In the relatively hypoxic centre of tumour masses this induction of *p53* apparently leads to apoptosis, so favouring the outgrowth and eventual domination of *p53* deficient cells. However, in some cell types, *p53* clearly does not couple injury to death, though it may still promote cell cycle arrest. One such tissue is liver. Normal murine hepatocytes fail to initiate apoptosis by a *p53*-dependent route after exposure to either gamma radiation or UV-C (which mimics many carcinogens in its effect on DNA). Perhaps significantly, hepatocellular tumours are not a feature of *p53*-deficient animals.

REFERENCES

Arends MJ, McGregor AH, Toft NJ et al 1993 Susceptibility to apoptosis is differentially regulated by *c-myc* and mutated *Ha-ras* oncogenes, and is associated with endonuclease availability. *Br J Cancer* **68**: 1127–1133
Boldin M, Goncharov TM, Goltsev YV et al 1996 Involvement of MACH, a novel MORT

1/FADD-ineracting protease, in *Fas/APO-1* and TNF receptor-induced cell death. *Cell* **85**: 803–815

Chapman RS, Whetton AD, Dive C 1994 The suppression of drug-induced apoptosis by activation of *v-abl* protein tyrosine kinase. *Cancer Res* **54**: 5131–5137

Clarke AR, Maandag ER, van Room M et al 1992 Requirements for a functional *Rb-1* gene in murine development. *Nature* **359**: 328–330

Clarke AR, Purdie CA, Harrison DJ et al 1993 Thymocyte apoptosis induced by *p53*-dependent and independent pathways. *Nature* **362**: 849–851

Clarke AR, Gledhill S, Hooper ML et al 1994 *p53* dependence of early apoptotic and proliferative responses within the mouse intestinal epithelium following γ-irradiation. *Oncogene* **9**: 1767–1773

Clem RJ, Hardwick JM, Miller LK 1996 Anti-apoptotic genes of baculoviruses. *Cell Death & Differentiation* **3**: 9–16

Debatin KM 1996 Disturbances of the CD95 (APO-1/*Fas*) system in disorders of lymphohaematopoietic cells. *Cell Death & Differentiation* **3**: 185–189

Dhein J, Walczak H, Westendorp MO et al 1995 Molecular mechanisms of APO-1/*Fas* (CD95)-mediated apoptosis in tolerance and AIDS. *Behring Inst Mitt* **9**: 13–20

Farrow SN, Brown R 1996 New members of the *bcl-2* family and their protein partners. *Curr Op Genet Devel* **6**: 45–49

Greenberg AH 1996 Activation of apoptosis pathways by granzyme B. *Cell Death & Differentiation* **3**: 269–274

Griffiths SD, Clarke AR, Healy LE et al 1996 Absence of *p53* promotes propagation of mutant cells following genotoxic damage. *Oncogene* (in press)

Haimovitz-Friedman A, Kan C-C, Enleiter D et al 1994 Ionizing radiation acts on cellular membranes to generate ceramide and initiate apoptosis. *J Exp Med* **180**: 525–535

Harrington EA, Bennett MR, Fanidi A et al 1994 *C-myc* induced apoptosis in fibroblasts is inhibited by specific cytokines. *EMBO J* **13**: 3286–3295

Hengartner MO 1996. Programmed cell death in invertebrates. *Curr Op Genet Devel* **6**: 34–38

Hengartner MO, Horvitz JR 1994 *C. elegans* survival gene *ced-9* encodes a functional homologue of the mammalian proto-oncogene *bcl-2*. *Cell* **76**: 665–676

Howes KA, Ransom N, Papermaster DS et al 1994 Apoptosis or retinoblastoma: alternative fates of photoreceptors expressing the HPV-16 E7 gene in the presence or absence of *p53*. *Genes Dev* **8**: 1300–1310

Jacobson MD, Raff MC 1995 Programmed cell death and *bcl-2* protection in very low oxygen. *Nature* **374**: 814–816

Kerr J F R, Wyllie A H, Currie A R 1972 Apoptosis: a basic biological phenomenon with wide-ranging implications in tissue kinetics. *Br J Cancer* **26**: 239–257

Krammer PH, Dhein J, Walezak H et al 1994 The role of APO-1-mediated apoptosis in the immune system, *Immunol Rev* **142**: 175–191

Liu H-J L, Eviner V, Predegart GC et al 1995 Activated H-*ras* rescues E1A-induced apoptosis and cooperates with E1A to overcome *p53*-dependent growth arrest. *Mol Cell Biol* **15**: 4535–4544

Lowe SW, Schmitt EM, Smith SW et al 1993 *p53* is required for radiation induced apoptosis in mouse thymocytes. *Nature* **362**: 847–849

Lowe SW, Jacks T, Housman DE et al 1994 Abrogation of oncogene-associated apoptosis allows transformation of *p53*-deficient cells. *Proc Natl Acad Sci USA* **91**: 2026–2030

Muzio M, Chinnaiyan AM, Kischkel FL et al 1996 FLICE, a novel FADD-homologous ICE/CED-3-like protease, is recruited to the CD95 (Fas/APO-1) death-inducing signalling complex. *Cell* **85**: 817–827

Nuñez G, Clarke MF 1994 The *bcl-2* family of proteins: regulators of cell death and survival. *Trends in Cell Biol.* **4**: 399–403

Pan H, Griep AE 1994 Altered cell cycle regulation in the lens of HPV-16 E6 or E7 transgenic mice: implications for tumor suppressor gene function in development. *Genes Dev* **8**: 1285–1299

Peter ME, Kischker FC, Hellbardt S et al 1996 CD95 (APO-1/*Fas*)-associated signalling proteins. *Cell Death & Differentiation* **3**: 161–170

Saenz-Robles MT, Symonds H, Chen J et al 1994 Induction versus progression of brain tumor development: differential functions for the pRB and *p53* targeting domains of simian virus 40 TAg. *Mol Cell Biol* **14**: 2686–2698

Shen Y, Shenk TE 1995 Viruses and apoptosis. *Curr Op Genet Devel* **5**: 105–111

Shimizu S, Eguchi Y, Kosaka H et al 1995 Prevention of hypoxia-induced cell death by *bcl-2* and *bcl-XL*. *Nature* **374**: 811–813

Skowronski EW, Kolesnick RN, Green DR 1996 *Fas*-mediated apoptosis and sphingomyelinase signal transduction: the role of ceramide as a second messenger for apoptosis. *Cell Death & Differentiation* **3**: 171–176

Slebos RJ, Lee MH, Plunkett BS et al 1994 *P53*-dependent G$_1$ arrest involves prb-related proteins and is disrupted by the human papillomavirus 16 E7 oncoprotein. *Proc Natl Acad Sci USA* **91**: 5320–5324

Strasser A, Harris AW, Jacks T et al 1994 DNA damage can induce apoptosis in proliferating lymphoid cells via *p53*-independent mechanisms inhibitable by *bcl-2*. *Cell* **79**: 329–340

Takahashi A, Earnshaw WC 1996 ICE-related proteases in apoptosis. *Curr Op Genet Devel.* **6**: 50–55

Tanaka N, Ishihara M, Lamphier MS et al 1996 Cooperation of the tumour suppressors IRF-1 and *p53* in response to DNA damage. *Nature* **382**: 816–818

Trauth BC, Klas C, Peters AMJ, Matzku S, Möller P, Valk W, Debatin K-M, Krammer PH. 1989 Monoclonal antibody mediated tumor regression by induction of apoptosis. *Science* **245**: 301–305

White E 1996 Life, death and the pursuit of apoptosis. *Genes Dev* **10**: 1–15

White AE, Livanos EM, Tlsty TD 1994 Differential disruption of genomic integrity and cell cycle regulation in normal human fibroblasts by the HPV oncoproteins. *Genes Dev* **8**: 666–677

Whyte M 1996 ICE/CED-3 proteases in apoptosis. *Trends in Cell Biology* **6**: 245–248

Wu J, Zhou T, He J et al 1993 Autoimmune disease in mice due to integration of an endogenous retrovirus in an apoptosis gene. *J Exp Med* **178**: 461–468

Wu X, Levine AJ 1994 *P53* and E2F cooperate to mediate apoptosis. *Proc Natl Acad Sci USA* **91**: 3602–3606

Wyllie A H, Kerr J F R, Currie A R 1980 Cell death: The significance of apoptosis. *Int. Rev Cytol* **68**: 251–306

Wyllie AH, Carder PJ, Clarke AR et al 1994 Apoptosis in carcinogenesis: the role of *p53*. Cold Spring Harbor Symposia on Quantitative Biology. 403–409

Xia Z, Dickens M, Raingeaud J et al 1995 Opposing effects of ERK and JNK-p38 MAP kinases on apoptosis. *Science* **270**: 1326–1331.

Yuan JY, Shaham S, Ledoux S et al 1993 The *C. elegans* cell death gene *ced-3* encodes apoptosis similar to mammalian interleukin-1β-converting enzyme. *Cell* **75**: 641–652

Zychlinsky A, Kenny B, Menard R et al 1994 IpaB mediates macrophage apoptosis induced by *Shigella flexneri*. *Mol Microbiol* **11**: 619–627

2

Prognostic markers and mechanisms of metastasis

D. Tarin

The phenomenon that some tumours can spread in the human body to form secondary colonies which grow and destroy distant organs was first recognised and termed metastasis by Jean-Claude Recamier in 1829. Since then, this remarkable deductive insight, which was formulated without any complicated methods of investigation, has exerted radical and far reaching effects on tumour biology and medicine. As a result, it is now universally accepted that metastasis is a common event which severely compromises the patient's chances of survival. Even when there are no clinically detectable metastases at the time of removal of the primary tumour, the prognosis is uncertain, because disseminated cells may be dormant or grow slowly in vital organs for several years.

Pathogenetically, metastasis is a pattern of tumour cell behaviour which results from failure of some of the most fundamental regulatory processes controlling body organisation in multicellular organisms. Normal tissue structure and function depend on strict localisation of different cell lineages in defined territorial domains and on tight regulation of cell turnover kinetics. Metastasis is, therefore, a striking manifestation of anomalous cell differentiation in which cells break these basic restrictions and embark on disorderly formation of new tissues which grow relentlessly in ectopic sites. This chapter presents evidence that this apparently random and unpredictable phenomenon is governed by coordinated but inappropriately activated genetic programmes normally concerned with physiological processes. From this evidence a new hypothesis is proposed, namely that in adults such programmes are usually operational only in defined populations of migratory white blood cells which follow precisely specified recirculatory pathways. Such complex inappropriate behaviour is probably not the product of a single malfunctioning gene, but of a coordinated, interactive hierarchy of genetic loci, which in a neoplastic setting could be regarded as the metastasis operon.

The following account assumes that readers are already familiar with general clinical and pathological aspects of tumour metastasis presented in recent reviews of this subject (Tarin 1992, 1995) and will focus on recent advances in clinically and scientifically relevant areas including early diagnosis, mechanisms of metastasis and prognostic markers.

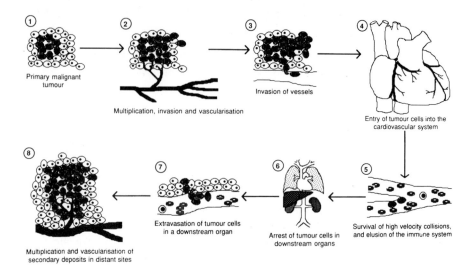

Fig. 2.1   The multistep process of metastasis

MECHANISMS OF METASTASIS

Current understanding of the spread of cancer in the human body (Darling & Tarin 1990) is based on much previous research which has established that:

- It is a stepwise phenomenon, summarised in Figure 2.1, capable of being undertaken by only a subpopulation of cells within the heterogeneous masses of cells in a tumour (Fidler & Kripke 1977, Fiedler 1978)

- It is highly selective and results in massive losses amongst the cells which set out on the venture (Fidler 1970, Weiss 1980, Juacaba et al 1989) and

- It is stably propagated over many generations among the cells which survive to form secondary tumour deposits (Fidler & Kripke 1977)

Hence it is likely to be genetically programmed (Tarin 1992, Hayle et al 1993) and to result from inappropriate expression of genes normally responsible for some similar or homologous activity of non-neoplastic cells. It is also known from many clinico-pathological studies that metastasis can occur by a number of anatomical pathways (Willis 1973, Tarin 1992) and that the distribution of tumour deposits tends to occur in non-random, organ-selective patterns that vary with the site and type of the primary tumour. Therefore, it appears to be subject to modulation by local environmental factors in the sites of tumour cell arrest, an interpretation also favoured by experimental data (Tarin et al 1984a,b, Horak et al 1986, Nicolson & Dulski 1986, Naito et al 1987). The advances to be discussed are consistent with and support this earlier framework of understanding.

The driving force of metastasis and how it is activated

Metastasis is a complex multistep process. The various individual phenotypic properties involved and their activation in a coordinated manner at the relevant stages in metastasis are therefore unlikely to be the sole, or even the primary factors responsible for this behaviour. The essential disturbance initiating and driving metastasis probably lies in the mis-regulation of a pleiotropic gene or operon which normally directs and coordinates the migration of cells which are patrolling the body via vascular routes on homeostatic or surveillance missions. It would be expected that this category of genes would be silent in sedentary cells. Hence, it is postulated that inappropriate activation of such a gene or genes, in tumours derived from cells which do not normally have such a patrolling function, could result in the emergence of metastatic behaviour.

When Fidler & Kripke (1977) isolated tumour cell clones with different metastatic capabilities from a common parent cell line, they clearly demonstrated the phenomenon of tumour cell heterogeneity and simultaneously showed that cell lineages with distinctive and heritable patterns of dissemination co-exist and propagate themselves in neoplasms. This was soon confirmed by others (Nicolson 1982, Poste 1982) and also verified in samples derived from fresh primary and secondary tumours (Tarin & Price 1979). It follows that the capability to metastasize is an inherent property of individual tumour cells and is reproduced with substantial reliability by their progeny. An attempt was made to transfer metastatic capability by transfection of high molecular weight DNA from highly metastatic human tumour cells into nonmetastatic or weakly metastatic mouse tumour cells. Figure 2.2 shows the design of the experiment. The purpose of arranging it so that the donor and recipient lines were of human and mouse origins respectively was that it would be possible to identify human DNA in the transfectants by the detection of human Alu repeat sequences.

A cell line was eventually produced that had greatly augmented metastatic properties (Hayle et al 1993). The transfected line (designated AH8 Test) not only colonised the lungs but also formed secondary tumours in several extrapulmonary sites including the skin, skeletal muscles, bone, liver, diaphragm, spleen and heart. There were no comparable effects when DNA from several non-metastatic or non-tumourigenic sources was used. Secondary transfection of metastatic capability with DNA obtained from a metastasis formed by the primary transfectant line was also accomplished. Concomitant transfer of human DNA through both transfection cycles in this experiment was confirmed by a variety of methods including Southern blot analysis, in situ hybridisation and Alu-PCR using primers recognising human-specific Alu repeat sequences. Finally, a 2858 base pair fragment containing human DNA was cloned from a genomic library of a cell line (AH8 LMC), derived from a metastasis, made by the original transfectants (Bao et al 1996). This clone contained human Alu repeats and had a novel sequence containing coding domains. In preliminary experiments involving reverse transcription of mRNA and amplification of the resulting cDNA with specific primers designed to anneal to one of the putative coding regions, there was evidence that it is expressed in fresh tissues from human malignant tumours and their metastases (unpublished observations). Further studies

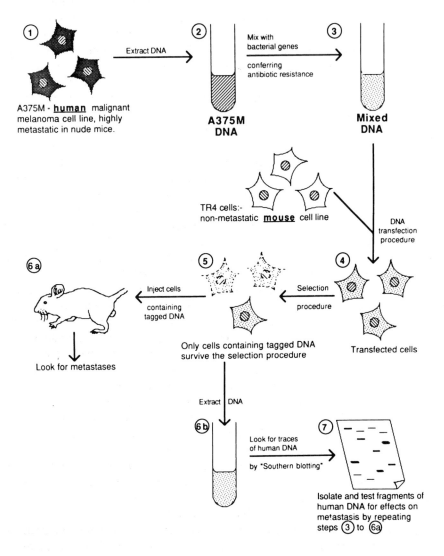

Fig. 2.2 Transfection of metastasis

involving cloning the rest of the gene and studying its expression in further fresh primary and secondary human tumours are now indicated. In particular, it will be interesting to know whether the fragment we have sequenced and other human DNA which we have cloned from the same genomic library are expressed in circulating white blood cells.

These observations indicate that components of the metastatic phenotype are heritable, are probably conserved in evolution (because genes transferred from humans are apparently functional in mouse cells), and are conferrable on tumour cells by transfer of genomic DNA. Also, it seems that whatever genetic activity is responsible for this new behaviour, it is not repressed by regulatory genes in the non-metastatic recipient cells. It must be noted, however, that transfected genes can be expressed in host cells in which the endogenous counterparts are inactive e.g. β globin in fibroblasts (Pellicer et al 1980). Stringent selection pressure was imposed on our transfectants by injecting them into animals and screening for metastases, from which new cell lines were derived for further work. Hence, cells in which relevant transfected genes were 'dominated' by host repressors would not have made metastases and thus may never have come to our attention. The existence of such repressor genes has been reported by Steeg et al (1988) who have cloned a sequence from the K1735 mouse melanoma (designated nm23) which they believe may have metastasis inhibitory activity. Subsequent studies by the same and other laboratories (Bevilacqua et al 1989, Barnes et al 1991, Hennessy et al 1991) indicated that the level of expression of the nm23 gene family has a good inverse correlation with the extent of spread of human breast cancer and may provide useful prognostic information on the course of the disease. However, other studies on human colon cancer (Cohn et al 1991, Haunt et al 1991) and on neuroblastoma (Hailat et al 1991) are contradictory and more information is needed to evaluate the precise relationship of nm23 function to the metastatic process.

The idea of balanced interaction between stimulatory (activator) and inhibitory (repressor) elements is attractive. In the transfection experiments described above, it is possible that a deranged regulatory complex, capable of pleiotropic control over numerous other genes lower in the hierarchy as well as on responses to local environmental conditions, took control of misregulated host cell genes, thereby imposing metastatic behaviour. Otherwise, it seems unlikely that a range of individual, abnormally functioning genes, necessary for such a complicated process, could have been collectively transferred through two rounds of transfection, as the experimental data indicate. These findings therefore suggest that the metastatic process is orchestrated by one or a few functionally inter-related controlling genetic elements, which are probably in close physical proximity. The most attractive candidate for this role is the group of genes which programmes the nomadic behaviour of white blood cells. These cells possess an exceptional degree of freedom to move around the body and to traverse other tissues, that is denied to other cell lineages, but it is predetermined, orderly and strictly controlled. The human DNA fragment recovered from the transfectants which were induced to become metastatic offers the possibility of a tool with which to unravel the complexities of normal and inappropriate long-distance cell migration.

Influence of the organ micro-environment on metastatic dissemination

In recent years it has become apparent that the non-neoplastic cells and tissues of the organ housing the primary tumour are not passive bystanders in the metastatic event. Figure 2.3 summarises the many interactive processes that exist between normal and neoplastic cells.

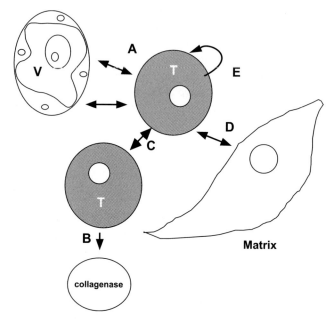

Fig. 2.3 Cell interactions in metastasis. T = tumour cells; F = host stromal cells; V = vascular channel lined by endothelium. A = tumour cell/matrix interaction; B = tumour cell lysing matrix; C = signalling between tumour cells; D = signalling between tumour and host normal cells; E = autocrine feedback loop

Effects of interactions with local non-neoplastic cells — orthotopic implantation experiments

Experiments involving inoculation of tumour cell lines derived from various organs including the breast (Price et al 1990) colon (Morikawa et al 1988, Breaslier et al 1987) kidney (Naito et al 1986) and prostate (Stephenson et al 1992) into nude mice by different routes have shown that metastatic behaviour is expressed more vigorously when the tumour cells grow initially in an orthotopic site (i.e. in the organ corresponding to that from which the tumour cells originated). Although subcutaneous inoculation of tumour cells is very convenient and growth of the resulting tumour can easily be monitored, some tumour cell lines which clearly have metastatic potential when implanted orthotopically do not metastasize at all from a subcutaneous location where they form a well circumscribed tumour surrounded by a dense fibrous capsule (Fidler 1990).

The nature of the influence exerted by the host organ in facilitating metastatic behaviour by cells which have the necessary intrinsic properties is unknown. However, recent experiments (Fabra et al 1992) involving co-culture of highly metastatic colon carcinoma cells with fibroblast monolayers derived from the colon, lung and skin produced data suggesting that the tumour cells only showed significant attachment and invasion through the monolayer when co-cultured with fibroblasts of orthotopic origin. Although these tumour cells produced a 68 kDa collagenase type IV (gelatinase) when cultured on plastic or on colonic or lung fibroblasts they did not do so when cultured on skin fibroblasts. This experiment illustrates how interactions between tumour cells and non-neoplastic stromal cells of the host organ can influence the expression of properties relevant to invasive and metastatic behaviour.

Effects of the local extracellular matrix (ECM)

In vivo, carcinoma cells are surrounded by cellular connective tissue composed of fibroblasts, endothelium and other cells in a dense network of extracellular matrix proteins which provides them with a three dimensional structural framework and influences their behaviour. The interdependency of these elements in pathological processes is illustrated by recent experimental observations which indicate that tumour growth and behaviour is influenced by non-cellular elements of the adjacent connective tissue matrix. It was found that a reconstituted basement membrane derivative termed Matrigel, composed mainly of laminin, collagen type IV, heparan sulphate proteoglycan and entactin, greatly enhances the ability of various types of malignant cells to form tumours (Fridman et al 1992, Bao et al 1994) and accelerates the growth rate of the resulting tumours. In addition, Matrigel facilitates not only the growth but also the metastasis of tumours formed by the human breast carcinoma line MDA-MB-435 in nude mice and by some of the clones derived from it (Bao et al 1994). Orthotopic inoculation into the mammary fat pad acts synergistically with Matrigel to facilitate all cell lines to rapidly produce large tumours, but does not induce non-metastatic clones to become metastatic, though the incidence and number of metastasis by metastatic clones is increased. Such results indicate that pulmonary metastasis after inoculation, either subcutaneously or into mammary fat pad, or with Matrigel, primarily depends on the intrinsic properties of tumour cells (Hayle et al 1993), i.e. on patterns of gene expression programming for metastatic behaviour, but it can be modulated by local micro-environmental factors. The mechanisms by which this effect is mediated deserve further investigation, to ascertain whether they might be vulnerable to pharmacological hindrance. This could have the dual clinical benefit of retarding the growth of secondary tumours as well as impeding further dissemination.

Interactions between different sub-populations of tumour cells

Interactions between metastatic and non-metastatic tumour cell populations co-existing in composite neoplasms can affect metastatic performance. This has been demonstrated by experiments utilising cell lineages marked with a dominant selectable genetic marker for neomycin resistance. Cells transfected with this gene integrate it into their genome and become indelibly marked with a label that replicates with the cell. The presence of the marker can be detected by several methods including survival of the cells in neomycin-containing culture medium, PCR and Southern blot hybridisation. As the site of integration is random in each transfected cell and stable over many cell generations in vitro and in vivo, its progeny can be recognised and distinguished from those of other neomycin-resistance tagged cells because they have a characteristic pattern of bands in Southern blots of their digested DNA when probed with the neomycin resistance gene.

Experiments using such tumour cell lines have produced surprising and thought-provoking results (Moffett et al 1992, Baban et al 1993). A single metastatic (M^+) clone was each time combined with a mixed polyclonal non-metastatic (M^-) population and both were distinctly and recognisably marked. This made it possible to ascertain the fates of clones with different metastatic capabilities during tumour progression and metastasis and to evaluate their relative contributions to the extent of disease.

It was found that metastatic and non-metastatic cell lineages co-existed in most of the primary tumours formed by these cell mixtures. A cell lineage which was invariably non-metastatic when growing on its own could, when grown to form a primary tumour in combination with cells from a metastatic clone, be found thriving in distant metastatic deposits with surprising frequency. In fact, occasional metastases from such mixed tumours contained no detectable cells of the metastatic lineage. These observations established beyond reasonable doubt that, in certain circumstances, non-metastatic cell lineages can in the presence of metastatic ones participate in the formation of secondary deposits.

Such endowment of a tumour cell lineage with a new, clinically significant, capability which it had not manifested before, by another coexisting cell population, could contribute to the geometric increase of the metastatic burden in the host. These effects of heterogeneous evolving clonal cell lineages upon each other during the lifetime of a tumour may influence not only its clinical behaviour but also its therapeutic susceptibilities.

The relocation of tumour cells to distant organs —
the vascular phase

Transit into and out of local vessels and passage through the basement membranes

Once tumour cells have activated the genetic programmes which are required for dissemination from the primary lesion, they spread outwards into the surrounding tissue releasing proteases, especially collagenases (Hashimoto et al 1973, Ogilvie et al 1985) and destroy much of the adjacent extracellular matrix (Tarin 1967, 1969, 1972) until they collide with local capillary blood vessels and lymphatics. The capillaries are ensleeved in basement membranes which are not readily breached by most normal cells. However, this membrane has to be traversed by cells programmed to disseminate via vascular channels or by lymphocytes circulating through the tissues on routine surveillance missions.

Basement membranes contain laminin and collagen type IV. The latter is selectively digested by a specific metalloprotease, gelatinase, otherwise known as collagenase IV. This is known to be secreted in elevated quantity by several types of tumour cells (Liotta et al 1979). It has also been suggested that this enzyme is secreted in greater quantity by cell lines which are highly metastatic than by ones which are not (Liotta et al 1980), and there is little doubt that various specialised collagenases are actively involved in tumour invasion and metastasis. Even so, the production of these lytic agents in tumours is spatially and temporally erratic, and there is no direct evidence that collagenase levels in individual lesions are of diagnostic or prognostic significance (Ogilvie et al 1985).

Laminin binds to specific receptors on the cell surface and to collagen IV molecules and it has been found to be very effective in increasing cell attachment to surfaces coated with collagen IV. It has therefore been suggested that circulating tumour cells with increased numbers of vacant laminin receptors have a greater chance of binding to the laminin, in any exposed sections of the basement membranes investing capillaries, and have enhanced chances of forming metastases. Some evidence favouring this interpretation has been provided by experiments which showed that there is a correlation between Dukes' stage of human colorectal cancer and degree of laminin receptor expression in the tumour tissue (Cioce et al 1991). In other studies it was found that if highly metastatic B16 melanoma cell lines were treated before intravenous inoculation with the receptor binding fragment of laminin or with antibodies to laminin, this resulted in reduced numbers of pulmonary metastases (Terranova et al 1982, Barsky et al 1984). It was also found that pretreatment with whole laminin increased metastatic colony formation and it was concluded that this was because the globular end regions of the molecule contained binding sites for collagen IV which promoted attachment of the cells to exposed basement membranes.

Interactions between tumour cells and basement membrane components can be rate limiting events in the migration of tumour cells to set up secondary colonies but they are only part of the process of entry into and exit from the circulation. Important interactions also occur with the vascular endothelium during transit. Little is known of the exact mechanisms by which tumour cells insinuate between apposed endothelial cells to gain access to the lumen but they appear to induce retraction of the latter and then to squeeze through the resulting gap. Once they are in the lumen, they detach from the wall and are carried away by the passing lymph or blood. Lymph ebbs and flows sluggishly and transit is gradual, erratic and slow, whereas blood flows in a laminated jet-stream throwing suspended cells against the walls of vessels and each other and exposing them to severe shear forces and collisions. Studies with labelled tumour cells (Fidler 1970), artificially released into the blood, have indicated that there is a rapid high mortality during and just after vascular transport, partly due to mechanical damage and partly to destruction by natural killer cells (Hanna 1982) and other mediators of non-specific immunity such as macrophages (Fidler 1985).

Arrest, attachment and exit from the circulation

Tumour cells which enter the lymph may be carried peripherally or centrally according to the vagaries of its ebb and flow and are arrested either in the lumen of the lymphatic channels, or in the subcortical sinus of the next most proximal lymph node. Those tumour cells which enter the blood stream directly arrive in the capillaries of the next organ downstream, in which many impact and die, but labelling studies (Fidler 1970, Potter et al 1983, Juacaba et al 1989) show that many pass through to the arterial side of the circulation which scatters them to all organs of the body within 15 minutes.

For a cell to succeed in producing a secondary tumour colony, it must then re-emerge from the vascular compartment, multiply in the parenchyma of the new host organ and induce the local mesenchymal and vascular endothelial cells to grow in and supply it with its metabolic needs. Normal adult cells do not seem able to colonise and flourish in ectopic sites after natural or experimentally induced dissemination via the circulation (Price et al 1982). Indeed, it is probably essential for the preservation of normal body organisation that accidentally shed normal cells cannot survive in other sites (Horak et al 1986). The cells of some human (Tarin et al 1984a) and animal (Tarin & Price 1979) tumours do not seem able to do so either, even when infused directly into the venous blood for several months. This raises two basic questions, namely: what are the special properties needed for a cell to enter, survive and grow in ectopic sites after vascular dissemination and, given that malignant cells soon reach all organs, why do they form tumours only in some and not in others?

Tumour cells passing through the capillary bed of an organ can become detained there either because they are in a cellular embolus which becomes lodged in the vessel, or as recent evidence suggests (Rice & Bevilacqua 1989, Bao et al 1993), because they encounter large adhesion molecules trailing in the fluid stream and happen to be displaying receptors to which they bind.

Such molecules and their ligands have been found to be important in the recirculatory traffic of leucocytes (Springer 1990). The increased presence of some of them on the surfaces of metastatically competent tumour cells suggests that these cells may have acquired such properties as a result of inappropriate activation of genetic programmes regulating the migration of normal leucocytes. Being also capable of unlimited multiplication and of releasing angiogenic factors and other cytokines required for initial primary tumour formation before dissemination, such tumour cells might be suitable candidates for seeding other sites and producing secondary tumour colonies. Candidate leucocyte/lymphocyte adhesion molecules recently reported to be markedly more expressed on metastatic tumour cells than on non-metastatic counterparts include the integrin VLA-4, the selectin Elam 1 and the glycoprotein CD 44.

In a study of VLA-4 expression in several human tumour cell lines using fluorescence activated cell analysis, immunocytochemistry and pathological evaluation of metastatic behaviour in vivo, there was evidence indicating differential expression of this molecule on metastatic cell populations compared with non-metastatic ones (Bao et al 1993). VLA-4 is known to be a receptor for at least two ligands, namely the inducible endothelial adhesion molecule VCAM-1 and the extracellular matrix component fibronectin, and is thought to be mechanistically important in the attachment and diapedesis of lymphocytes. In particular, VLA-4 has been shown to be a receptor used by lymphocytes homing to Peyer's patches (Holzmann & Weissman 1989). VCAM-1 is expressed on vascular endothelial cells stimulated by cytokines such as IL-1 and TNFα, but is not produced constitutively at high level in most normal endothelia (Osborn et al 1989). However, it is expressed on bone marrow cells and it has recently been reported (Matsuura et al 1996) that transfection of a Chinese hamster ovary cell line, which normally metastasises to the lungs, with the VLA-4 gene in a high expression vector, resulted in bone metastases. Furthermore, unpolymerised fibronectin is present in solution in the plasma and its insoluble fibrous form is an important constituent of the extracellular matrix coating cell surfaces and anchoring them to the substratum. Hence, tumour cells displaying VLA-4 could, under appropriate circumstances, have a greater capacity to attach themselves to the lining of small capillaries, compared with tumour cells without such surface properties. It follows that VLA-4 may be an important molecular participant in the metastatic process.

Some recent in vitro studies (Lauri et al 1991, Martin-Padura et al 1991) also implicated VLA-4 integrin and its counter-receptor VCAM-1/INCAM 110 in the attachment of tumour cells to vascular endothelium and documented heterogeneity of VLA-4 expression among clones derived from a human melanoma metastasis. Evidence was provided that this expression correlated with the extent of adhesion of tumour cells to cytokine stimulated endothelial cells and that this could be blocked or reduced by monoclonal antibodies to VLA-4 and VCAM-1. Antibodies to other cell attachment receptors, such as ELAM-1, ICAM-1 and VLA-5 and to fibronectin, were ineffective in reducing cell binding in this assay. Similarly, Rice & Bevilacqua (1989) reported that treatment of IL-1 stimulated endothelial cells with an antibody to INCAM110, which is believed to be identical to VCAM-1 (Hemler 1990), markedly inhibited the binding of a number of melanoma cell lines to them. However, this antibody did not significantly reduce attachment of HT-29 colon carcinoma cells, though in separate assays with this cell line, an antibody to the selectin ELAM-1 was effective. These data have been confirmed and extended by Lauri et al (1991). Such observations raise the possibility that different carcinoma cell lines express different adhesion receptors and that this may affect the distribution of their metastases in vivo.

Some time ago, Butcher and colleagues (reviewed in Picker et al 1989) reported that some CD44 epitopes, recognised by the Hermes-3 mAb, function as lymph node receptors or 'homing' molecules which enable circulating lymphocytes to recognise and circulate through regional lymph nodes. Further monclonal antibodies to this antigen later became available and Stamenkovic et al (1991) used one of them to isolate and clone a complementary DNA (cDNA) sequence coding for the standard polypeptide backbone of this protein. Since then it has been established that CD44 is a large gene which can produce a family of diverse protein isoforms by alternative splicing (Hofmann et al 1991, Screaton et al 1992, Tolg et al 1993).

More recent work by two other groups (Birch et al 1991, Sy et al 1991) suggested that the CD44 gene, and particularly the 80–90 kD protein which it produces, plays a role in metastasis of certain human tumour cell lines when they are implanted in nude mice. Meanwhile, Gunthert et al (1991) had obtained results indicating that a newly identified variant isoform of glycoprotein CD44, is required for metastatic behaviour of rat pancreatic adenocarcinoma cells. Using an antibody raised to a metastatic clone of this tumour cell line, they isolated a cDNA sequence corresponding to this new variant form of rat CD44 glycoprotein and found that it contained previously unidentified exons. Re-introduction of a specially constructed piece of DNA designed to over-express this particular sequence, unique to the metastatic counterpart, into a non-metastatic clone of the same rat tumour cell line, induced metastatic behaviour (Gunthert et al 1991, Rudy et al 1993). This observation, although impressive, has not yet been independently confirmed by another laboratory. Also, it has recently been reported that deletion of both alleles of the CD44 gene in a metastatic mouse lymphoma cell line did not abrogate its metastatic capabilities (Driessens et al 1995).

In view of these findings, it became important to know whether metastatic human tumours and ones without clinically detectable metastases differentially express CD44 products, particularly the new variant sequence. Analysis of the pattern of expression of this gene in a series of human breast, bladder and colon carcinomas using the technique of reverse transcription followed by the polymerase chain reaction (RT-PCR) provided surprising results (Matsumura & Tarin 1992). All samples of neoplastic tissue showed gross over-expression

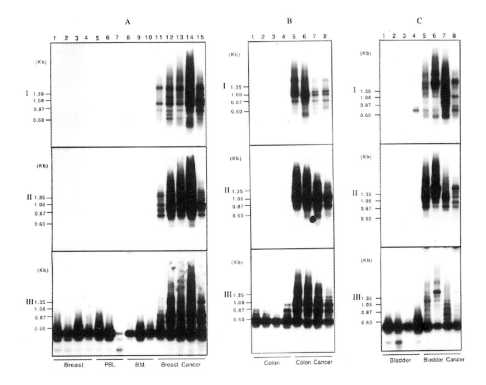

Fig. 2.4 Autoradiograph of filters hybridised with probes for exon 7 (v2), exon 11 (v6) and standard form CD44 in rows I, II and III respectively after amplification with primers P1 and P4. **Panel A** shows results for normal breast tissue (lanes 1–4), peripheral blood leucocytes (PBL) from healthy volunteers (lanes 5–7), sternal bone marrow (BM) from patients with heart disease (lanes 8–10), and breast cancer tissue (lanes 11–15); **Panel B** shows non-neoplastic colon tissue in lanes 1–4, normal tissue in lanes 1 and 3 and inflamed colonic mucosa, from Crohn's disease in lane 2 and ulcerative colitis in lane 4 and tissue from primary colonic cancer in lanes 5–8; **Panel C** shows normal bladder tissue (lanes 1–4) and primary bladder cancer tissue (lanes 5–8). Note the overexpression of CD44 gene products in cancer samples resulting in long dense smears not seen in normal counterparts. (Reproduced with permission from Matsumura et al 1994.)

of several alternatively-spliced products of the CD44 gene and none of the samples from non-neoplastic tissue did so (Fig. 2.4). Also, the differences in pattern between metastatic tumours and ones without any clinical indication of metastasis were obvious (Matsumura & Tarin 1992), thereby providing a potentially useful diagnostic and prognostic marker which is being evaluated. Small quantities of one or two variant isoforms can be detected in most non-neoplastic tissues and so it is important to recognise that alternatively spliced versions of the CD44 molecule are not exclusively associated with lymphocyte migration or with neoplasia and metastasis. New evidence indicates that the

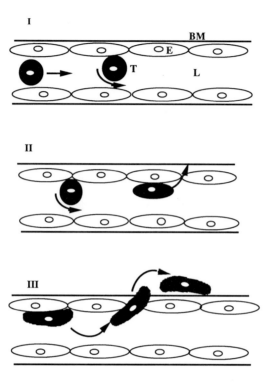

Fig. 2.5 Growth and survival in the new organ environment. After the disseminated tumour cell has hooked itself out of the passing stream of fluid, it must execute a number of complex manoeuvres to reach the interior of a new organ.

several isoforms of the CD44 family of proteins are involved in many different processes in normal tissues including adhesion to substrates, hyaluronate endocytosis and metabolism, drug uptake and metabolism, signal transduction and growth factor feedback loops.

Thus, there is reason for concluding that a number of integrin and other cell adhesion molecules involved in lymphocyte traffic contribute mechanistically to the process of tumour metastasis, either synergistically or individually, according to cell type and/or the stage of the process. It is possible that the presence of some such molecules on the surfaces of metastatic tumour cells is coincidental, but the results of the transfection experiments of Chan et al (1991), Gunthert et al (1991) and of Rudy et al (1993) suggest otherwise. Further studies now in progress should clarify this issue.

The above evidence that cell surface determinants which are normally involved in lymphocyte traffic may play a role in metastasis is valuable and attractive, because it suggests a normal cellular activity which might be the prototype for this aspect of neoplastic behaviour. This in turn indicates new avenues for investigating how the abnormal behaviour originates.

Growth and survival in the new organ environment

After the disseminated tumour cell has hooked itself out of the passing stream of fluid, it must execute a number of complex manoeuvres to reach the interior of a new organ (Fig. 2.5). The picture here is incomplete but the available evidence indicates that, again, it uses some of the same mechanisms used by leuko/lymphocytes. Hence the tumour cell needs to ratchet-in the trailing endothelial adhesion molecule to which it initially becomes attached and latch firmly onto the endothelial surface, so that it may roll along with the flow until it engages tighter binding receptors to flatten its profile. The tumour cell thereby reduces the risk of being sheared off, after which it can induce endothelial cell retraction and pull itself through the discontinuity in the lining between retracting endothelial cells using VLA 4 and laminin receptors, lyse the basement membrane by focal secretion of collagenase IV and crawl through the resulting gap. Even if, and when it has accomplished these feats, the tumour cell still has to multiply and communicate with surrounding indigenous cells to attract a supporting mesenchymal framework and a vascular supply. If it fails to do this it remains inert and dormant or dies. Direct evidence of the presence of such latent cells was reported in the tissues of a patient with inoperable ovarian carcinoma who had been treated palliatively for recurrent massive ascites by insertion of a peritoneo-venous shunt (Tarin et al 1984 a,b). This remained in place for two and a half years, during which time many millions of viable tumour cells were infused directly into the blood, but no haematogenous metastases could be detected in any organ at autopsy, although individual tumour cells could be seen leaving the pulmonary capillaries and lying free in the interstitial tissues of the lungs. Other patients in that study (Tarin et al 1984a) did develop metastases after shunt therapy but only in some organs, notably ones which were clinically involved before shunting, confirming Paget's seed and soil hypothesis (Paget 1889). The remaining organs remained metastasis-free despite having been infused continuously with blood containing millions of viable metastasis-competent cells for several months.

These findings in humans were in close agreement with earlier studies on naturally-occurring murine mammary tumours (Tarin & Price 1981). Using homologous techniques of intravascular infusion of tumour cells, it was demonstrated that cells from such tumours, known to be capable of forming metastases in the lungs, would not necessarily form haematogenous deposits in other organs, such as the liver, bones or brain even if injected directly into the supplying vessels (Juacaba et al 1983). Further supporting data were provided by Hart & Fidler (1980) with a transplantable mouse tumour (B16 melanoma) and Kinsey (1960) with the Cloudman melanoma in rats. Both studies showed that the cells from many tumours grow preferentially in certain organs after vascular dissemination.

The findings in all three species are therefore mutually complementary and imply that microenvironmental influences in the sites where tumour cells lodge can modulate whether cells with proven metastatic capability, can express this potential. The clinical significance of this knowledge is that metastasis is not an inevitable consequence of tumour cell dissemination.

Subsequent work (Horak et al 1986, Nicolson & Dulski 1986, Naito et al 1987) suggested that these effects may be exerted, at least in part, by soluble factors released by the constituent cells of each organ. Co-culturing mouse mammary tumour cells, which normally form only pulmonary metastases, with fragments of liver or thyroid resulted in the death of the tumour cells, whereas co-culture with pieces of lung resulted in increased survival and adherence of the tumour cells to the substratum (Horak et al 1986). These effects could be transferred from one culture to another, with cell-free media 'conditioned' by the added organs. The findings in vitro were thus in good agreement with in vivo observations on the common distribution patterns of metastases of this tumour (Juacaba et al 1983). Similar results were reported by other groups and by Cavanaugh & Nicolson (1989) who isolated and purified a protein from lung tissue which they believed facilitates growth of metastatic tumour cells in that tissue.

Studies, by Cornil et al (1991) Lu et al (1992), and Lu & Kerbel (1993), indicated that the growth of tumour cell lines derived from early human malignant melanomas was inhibited by co-culture with irradiated normal dermal fibroblasts or culture medium from such cells. In contrast, cell lines derived from patients with advanced melanoma (deemed metastasis-competent) were stimulated by dermal fibroblasts and their medium (Cornil et al 1991). Lu et al (1992) have since provided evidence that the inhibitor secreted by fibroblasts is interleukin 6 (IL-6) and that the inversion of the response to this cytokine observed in advanced melanoma cell lines is associated with synthesis and secretion of IL-6 by these lines themselves. It was suggested that such changes in the responses of tumour cells to local tissue environmental factors may provide certain clones with a proliferative advantage and thereby facilitate progression of disease (Lu & Kerbel 1993). Other experiments (Kerbel 1992) indicated that more aggressive and metastatic clones in a tumour may sometimes release another inhibitory cytokine, TGFβ, to which they had become insensitive but to which less malignant sister clones were still responsive, thereby giving themselves a potential advantage in competition for local resources.

Fig. 2.6 (Facing page) Distribution of CD44 mRNA (**a,b & d**) and protein isoforms (**f,g,h & i**) in normal colonic mucosa and in colonic carcinomas visualised by dark field microscopy of in situ hybridisation and by immunohistochemistry. (**a**) Normal colonic mucosa showing low abundancy of CD44 standard form mRNA in the epithelium and in stromal cells demonstrated by the silver grains. (**b–c**) Colonic adenoma showing high abundancy of CD44 variant mRNA in the epithelium of the tumour but not in the stroma. (**d–e**) Invading islands of colonic carcinoma cells showing very high abundancy of CD44 mRNA in tumour cells but not in adjacent muscle. (**f**) Colonic mucosa stained with monoclonal antibody Hermes 3 showing low amount of CD44 standard protein in epithelium, but plentiful amount in stromal cells. (**g**) Elevated CD44 standard protein in invading colon carcinoma cells. (**h**) Patches of elevated CD44 variant 2 (exon 7) peptide in colon carcinoma cells. (**i**) Heavy overexpression of CD44 variant 6 (exon 11) peptide, predominantly in cell membranes of invading colon carcinoma cells. (Reprinted with permission from Gorham et al 1996.)

At present, not much more detail is known about the interactive signals that pass between colonising tumour cells and local host tissues but the available information strongly indicates that further investigation on cytokines and angiogenic factors in metastatic deposits and the tumours that generated such deposits will prove scientifically and clinically worthwhile.

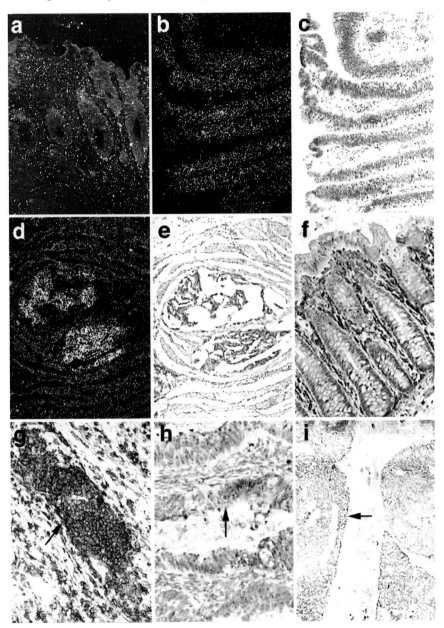

Fig. 2.6 (see opposite page for details)

CLINICAL APPLICATIONS: EARLY DIAGNOSIS AND EVALUATION OF PROGNOSIS

Most cancers can be cured by surgical resection, if diagnosed at an early stage (Kantoff 1990), before significant tumour cell migration has occurred via draining veins and lymphatics. Therefore, a search is continuing for new markers by which cancers can be detected early in their life history so that they can be removed whilst still localised and easily resected or destroyed. Ideally, to ensure good patient compliance, these markers should be measurable by simple non-invasive tests on specimens such as urine, stools, sputum and blood. Examination of the stool for occult blood (Winawer et al 1991) and urine cytology (Matzkin et al 1992) have limitations such as lack of specificity or sampling difficulties and are, in some cases, labour intensive. Radio-immunoassay for tumour markers, such as CEA, is not suitable for detecting cancer in its early stages because the sensitivity or specificity of the ones so far reported are insufficient for identification of very small tumours. However, such measures can sometimes be useful for assessment of prognosis and for monitoring patients for increasing tumour burden or recurrence (Hedin et al 1983). These circumstances continue to drive the search for markers which could be helpful for the early diagnosis of tumours and for the assessment of their metastatic potential.

New methods for early tumour diagnosis

CD44 gene expression

Many studies have demonstrated disorganised overexpression of the CD44 gene in various human cancers and this abnormality has emerged as an interesting candidate marker for early cancer diagnosis. Recently, the family of cell surface glycoproteins encoded by this gene has attracted increased scutiny because of rising interest in the mode of assembly of such a variety of products from a single locus and the diverse cellular functions in which it appears to be involved. The gene is composed of two groups of exons, one which is constantly expressed on most cell types, called the standard form, CD44s, and another, designated CD44v, the products of which can be assembled in various combinations by alternative mRNA splicing (Dougherty et al 1991, Hofmann et al 1991, Screaton et al 1992, Tolg et al 1993). By post-translational modifications, including glycosylation, these can be further modified to result in a polymorphic family of trans-membrane proteins (Jalkanen et al 1988, Stamenkovic et al 1989, Brown et al 1991, Rudy et al 1993). Details of the mechanisms regulating this synthetic activity in different cells and tissues are currently unknown. Also, there is, so far, very little information on the structure and functions of the many isoforms which can potentially be produced by this gene. However, the CD44 family has been implicated by many laboratories in numerous important and separate cellular activities (recently reviewed by Lesley et al 1993).

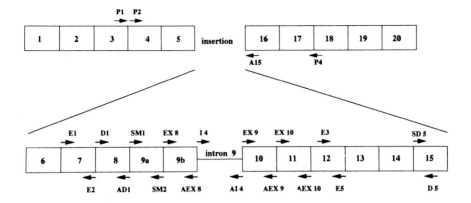

Fig. 2.7a Map of a CD44 cDNA molecule showing the position of intron 9 and of the primers used to generate various probes.

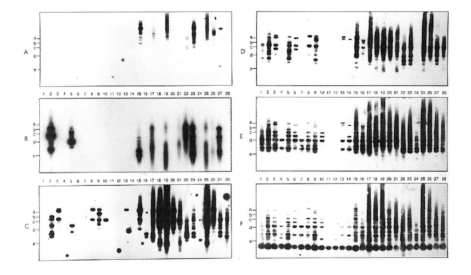

Fig. 2.7b Southern hybridisation of urinary samples amplified with primers P1 and P4 (*see* map in Fig. 2.7a). Tracks **1–14** show the results with urine samples from tumour-free people. Tracks **15–28** show the results with urine samples from bladder cancer patients. In these PCR studies, 35 cycles were performed. Panels **A, B, C, D, E** and **F** show the same filter hybridised with probes for intron 9, exon 9a, exon 7, exon 12, exon 15 and for the standard form of CD44, respectively. The filter was stripped between each hybridisation. (Reprinted with permission from Matsumura et al 1995.)

The involvement of CD44 proteins in a much wider variety of biological and pathological processes subsequently emerged when other groups, working on tumours, reported abnormal expression of new variant CD44 isoforms in cell lines and in fresh surgical biopsy samples of several different human tumours (Stamenkovic et al 1989, 1991, Gunthert et al 1991, Jackson et al 1992, Matsumura & Tarin 1992, Harn et al 1995). These early reports have been corroborated by many more, reviewed by Tarin et al (1995), and from all this work it has emerged that the defective expression of this locus in neoplasia does not characteristically involve a single exon or a particular combination of exons. Instead, it is the disorganised *pattern* of expression which is so distinctive. Subsequent immunohistochemical and *in situ* hybridisation studies have also confirmed that the over-abundant CD44v transcripts and proteins in tumour tissues are localised only in cancer cells (Fig. 2.6) and not in the surrounding inflammatory cells (Gorham et al 1996), suggesting that these gene products could be clinically useful markers for malignant cells in diagnostic biopsies and fluid samples. As small quantities of one or two small variant isoforms can be detected in non-neoplastic epithelium it is important to emphasise that alternatively spliced versions of the CD44 molecule are not exclusively associated with lymphocyte migration or with neoplasia and metastasis, though they may be implicated in all these processes.

Subsequent studies demonstrated that analysis of body fluids, tissues and waste products (urine and stools) for signs of abnormal CD44 gene activity can signal the presence of small numbers of exfoliated cancer cells from tumours in the corresponding organs. Thus, CD44 mRNA extracted from urine cell pellets and amplified with the polymerase chain reaction showed numerous abnormal CD44 transcripts and a dense intervening smear (see Fig. 2.7b) in 40 of 44 patients with bladder cancer (sensitivity 91%), but not in 38 of 46 people with no urinary symptoms or evidence of neoplasia (specificity 83%) (Matsumura et al 1994). Western blot analysis revealed several high molecular weight CD44 isoforms >160kD, in urine cell-lysates from 33 of 44 patients (sensitivity =75%) with histologically-proven bladder cancer and in 2 of 3 patients with severe epithelial dysplasia but in none of 41 asymptomatic volunteers (specificity 100%).

It is interesting to note that samples from 66% of patients with very early stage tumours (pTaG1) and severe epithelial dysplasia showed the abnormal CD44 protein pattern seen in more advanced bladder malignancy (Sugiyama et al 1995). Abnormalities in CD44 expression have also been reported in colonic adenomas, which are recognised precursor lesions for colorectal cancer (Heider et al 1993, Gorham et al 1996). This suggests that the disturbances in the activity of this gene begin very early in the neoplastic process and this may prove to be clinically useful in diagnosis.

With RT-PCR/Southern hybridisation analysis, distinctive large molecular weight amplicons can be visualised in extracts from tumour cell-containing samples, although long dense smears are the more usual indications of severely disturbed CD44 gene transcription (Figs 2.4 and 2.7b). A possible explanation for this highly characteristic abnormality could be that the over-abundant transcripts produced by the CD44 gene in tumour cells contain immature or defective mRNA species of a wide range of sizes, possibly with retained intron sequences and that these might crowd the gels, causing the signals to fuse into a smear. A probe was therefore designed for the smallest intron of the gene (Fig. 2.7a) and used to test this hypothesis (Matsumura et al 1995). In studies involving hybridisation with a probe for intron 9, only 1 (2.5%) of 41 normal samples gave a positive signal (97.5% specificity). On the other hand, samples from 18 of 30 patients with bladder cancer showed positive bands and smear patterns (60% sensitivity). It should be noted that two tumour urine samples which showed a smear pattern with intron 9 (e.g. lane 15, Fig. 2.7b) were from patients with very early stage (pTaG1) bladder cancer (Matsumura et al 1995). Further studies have shown that this and other introns, from both the standard and the variant regions, can also be detected in the over-abundant CD44 transcripts present in several other types of tumours including colorectal (Yoshida et al 1995), gastric (Higashikawa et al 1996) and breast carcinomas (Bolodeoku et al 1996).

CD44 abnormalities for detection of neoplasia compare favourably with data on other molecular markers. For example, p53 gene mutations were detected in 1-7% of exfoliated cells in the urine of three patients with bladder cancer (Sidransky et al 1991) whilst H-ras gene mutations were observed in the urinary cells of 10 of 21 patients with the same condition (Haliassos et al 1992) and K-ras mutations were found in DNA retrieved from stool samples from 8 of 9 cases of colorectal cancer (Sidransky et al 1992). These studies on other potential markers were conducted on relatively small numbers of patients, but demonstrate that diagnosis of neoplasia by molecular genetic analysis of minute clinical samples is feasible and that new tools for accurate non-invasive cancer diagnosis are on the horizon. This conclusion is supported by the summation of our results, cited above, which demonstrates that abnormalities of CD44 expression were detected in exfoliated cells in the urine from 96 of 121 patients with bladder cancer. It would be premature to claim that abnormal CD44 gene products, particularly the retained introns, constitute the best analytes for colorectal cancer detection, but the results do show that they are very promising candidates and provide the incentive for further work.

Telomerase

Other genes which might deserve consideration as candidate molecular diagnostic or prognostic markers, once the technical procedures for obtaining suitable yields of exfoliated cells from stools and other clinical samples, such as sputum, have been solved, include p53 (Hollstein et al 1991), APC (Kinzler et al 1991a), Ki-ras (Fearon & Vogelstein, 1990), MCC (Kinzler et al 1991b), DCC (Fearon et al 1990) replication error repair genes (Leach et al 1993), microsatellite markers (Mao et al 1996) and telomerase (Kim et al 1994, Rhyu 1995).

Telomeres are specialised regions at the ends of eukaryotic chromosomes in which the DNA is composed of multiple tandem repeats. They are believed to protect the ends of the chromosomes from fusion and recombination events by attachment of the chromosome to the nuclear matrix near the nuclear membrane (Flint et al 1994, Collins et al 1995, Shay et al 1995). Somatic cell telomeres are progressively shortened with each cell division and this appears to correlate with exit from the cell cycle, senescence and eventual cell death. Cells that can overcome this limitation have the potential for prolonged survival and indefinite proliferation. Telomerase is a ribonucleoprotein that can compensate for the loss of about 40-200 base pairs of the DNA sequence at the end (the telomere) of each chromosome that ordinarily occurs at each cell division (Greider & Blackburn 1987, Morin 1989). This repair is achieved by the direct synthesis of TTAGGG tandem repeats in each telomeric region to re-extend it to its original length. The enzyme is active in embryonic cells but undetectable in normal adult somatic cells and recent data indicate that it is reactivated in immortal cancer cells. Somatic cells do not have telomerase activity and stop dividing to become senescent when the telomeres of their chromosomes have shortened to a critical length. Therefore, it has been postulated that the synthesis of DNA at the ends of the chromosome by telomerase, may be necessary to sustain the indefinite proliferation of malignant cells (Counter et al 1992, Counter et al 1994, Greider 1994, Rhyu 1995, Shay et al 1995).

Recently, Kim et al (1994) developed an extremely sensitive assay for this enzyme based upon the polymerase chain reaction. They termed this the telomeric repeat amplification protocol (TRAP) and used it to demonstrate that 98 of 100 immortal and none of 22 mortal cell populations in vitro were positive for telomerase activity. More importantly, from a diagnostic perspective, 90 of 101 biopsies from 12 different tumour types were also positive for telomerase activity. This enzyme has since been detected in tissue samples from neuroblastomas (Hiyama et al 1995a), lung carcinomas (Hiyama et al 1995b), hepatocellular carcinomas (Tahara et al 1995a), gastric and colon carcinomas (Chadeneau et al 1995, Hiyama et al 1995c, Tahara et al 1995b) and brain tumours (Langford et al 1995) but not in corresponding normal tissues. Telomerase activity is also present in breast (Sugino et al 1996) and bladder carcinomas (Yoshida et al 1996) and can be found in fine needle aspirates and urine samples, respectively, from patients with these conditions.

This indicates that the telomerase assay could become a useful new modality for supplementing microscopic cytopathology in the detection of cancer cells in small tissue biopsies, fine needle aspirates and non-invasively obtained body fluids such as urine.

Evaluation of prognosis

Statistical associations have been shown between some clinical and molecular properties of tumours and survival of the host which, in general, correlate with the presence of metastases, but the ultimate goal of accurately evaluating the prognosis of individual patients, so that their treatment can be tailored accordingly, is still out of reach. Research is continuing and, meanwhile, the following are considered to be of some help.

Clinical prognostic indicators

> Size
> Grade
> Vascular invasion
> Lymph node status

And the following are some interesting new candidates which may prove to be useful additional prognostic indicators:

Molecular and other markers

> c-met
> CD44
> nm23
> EGFR
> ER
> Angiogenesis factors
> Degree of neovascularisation
> MAGNA
> (an acronym for Metastasis Associated Gene or Nucleic Acid)

The evidence for the traditional clinical prognostic indicators is discussed in relation to tumours of the individual organs in several textbooks (see, for example, Peckham et al 1995) and original papers. The reader is referred to these for details.

Many of the new candidate molecules which may become useful prognostic markers have been extensively investigated by Tahara and colleagues and are discussed in some excellent recent reviews (Tahara 1993, 1995). In a new scheme which he has pioneered, a panel of molecular genetic markers are used in routine diagnostic practice to provide an individual profile of a patient's tumour (Tahara 1995).

c-met

Recent evidence has indicated that the pattern and level of expression of this oncogene, which encodes the receptor for hepatocyte growth factor (HGF), is changed in tumours of the stomach compared with normal gastric mucosa. Kuniyasu et al (1993) reported that a 6 kilobase transcript, which is rarely and only slightly expressed in non-neoplastic mucosa, was expressed at high levels in 52% of gastric carcinomas and was closely correlated with depth of invasion, tumour staging and lymph node metastasis. Pisters et al (1995) using immunohistochemistry to study prostatic biopsies found positive staining for the protein encoded by this gene in 84% of primary cancers versus 18% of benign prostatic hyperplasias, 4 of 4 lymph node metastases, 23 of 23 bone marrow metastases and 1 of 3 metastases in other sites. The expression of this locus on chromosome 7q in malignancy is therefore of considerable interest and deserves more investigation.

CD44

Several groups have reported that overexpression of splice variants containing epitopes encoded by exon 11 (v6) of this gene assessed by immunohistochemistry correlates with poor prognosis in patients with colorectal (Mulder et al 1994) and breast carcinomas (Kaufmann et al 1995) non-Hodgkin's lymphoma (Koopman et al 1993) and other neoplasms (Tarin et al 1995) as judged by more advanced tumour stage, presence of metastases or shorter survival time. Results obtained by other groups using RT-PCR (Tarin & Matsumura 1992, Finn et al 1994, Lee et al 1995) and Northern blotting (Takeuchi et al 1995) support these conclusions. On the other hand, a few reports describing either lack of any such correlation in breast cancer (Friedrichs et al 1995), or down-regulation of CD44 isoforms in pulmonary adenocarcinomas (Clarke et al 1995) have also been published). Collectively, however, the majority of available evidence currently indicates that there are meaningful associations between abnormal expression of alternatively spliced CD44 isoforms, tumour metastasis and reduced survival.

There are considerable difficulties in trying to evaluate and compare the local staining intensities and overall distribution of immunoreactivity and at least some of the apparent discrepancies described above may reflect problems in methodology and assessment , as well as differences in fixation, tissue processing and observer interpretation. Immunohistochemical evaluation of CD44 expression in archival tissue is therefore not an optimal method for the evaluation of the prognosis in a given individual. For a more accurate knowledge of the prognostic potential of this marker it will be necessary to use more objective and quantitative measurements. However, prospective studies using such new methods will take considerable time. Using quantitative techniques, Takeuchi et al (1995) demonstrated a significant association between overexpression of exons 13-15 (v8-10) and colorectal cancer metastasis, and Guo et al (1994) suggested that the level of soluble CD44 proteins in the blood may serve as an indicator of tumour burden and metastasis in colonic and gastric cancer.

Oestrogen receptors and the Epidermal Growth Factor Receptor (EGFR)

Oestrogen receptor status and level of expression of certain other markers, such as EGFR and the neu oncogene have been reported (Harris et al 1989) to be useful extra discriminators for judging which patients, with *node-negative* breast cancer at the time of diagnosis, might have earlier progression of disease, shorter survival and poorer response to hormone therapy.

Degree of neovascularisation

Some recent studies (Bosari et al 1992, Macchiarini et al 1992, Weidner et al 1992) have suggested that there is a direct correlation between the number of capillaries visible in histological sections of tumours and their metastatic behaviour. These reports indicate that counting the number of capillaries/mm^2 in the most highly vascularised areas of a tumour section can provide an important independent variable which predicts the prognosis of patients with lung cancer (Macchiarini et al 1992) and breast cancer (Bosari et al 1992, Weidner et al 1992).

Angiogenesis factors

Studies analysing the patterns of expression of growth factors known to promote angiogenesis (see for example O'Brien et al 1995) show that they are produced in different stages of invasion and dissemination and may predict future recurrence and aggressive behaviour.

MAGNA

Preliminary evidence suggests that a putative coding region within this recently isolated DNA fragment (Hayle et al 1993, Bao et al 1996) is expressed to a much higher degree in tumours and their metastatic deposits than in non-metastatic neoplasms or non-neoplastic tissue counterparts. If this is confirmed, detection of such gene expression in a tumour might prove to be a useful early warning of potential metastatic spread.

This overview of clinical and biological aspects of tumour metastasis is intended to convey a sense of wonder and interest in a phenomenon which is both an intractable clinical problem and a rich source of information on how the multicellular community constituting a healthy metazoön organism interacts to sustain its complex structural integrity. Modern molecular pathology has provided us with the tools for unravelling the genetic programmes driving this process. The pursuit of the putative metastasis operon is the next great challenge in this field and the clinical and scientific benefits of undertaking it are likely to be significant.

REFERENCES

Baban D, Matsumura Y, Kocialkowski S et al 1993 Studies on relationships between metastatic and non-metastatic tumor cell populations using lineages labeled with dominant selectable genetic markers. Int J Dev Biol 37: 237–243

Bao L, Pigott R, Matsumura Y et al 1993 Correlation of VLA-4 integrin expression with metastatic potential in various human tumour cell lines. Differentiation 52: 239–246

Bao L, Matsumura Y, Baban D et al 1994 Effects of inoculation site and Matrigel on growth and metastasis of human breast cancer cells. Br J Cancer 70: 228–232

Bao L, Cowe E, Tarin D 1996 Characteristics of human DNA recovered from cells induced to become metastatic by transfection. Submitted

Barnes R, Masood S, Barker E et al 1991 Low nm23 protein expression in infiltrating ductal breast carcinomas correlates with reduced patient survival. Am J Pathol 139: 245–250

Barsky S H, Rao C N, Williams J E et al 1984 Laminin molecular domains which alter metastasis in a murine model. J Clin Invest 74: 843–848

Bevilacqua G, Sobel M E, Liotta L A et al 1989 Association of low nm23 RNA levels in human primary infiltrating ductal breast carcinomas with lymph node involvement and other histopathological indicators of high metastatic potential. Cancer Res 49: 5185–5190

Birch M, Mitchell S, Hart I R 1991 Isolation and characterization of human melanoma cell variants expressing high and low levels of CD44. Cancer Res 51: 6660–6667

Bolodeoku J, Yoshida K, Sugino T et al 1996 Accumulation of immature intron-containing CD44 gene transcripts in breast cancer tissues. Molecular Diagnosis 1: 175–181

Bosari S, Lee A K, DeLellis R A et al 1992 Microvessel quantitation and prognosis in invasive breast carcinoma. Hum Pathol 23: 755–761

Bresalier R S, Raper S E, Hujanen E S et al 1987 A new animal model for human colon cancer metastasis. Int J Cancer 39: 625–630

Brown R A, Bouchard T, St John T et al 1991 Human keratinocytes express a new CD44 core protein (CD44E) as a heparan-sulphate intrinsic membrane proteoglycan with additional exons. J Cell Biol 113: 207–221

Cavanaugh P G, Nicolson G L 1989 Purification and some properties of a lung-derived growth factor that differentially stimulates the growth of tumor cells metastatic to the lung. Cancer Res 49: 3928–3933

Chadeneau C, Hay K, Hirte H W et al 1995 Telomerase activity associated with acquisition of malignancy in human colorectal cancer. Cancer Res 55:2533–2536

Chan B M C, Matsuura N, Takada Y et al 1991 In vitro and in vivo consequences of VLA-2 expression on rhabdomyosarcoma cells. Science 251: 1600–1602

Ciocc V, Castronovo V, Shmookler B M et al 1991 Increased expression of the laminin receptor in human colon cancer. J Natl Cancer Inst 83: 29–36

Clarke M R, Landreneau R J, Resnick N M et al 1995 Prognostic significance of CD44 expression in adenocarcinoma of the lung. J Clin Pathol: Mol Pathol 48: M200–M204

Cohn K H, Wang F, Desoto-Lapaix F et al 1991 Association of nm23-H1 allelic deletions with distant metastases in colorectal carcinoma. Lancet 338: 722–724

Collins K, Kobayashi R, Greider C W 1995 Purification of tetrahymena telomerase and cloning of genes encoding the two protein components of the enzyme. Cell 81: 677–686

Cornil I, Theodorescu D, Man S et al 1991 Fibroblast cell interactions with human melanoma cells affect tumor cell growth as a function of tumor progression. Proc Natl Acad Sci USA 88: 6028–6032

Counter C M, Avilion A A, LeFeuvre C E et al 1992 Telomere shortening associated with chromosome instability is arrested in immortal cells which express telomerase activity. EMBO J 11: 1921–1929

Counter C M, Hirte H W, Bacchetti S et al 1994 Telomerase activity in human ovarian carcinoma. Proc Natl Acad Sci USA 91: 2900–2904

Darling D, Tarin D 1990 The spread of cancer in the human body. New Scientist 1726:50–53

Dougherty G J, Landsdorp P M, Cooper D L et al 1991 Molecular cloning of CD44R1 and CD44R2, two novel isoforms of the CD44 lymphocytes 'homing' receptor expressed by hemopoietic cells. J Exp Med 174: 1–5

Driessens M H E, Stroeken P J M, Erena N F R et al 1995 Targeted disruption of CD44 in MDAY-D2 lymphosarcoma cells has no effect on subcutaneous growth or metastatic capacity. J Cell Biol 131: 1849–1855

Fabra A, Nakajima M, Bucana C D et al 1992 Modulation of the invasive phenotype of human colon carcinoma cells by organ specific fibroblasts of nude mice. Differentiation 52: 101–110

Fearon E R, Vogelstein B 1990 A genetic model for colorectal tumorigenesis. Cell 61: 759–767

Fearon E R, Cho K R, Nigro J M et al 1990 Identification of a chromosome 18q gene that is altered in colorectal cancers. Science 247: 49–56

Fidler I J 1970 Metastasis: Quantitative analysis of distribution and fate of tumor emboli labelled with 125 1-5-Iodo-2'-deoxyuridine. J Natl Cancer Inst 45: 773–782

Fidler I J 1978 Tumour heterogeneity and the biology of cancer invasion and metastasis. Cancer Res 38: 2651–2660

Fidler I J 1985 Macrophages and metastasis — A biological approach to cancer therapy. Cancer Res 45: 4714–4726

Fidler I J 1990 Critical factors in the biology of human cancer metastasis. Cancer Res 50: 6130–6138

Fidler I J, Kripke M L 1977 Metastasis results from pre-existing variant cells within a malignant tumour. Science 197: 893–895

Finn L, Dougherty G, Finley G et al 1994 Alternative splicing of CD44 pre-mRNA in human colorectal tumors. Biochem Biophys Res Commun 200: 1015–1022

Flint J, Craddock C F, Villegas A et al 1994 Healing of broken human chromosomes by addition of telomeric repeats. Am J Hum Genet 55: 505–512

Fridman R, Sweeney T M, Zain M et al 1992 Malignant transformation of NIH-3T3 cells after subcutaneous co-injection with a reconstituted basement membrane (Matrigel). Int J Cancer 51: 740–744

Friedrichs K, Franke F, Lisboa B-W et al 1995 CD44 isoforms correlate with cellular differentiation but not with prognosis in human breast cancer. Cancer Res 55: 5425–5433

Goodison S, Tarin D 1996 Transcript retention of CD44 intron 18 in colorectal cancer. Submitted

Gorham H, Sugino T, Woodman A C et al 1996 Cellular distribution of CD44 gene transcripts in colorectal carcinomas and in normal colonic mucosa. J Clin Pathol 49: 482–488

Greider C W 1994 Mammaliam telomere dynamics: healing, fragmentation, shortening and stabilization. Curr Op Gen Develop, 4: 203–211

Greider C W, Blackburn E H 1987 The telomere terminal transferase of Tetrahymena is a ribonucleoprotein enzyme with two kinds of primer specificity. Cell 51: 887–898

Gunthert U, Hofmann M, Rudy W et al 1991 A new variant of glycoprotein CD44 confers metastatic potential to rat carcinoma cells. Cell 65: 13–24

Guo Y-J, Liu G, Wang X et al 1994 Potential use of soluble CD44 in serum as indicator of tumor burden and metastasis in patients with gastric or colon cancer. Cancer Res 54: 422–426

Hailat N, Keim D.R, Melhem R F et al 1991 High levels of p19/nm23 protein in neuroblastoma are associated with advanced stage disease and with N-myc gene amplification. J Clin Invest 88: 341–345

Haliassos A, Liloglou T, Likourinas M et al 1992 H-ras oncogene mutations in the urine of patients with bladder tumours: description of a non-invasive method for the detection of neoplasia. Int J Oncol 1: 731–734

Hanna N 1982 Role of natural killer cells in control of cancer metastasis. Cancer Metastasis Rev 1: 45–65

Harn H-J, Ho L-I, Chang J-Y et al 1995 Differential expression of the human metastasis adhesion molecule CD44V in normal and carcinomatous stomach mucosa of Chinese subjects. Cancer 75: 1065–1071

Harris A L, Nicholson S, Sainsbury J R et al 1989 Epidermal growth factor receptors in breast cancer: association with early relapse and death, poor response to hormones and interactions with neu. J Steroid Biochem 34: 123–131

Hart I R, Fidler I J 1980 The role of organ selectivity in the determination of metastatic patterns of B16 melanoma. Cancer Res 40: 2281–2287

Hashimoto K, Yamanishi Y, Maeyens E et al 1973 Collagenolytic activities of squamous-cell carcinoma of skin. Cancer Res 33: 2790–2801

Haunt M, Steeg P S, Willson J K V et al 1991 Induction of nm23 gene expression in human colonic neoplasms and equal expression in colon tumors of high and low metastatic potential. J Natl Cancer Inst 83: 712–716

Hayle A J, Darling D L, Taylor A R et al 1993 Transfection of metastatic capability with total genomic DNA from metastatic human and mouse tumour cell lines. Differentiation 54: 177–189

Hedin A, Carlsson L, Berglund A et al 1983 A monoclonal antibody-enzyme immunoassay for serum carcinoembryonic antigen with increased specificity for carcinomas. Proc Natl Acad Sci USA 80: 3470–3474

Heider K-H, Hofmann M, Hors E et al 1993 A human homologue of the rat metastasis-associated variant of CD44 is expressed in colorectal carcinomas and adenomatous polyps. J Cell Biol 120: 227–233

Hemler ME 1990 VLA proteins in the integrin family: Structures, functions and their role on leukocytes. Annu Rev Immunol 8: 365–400

Hennessy C, Henry J A, May F E B 1991 Expression of the antimetastatic gene nm23 in human breast cancer: An association with good prognosis. J Natl Cancer Inst 83: 281–285

Higashikawa K, Yokozaki H, Ue T et al 1996 Evaluation of CD44 transcription variants in human digestive tract carcinomas and normal tissues. Int J Cancer 66: 11–17

Hiyama E, Hiyama K, Yokoyama T et al 1995a Correlating telomerase activity levels with human neuroblastoma outcome. Nature Med 1: 249–255

Hiyama K, Hiyama E, Ishioka S et al 1995b Telomerase activity in small-cell and non-small-cell lung cancers. J Natl Cancer Inst 87: 895–902

Hiyama E, Yokoyama T, Tatsumoto N et al 1995c Telomerase activity in gastric cancer. Cancer Res 5: 3258–3262

Hofmann M, Rudy W, Zoller M et al 1991 CD44 splice variants confer metastatic behaviour in rats: Homologous sequences are expressed in human tumor cell lines. Cancer Res 51: 5292–5297

Hollstein N, Sidransky D, Vogelstein B et al 1991 p53 mutations in human cancers. Science 253: 49–53

Holzmann B, Weissman IL 1989 Peyer's patch-specific lymphocyte homing receptors consist of a VLA-4-like α chain associated with either of two integrin β chains, one of which is novel. EMBO J 8:1735–1741

Horak E, Darling D L, Tarin D 1986 Analysis of organ-specific effects on metastatic tumor formation by studies in vitro. J Natl Cancer Inst 76: 913–922

Jackson D G, Buckley J, Bell J I 1992 Multiple variants of the human lymphocyte homing receptor CD44 generated by insertions at a single site in the extracellular domain. J Biol Chem 267: 4732–4739

Jalkanen S, Jalkanen M, Bargatze R et al 1988 Biochemical properties of glycoproteins involved in lymphocyte recognition of high endothelial venules in man. J Immunol 141: 1615–1623

Juacaba S F, Jones L D, Tarin D 1983 Organ preferences in metastatic colony formation by spontaneous mammary carcinomas after intra-arterial inoculation. Invasion Metastasis 3: 221–233

Juacaba S F, Horak E, Price J E et al 1989 Tumour cell dissemination patterns and metastasis of murine mammary carcinoma. Cancer Res 49: 570–575

Kantoff P W 1990 Bladder cancer. Curr Probl Cancer 14: 233–292

Kaufmann M, Heider K-H, Sinn H-P et al 1995 CD44 variant exon epitopes in primary breast cancer and length of survival. Lancet 345: 615–619

Kerbel R S 1992 Expression of multi-cytokine resistance and multi-growth factor independence in advanced stage metastatic cancer. Am J Pathol 141: 519–524

Kim N W, Piatyszek M A, Prowse K R 1994 Specific association of human telomerase activity with immortal cells and cancer. Science 266: 2011–2015

Kinsey D L 1960 An experimental study of preferential metastasis. Cancer 13: 674–676

Kinzler K W, Nilbert M C, Su L-K 1991a Identification of FAP locus genes from chromosome 5q21. Science 253: 661–665

Kinzler K W, Nilbert M C, Vogelstein B et al 1991b Identification of a gene located at chromosome 5q21 that is mutated in colorectal cancers. Science 251: 1366–1370

Koopman G, Heider K-H, Horst E et al 1993 Activated human lymphocytes and aggressive non-Hodgkin's lymphomas express a homologue of the rat metastasis-associated variant of CD44. J Exp Med 177: 897–904

Kuniyasu H, Yasui W, Yokozaki H et al 1993 Aberrant expression of c-met mRNA in human gastric carcinomas. Int J Cancer 55: 72–75

Langford L A, Piatyszek M A, Xu R et al 1995 Telomerase activity in human brain tumours. Lancet. 346: 1267–1268

Lauri D, Needham L, Dejana E 1991 Tumor cell adhesion to the endothelium. In: Gordon JL (ed) Vascular endothelium: Interactions with circulating cells. Elsevier, Amsterdam, pp 111–128

Leach F S, Nicolaides N C, Papadopoulos N et al 1993 Mutations of a *muts* homolog in hereditary nonpolyposis colorectal cancer. Cell 75: 1215–1225

Lee J-H, Kang Y-S, Kim B-G et al 1995 Expression of the CD44 adhesion molecule in primary and metastatic gynecologic malignancies and their cell lines. Int J Gynecol Cancer 5: 193–199

Lesley J, Hyman R, Kincade PW 1993 CD44 and its interaction with the extracellular matrix. Adv Immunol 54: 271–335

Liotta L A, Abe S, Robey P G et al 1979 Preferential digestion of basement membrane collagen by an enzyme derived from a metastatic murine tumor. Proc Natl Acad Sci USA 76: 2268–2272

Liotta L A, Tryggvason K, Garbisa S et al 1980 Metastatic potential correlates with enzymatic degradation of basement membrane collagen. Nature 284: 67–68

Lu C, Vickers M F, Kerbel R S 1992 Interleukin 6: A fibroblast-derived growth inhibitor of human melanoma cells from early but not advanced stages of tumor progression. Proc Natl

Acad Sci USA 89: 9215–9219

Lu C, Kerbel R S 1993 Interleukin-6 undergoes transition from paracrine growth inhibitor to autocrine stimulator during human melanoma progression. J Cell Biol 120: 1281–1288

Macchiarini P, Gontanini G, Hardin M J et al 1992 Relation of neovascularisation to metastasis of non-small-cell lung cancer. Lancet 340:145–146

Mao L, Schoenberg M P, Scicchitano M et al 1996 Molecular detection of primary bladder cancer by microsatellite analysis. Science 271: 659–662

Martin-Padura I, Mortarini R, Lauri D et al 1991 Heterogeneity in human melanoma cell adhesion to cytokine activated endothelial cells correlates with VLA-4 expression. Cancer Res 51: 2239–2241

Matsumura Y, Tarin D 1992 Significance of CD44 gene products for cancer diagnosis and disease evaluation. Lancet 340: 1053–1058

Matsumura Y, Hanbury D, Smith J et al 1994 Non-invasive detection of malignancy by identification of unusual CD44 gene activity in exfoliated cancer cells. BMJ 308: 619–624

Matsumura Y, Sugiyama M, Matsumura S et al 1995 Unusual retention of introns in CD44 gene transcripts in bladder cancer provides new diagnostic and clinical oncological opportunities. J Pathol 177: 11–20

Matsuura N, Puzon-McLaughlin W, Irie A et al 1996 Induction of experimental bone metastasis in mice by transfection of integrin $\alpha4\beta1$ into tumor cells. Am J Pathol 148:55–61

Matzkin H, Moinuddin S M, Soloway M S 1992 Value of urine cytology versus bladder washing in bladder cancer. Urology 39: 201–203

Moffett B F, Baban D, Bao L et al 1992 Fate of clonal lineages during neoplasia and metastasis studied with an incorporated genetic marker. Cancer Res 52: 1737–1743

Morikawa K, Walker S M, Nakajima M et al 1988 Influence of organ environment on the growth, selection, and metastasis of human colon carcinoma cells in nude mice. Cancer Res 48: 6863–6871

Morin G B 1989 The human telomere terminal transferase enzyme is a ribonucleoprotein that synthesizes TTAGGG repeats. Cell 59: 521–529

Mulder J-W R, Kruyt M, Sewnath M et al 1994 Colorectal cancer prognosis and expression of exon-v6-containing CD44 proteins. Lancet 344: 1470–1472

Naito S, von Eschenbach A C, Giavazzi R et al 1986 Growth and metastasis of tumor cells isolated from a human renal cell carcinoma implanted into different organs of nude mice. Cancer Res 46: 4109–4115

Naito S, Giavazzi R, Fidler I J 1987 Correlation between the in vitro interactions of tumour cells with an organ microenvironment and metastasis in vivo. Invasion Metastasis 7: 126–129

Nicolson G L 1982 Cancer metastasis: organ colonization and the cell-surface properties of malignant cells. Biochim Biophys Acta 695: 113–176.

Nicolson G L, Dulski K M 1986 Organ specificity of metastatic tumor colonization is related to organ-selective growth properties of malignant cells. Int J Cancer 38: 289–294

O'Brien T, Cranston D, Fuggle S et al 1995 Different angiogenic pathways characterize superficial and invasive bladder cancer. Cancer Res 55: 510–513

Ogilvie D J, Hailey J A, Juacaba S F et al 1985 Collagenase secretion by human breast neoplasms: A clinicopathologic investigation. J. Natl Cancer Inst 74:19–27

Osborn L, Hession C, Tizard R et al 1989 Direct expression cloning of vascular cell adhesion molecule 1, a cytokine-induced endothelial protein that binds to lymphocytes. Cell 59: 1203–1211

Paget S 1889 The distribution of secondary growths in cancer of the breast. Lancet i, 571–573

Peckham M, Pinedo H M, Veronesi U 1995 Oxford Textbook of Oncology, Oxford University Press, Oxford

Pellicer A, Robins D, Wold B et al 1980 Altering genotype and phenotype by DNA-mediated gene transfer. Science 209: 1414–1422

Picker L J, Nakache M, Butcher E C 1989 Monoclonal antibodies to human lymphocyte homing receptors define a novel class of adhesion molecules on diverse cell types. J Cell Biol 109: 927–937

Pisters L L, Troncoso P, Zhau H E et al 1995 c-met proto-oncogene expression in benign and malignant human prostate tissues. J Urol 154: 293–298

Poste G 1982 Experimental systems for analysis of the malignant phenotype. Cancer Metastasis Rev 1:141–199

Potter K M, Juacaba S F, Price J E et al 1983 Observations on organ distribution of fluorescein labelled tumour cells released intravascularly. Invasion Metastasis 3: 221–233

Price J E, Carr D, Jones L D et al 1982 Experimental analysis of factors affecting metastatic spread using naturally occurring tumours. Invasion Metastasis 2: 77–112

Price J E, Polyzos A, Zhang R D et al 1990 Tumorigenicity and metastasis of human breast carcinoma cell lines in nude mice. Cancer Res 50: 717–721

Rhyu M S 1995 Telomeres, Telomerase, and Immortality. J Natl Cancer Inst 87: 884–896

Rice G E, Bevilacqua M P 1989 An inducible endothelial cell surface glycoprotein mediates melanoma adhesion. Science 246: 1303–1306

Rudy W, Hofmann M, Schwartz-Albiez R et al 1993 The two major CD44 proteins expressed on a metastatic rat tumor cell line are derived from different splice variants: Each one individually suffices to confer metastatic behaviour. Cancer Res 53: 1262–1268

Screaton G R, Bell M V, Jackson D G et al 1992 Genomic structure of DNA encoding the lymphocyte homing receptor CD44 reveals at least 12 alternatively spliced exons. Proc Natl Acad Sci USA 89: 12160—12164

Shay J W, Werbin H, Wright W E 1995 You haven't heard the end of it: Telomere loss may link human aging with cancer. Can J Aging 14: 511–524

Sidransky D, von Eschenbach A, Tsai Y C et al 1991 Identification of p53 gene mutations in bladder cancers and urine samples. Science 252: 706–709

Sidransky D, Tokino T, Hamilton S R et al 1992 Identification of ras oncogene mutations in the stool of patients with curable colorectal tumors. Science 256: 102–105

Springer T A 1990 Adhesion receptors of the immune system. Nature 346: 425–434

Stamenkovic I, Amiot M, Pesando JM et al 1989 A lymphocyte molecule implicated in lymph node homing is a member of the cartilage link protein family. Cell 56: 1057–1062

Stamenkovic I, Aruffo A, Amiot M et al 1991 The hematopoietic and epithelial forms of CD44 are distinct polypeptides with different adhesion potentials for hyaluronate-bearing cells. EMBO J 10: 343–348

Steeg P S, Bevilacqua G, Kopper L et al 1988 Evidence for a novel gene associated with low tumor metastatic potential. J Natl Cancer Inst 80: 200–204

Stephenson R A, Dinney C P N, Gohji K et al 1992 Metastatic model for human prostate cancer using orthotopic implantation in nude mice. J Natl Cancer Inst 84: 951–957

Sugino T, Yoshida K, Bolodeoku J et al 1996 Telomerase activity in human breast cancer and benign breast lesions: Diagnostic applications in clinical specimens including fine needle aspirates. Int J Cancer 69: 301–306

Sugiyama M, Woodman A, Sugino T et al 1995 Non-invasive detection of bladder cancer by identification of abnormal CD44 proteins in exfoliated cancer cells in urine. J Clin Pathol: Mol Pathol 48: M142–M147

Sy M S, Guo Y-J, Stamenkovic I 1991 Distinct effects of two CD44 isoforms on tumor growth in vivo. J Exp Med 174: 859–866

Tahara E 1993 Molecular mechanism of stomach carcinogenesis. J Cancer Res Clin Oncol 119: 265–272

Tahara E 1995 Genetic alterations in human gastrointestinal cancers. The application to molecular diagnosis. Cancer 75: 1410–1417

Tahara H, Nakanishi T, Kitamoto M et al 1995a Telomerase activity in human liver tissues: Comparison between chronic liver disease and hepatocellular carcinomas. Cancer Res 55: 2734–2736

Tahara H, Kuniyasu H, Yasui W et al 1995b Telomerase activity in preneoplastic and neoplastic gastric and colorectal lesions. Clinical Cancer Res 1: 1245–1251

Takeuchi K, Yamaguchi A, Urano T et al 1995 Expression of CD44 variant exons 8–10 in colorectal cancer and its relationship to metastasis. Jpn J Cancer Res 86: 292–297

Tarin D 1967 Sequential electron microscopical study of experimental mouse skin carcinogenesis. Int J Cancer 2: 195–211

Tarin D 1969 Fine structure of murine mammary tumours: the relationship between epithelium and connective tissue in neoplasms induced by various agents. Br J Cancer 23: 417–425

Tarin D 1972 Morphological studies on the mechanism of carcinogenesis. In: Tarin D (ed) Tissue interactions in carcinogenesis Academic Press, London pp227–289.

Tarin D 1992 Tumour metastasis. In: McGee J O'D, Wright N A, Isaacson P G (eds) Oxford Textbook of Pathology. Oxford University Press, Oxford pp607–633

Tarin D 1995 Cancer metastasis In: Peckham M, Pinedo B, Veronesi U (eds) Oxford Textbook of Oncology, Oxford University Press, Oxford pp118–132

Tarin D, Price J E 1979 Metastatic colonization potential of primary tumour cells in mice. Br J Cancer 39: 740–754

Tarin D, Price J E 1981 Influence of microenvironment and vascular anatomy on 'metastatic' colonization potential of mammary tumors. Cancer Res 41: 3604–3609

Tarin D, Matsumura Y 1992 Significance of CD44 gene products for cancer diagnosis and disease evaluation. Lancet 340: 1053–1058

Tarin D, Price J E, Kettlewell M G W et al 1984a Mechanisms of human tumor metastasis studied in patients with peritoneovenous shunts. Cancer Res 44: 3584–3592

Tarin D, Vass A C R, Kettlewell M G W et al 1984b Absence of metastatic sequelae during long-term treatment of malignant ascites by peritoneo-venous shunting: a clinicopathological report. Invasion Metastasis 4: 1–12

Tarin D, Bolodeoku J, Hatfill S J et al 1995 The clinical significance of malfunction of the CD44 locus in malignancy. J Neuro-Oncol 26: 209–219

Terranova V P, Liotta L A, Russo R G et al 1982 Role of laminin in the attachment and metastasis of murine tumor cells. Cancer Res 42: 2265–2269

Tolg C, Hofmann M, Herrlich P et al 1993 Splicing choice from ten variant exons establishes CD44 variability. Nucleic Acids Res 21: 1225–1229

Weidner N, Folkman J, Pozza F et al 1992 Tumor angiogenesis: a new significant and independent prognostic indicator in early-stage breast carcinoma. J Natl Cancer Inst 84: 1875–1887

Weiss L 1980 Cancer cell traffic from the lungs to the liver: an example of metastatic inefficiency. Int J Cancer 25: 385–392

Willis R A 1973 The spread of tumours in the human body. 3rd ed. London: Butterworth

Winawer S J, Schottenfield D, Frehinger B S 1991 Colorectal cancer screening. J Natl Cancer Inst 83: 243–253

Yoshida K, Bolodeoku J, Sugino T et al 1995 Abnormal retention of intron 9 in CD44 gene transcripts in human gastrointestinal tumors. Cancer Res 55: 4273–4277

Yoshida K, Sugino T, Tahara H et al 1996 Telomerase activity in bladder carcinoma and its implications for non-invasive diagnosis by detection of exfoliated cancer cells in urine. Cancer: In Press

3

Pulmonary lymphoproliferative disorders

A. G. Nicholson   B. Corrin

Pulmonary lymphoproliferative disease comprises a spectrum of disorders. Involvement of the lung by nodal lymphomas (Berkman & Breuer 1993), angioimmunoblastic lymphadenopathy (Iseman et al 1976, Zylak et al 1976), plasmacytomas (Joseph et al 1993) and Castleman's disease (Mohamedani & Bennett 1985) have all been described, sometimes with pulmonary presentation. However, this chapter concentrates on those disorders in which pulmonary disease is the predominant feature. These have most commonly been termed primary pulmonary lymphoma, 'pseudolymphoma', lymphoid interstitial pneumonitis, follicular bronchiolitis and lymphomatoid granulomatosis.

Since the time of their initial descriptions, there has been much discussion about the nature of these conditions and how they relate to each other. Other terms, such as nodular and diffuse pulmonary lymphoid hyperplasia, benign lymphocytic angiitis and granulomatosis and angiocentric immunoproliferative lesions have subsequently been introduced, but have done little to delineate the nature of the disorders.

However, the recognition of extranodal lymphomas, together with the use of cytogenetics and molecular biology for their investigation has meant that the true nature of these lymphoid infiltrates is slowly being uncovered. In this chapter we review these findings and suggest how the various disorders can be distinguished histologically.

NEOPLASTIC LYMPHOPROLIFERATIVE INFILTRATES OF THE LUNG

'Pseudolymphoma'

Saltzstein (1963) distinguished pulmonary lymphoma from pseudolymphoma (also known as nodular lymphoid hyperplasia), regarding the latter as a reactive lesion analogous to pseudolymphoma seen elsewhere in the body such as eye and stomach. This was based on the histological features of a mixed infiltrate of mature lymphocytes and other inflammatory cells sometimes interspersed with germinal centres and a clinically indolent behaviour with localisation of the lesion to the lung and absence of lymph node involvement. However, the application of immunohistochemical techniques has shown that many pseudolymphomas are monoclonal B-cell proliferations (Weiss et al

1985, Addis et al 1988, Li et al 1990, Nicholson et al 1995a). Further evidence of monoclonality has come from Southern blot analysis (Shiota et al 1993) and from studies using the polymerase chain reaction (Nicholson et al 1995a). Although some still regard pseudolymphoma as a rare rather than non-existent reaction (Koss 1995), most workers now believe them to be low-grade B-cell non-Hodgkin's lymphomas (Addis et al 1988, Li et al 1990, Nicholson et al 1995a).

Pulmonary B-cell lymphomas of mucosa-associated lymphoid tissue (MALT) origin

Pulmonary lymphomas are rare but several series have now been published. The early cases were categorised according to nodal lymphoma classifications (Koss et al 1983, L'Hoste et al 1984, Turner et al 1984, Kennedy et al 1985), but more recently it has been recognised that most arise in MALT (Addis et al 1988, Li et al 1990, Cordier et al 1993, Fiche et al 1995, Nicholson et al 1995a). The low-grade tumours have the characteristic histology of MALT lymphomas and, although high grade pulmonary lymphomas have no distinctive features, it is thought that a significant number of these also arise from MALT; this view is supported by the occasional presence of low-grade areas in high grade tumours (Isaacson 1990, Li et al 1990, Nicholson et al 1995a).

Pulmonary B-cell lymphoma of MALT origin preferentially spreads to other mucosal sites; likewise other MALT lymphomas may spread to the lung (Cordier et al 1993, Nicholson et al 1995a). There is a relative lack of nodal involvement, but when it occurs the features are those of marginal zone or monocytoid B-cell lymphomas (Ngan et al 1991, Ortiz-Hidalgo & Wright 1992). This apparent 'homing-in' relates to the existence of a common mucosal immune system, in line with evidence from animal experiments. These have shown IgA responses in respiratory tissues after intestinal antigenic stimulation, and preferential repopulation of the lung by pulmonary lymphocytes removed from this site, and then re-introduced into the body (Rudzik et al 1975, McDermott & Bienenstock 1979).

Pathogenesis

The bronchial MALT from which these tumours originate was first described in rabbits, an animal species in which it is always present (Bienenstock et al 1973a, 1973b, Pabst & Gehrke 1990). However, bronchial MALT is less common in higher animals (Pabst & Gehrke 1990). It is not thought to be a normal constituent of the human bronchus, but develops as a response to various antigenic stimuli (Pabst 1992, Gould & Isaacson 1993, Holt 1993, Richmond et al 1993) as it does in the stomach where there is evidence that gastric lymphoma arises from MALT acquired as a result of *Helicobacter pylori* infection (Wotherspoon et al 1991). In the lung, the situation is less clear cut. Smoking causes an increased incidence of bronchial MALT (Richmond et al 1993) and pulmonary lymphoma is described in patients with autoimmune disorders (Kamel et al 1994), some of whom have associated fibrosing alveolitis. Immunoblastic transformation in lymphoid interstitial pneumonitis has also been described (Kradin et al 1982). Increased turnover of B-cells in patients with autoimmune diseases may contribute to lymphomagenesis and immunosuppressive therapy may be a possible additional factor (Symmons 1985, Frizzera 1994).

Cytogenetic studies on MALT lymphomas, including cases from the lung, have shown t(1;14) translocations in a small proportion of cases, though the most common abnormality has been trisomy of chromosome 3. Trisomies of chromosomes 7, 12 and 18 have also been identified. The underlying genetic mechanism remains obscure but the proto-oncogene bcl-6, interleukin-5 and certain tumour suppressor genes, all of which have been localised at least in part to chromosome 3, have been suggested as possible factors. The high incidence of trisomy 3 in both MALT lymphomas and marginal zone lymphomas supports the view that MALT lymphomas are distinct from other types of low-grade non-Hodgkin's lymphoma (Wotherspoon et al 1990, Wotherspoon et al 1992, Wotherspoon et al 1995).

Clinical findings

Patients with MALT lymphomas tend to be over 40 years of age and there is a slight male preponderance. Patients rarely present below the age of 30 years, unless their immune responses are impaired. The most common presentation in low-grade disease is the chance discovery of an asymptomatic mass on routine chest X-ray. The most common pulmonary symptoms are cough, dyspnoea, chest pain and haemoptysis. High grade lymphomas are nearly always symptomatic. Previous or synchronous MALT lymphoma at other extranodal sites is not uncommon, and there is often a monoclonal gammopathy. Some patients complain of 'B' symptoms (fever, weight loss, night sweats). Imaging shows either unilateral or bilateral disease, with isolated or multiple opacities, diffuse infiltration, reticulonodular shadowing and pleural effusions. Air bronchograms are a characteristic feature, though they are not specific. Spirometry in the majority of cases is normal but may show both obstructive and restrictive ventilatory defects. Broncho-alveolar lavage and fine-needle aspiration have occasionally been successful, but bronchoscopic or open lung biopsy and resection have been the commonest definitive diagnostic procedures (Davis & Gadek 1987, Sprague & Deblois 1989, Li et al 1990, Cordier et al 1993, Nicholson et al 1995a).

Pathology

Macroscopic descriptions are limited, but in our personal experience the commonest appearances are solitary or multiple cream coloured nodules

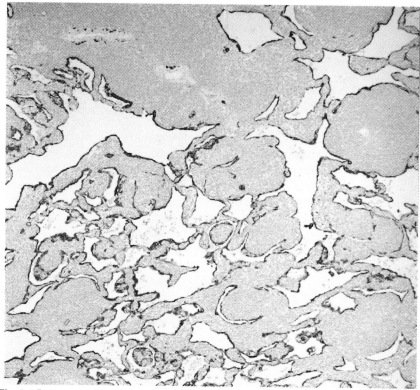

Fig. 3.1 Low power view of pulmonary infiltration by low grade lymphoma of MALT origin. Cytokeratin staining highlights the alveolar architecture, showing how the infiltrate spreads through the interstitium. Immunoperoxidase × 45.

which may become confluent and sometimes extend to involve the entire lung.

The morphological, immunohistochemical and cytogenetic features have been described by Li et al (1990), Wotherspoon et al (1990), Wotherspoon et al (1992), Fiche et al (1995), Nicholson et al (1995a) and Wotherspoon et al (1995). Low-grade tumours are composed of centrocyte-like, lymphocyte-like or monocytoid cells, all of which are thought to be variations of the same neoplastic cell (Isaacson 1990). In resection specimens, and to a lesser extent in open lung biopsies, the tumours show a characteristic pattern of spread. At their periphery, they infiltrate along bronchovascular bundles and interlobular septa, where they may appear as isolated nodules. Subsequent expansion and destruction of the alveolar walls with filling of the alveolar spaces give rise to confluent nodules that eventually form a mass (Fig. 3.1), within which foci of hyaline sclerosis are often seen. Vessels and airways tend to be spared in the masses, which explains the radiological feature of air bronchograms. Other features of MALT lymphomas, such as colonisation of germinal centres and lymphoepithelial lesions, are often seen (Fig. 3.2).

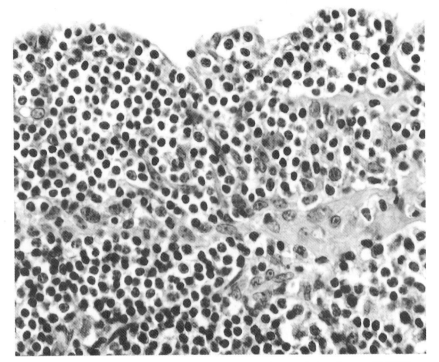

Fig. 3.2 Lymphoepithelial lesion of bronchial mucosa in a low grade lymphoma of MALT origin. H&E × 400.

This pattern of spread is not seen in high grade tumours, in which the infiltrate is more diffuse and destructive. Vascular infiltration, pleural involvement and granuloma formation are not uncommon in both low and high grade disease, but are of no prognostic significance. Necrosis is virtually confined to high grade tumours.

Immunohistochemistry shows that the neoplastic cells are of B-cell phenotype with a variable reactive T-cell population in the background (Fig. 3.3). Light chain restriction is observed in 30–70% of cases. The lymphoepithelial lesions and the destructive nature of the infiltrate are demonstrable by staining for cytokeratins.

Amplification of the immunoglobulin heavy chain gene by the polymerase chain reaction (PCR) has shown monoclonality in 60% of low grade lymphomas, but only occasionally in high grade disease.

Staging, treatment and survival

Staging as either Ie (unilateral or bilateral pulmonary involvement) or IIe (Stage Ie plus hilar/mediastinal involvement) is recommended. However, it is

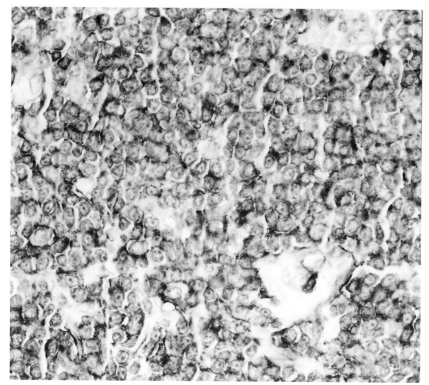

Fig. 3.3 CD20 staining shows a diffuse B-cell infiltrate in a low grade lymphoma of MALT origin. Immunoperoxidase × 400.

almost impossible to relate stage to therapy as cases are sporadic and treatment has varied over the years. Resection has produced prolonged remission (Uppal & Goldstraw 1992), but in bilateral or unresectable unilateral low-grade disease, the treatment has been similar to that used in advanced nodal lymphomas.

At present, a 'wait and watch' policy is perhaps best for patients with low grade pulmonary lymphoma, but when they develop symptoms (either local or systemic), chemotherapy may be started with either single drug treatment such as chlorambucil or combination chemotherapy (e.g. cyclophosphamide, vincristine, adriamycin and prednisolone) (Portlock 1982, Horning & Rosenberg 1984). Treatment varies, depending on the patient's age, personal wishes and the degree of remission considered optimum. Most patients with high grade lymphoma, however, require combination chemotherapy from the outset. Patients with localised disease respond well to CHOP-based regimens with 5-year survival rates of 80% or over (Miller & Jones 1983, Longo et al 1989). Local radiotherapy alone has been assessed in high grade lymphomas, giving inferior results with 5-year survival rates of 65% for stage I and Ie disease and 25% for stage II and IIe disease (Jones et al 1973).

If a biopsy diagnosis can be made without resection, the treatment of choice, if deemed appropriate, is chemotherapy for this offers a high response rate, although a controlled study comparing surgery with chemotherapy has yet to be set up. Clearly, if the diagnosis follows resection, the patient should be staged and postoperative chemotherapy, again if deemed appropriate, instigated. Five-year survival is quoted at 84–94% for low grade lymphomas, and 0–60% for high grade tumours.

Lymphomatoid granulomatosis

Lymphomatoid granulomatosis was first described by Liebow et al (1972) as an angiocentric and angiodestructive lymphoreticular proliferation. Subsequent reports documented that many patients went on to develop T-cell lymphomas (Katzenstein et al 1979, Colby & Carrington 1982, Pisani & DeRemee 1990), but it is still unclear whether these infiltrates are malignant from the outset. Some cases show undoubted histological evidence of neoplasia but others lack the necessary features.

The term angiocentric immunoproliferative lesion (AIL) was introduced in the 1980s to include both lymphomatoid granulomatosis and polymorphic reticulosis (also known as lethal mid-line granuloma). Polymorphic reticulosis shows morphological and clinical similarities to lymphomatoid granulomatosis but affects the upper airways (Jaffe 1984). Lipford et al (1988) introduced a grading system (1 to 3) for AIL, primarily based on the degree of lymphocytic atypia, but with necrosis and the polymorphic/monomorphic nature of the infiltrate also taken into consideration. Grade 3 lesions are synonymous with angiocentric lymphomas, grade 2 lesions equate quite well with lymphomatoid granulomatosis and grade 1 lesions with benign lymphocytic angiitis and granulomatosis, an entity initially described by Saldana et al (1977). Lipford et al (1988) found that 3 of 9 grade one lesions and 4 of 6 grade two lesions progressed to lymphoma.

Aetiology

The cases reported by Lipford et al (1988) were of T-cell phenotype and some were said to be analogous to T-cell lymphomas. In a further series also documenting a T-cell phenotype, rearrangements of the T-cell receptor genes could be found in only one case (Medeiros et al 1991). Guinee et al (1994) showed that the atypical lymphoid cells of pulmonary lymphomatoid granulomatosis were of B-cell phenotype and expressed Epstein-Barr virus (EBV) antigens; using PCR, monoclonal patterns could be shown in immunoglobulin heavy chain gene rearrangement. More recently, it has been shown that lymphomatoid granulomatosis is a mixture of B-cell and T-cell non-Hodgkin's lymphomas, indicating immunophenotypic diversity (Myers et al 1995). Furthermore, CD56-positive haematolymphoid malignancies (CD56 being a cluster differentiation group of antibodies that mark natural killer cells), may also involve the lung and it has been suggested that these, too, fall into the AIL spectrum (Wong et al 1992).

Thus, there is evidence that many cases of lymphomatoid granulomatosis and AIL are malignant from the outset, but there is a range of lymphoreticular tumours which can produce the characteristic histological pattern of AIL/lymphomatoid granulomatosis when they involve the lung.

Several studies have demonstrated the association of AIL with EBV (Veltri et al 1982, Katzenstein & Peiper 1990, Medeiros et al 1992, Guinee et al 1994, Tanaka et al 1994, Myers et al 1995). In one series, 80% of AILs were found to be positive for EBV, whilst other pulmonary lymphomas were consistently negative (Tanaka et al 1994). A Southern blot analysis showed clonal EBV in 2 of 8 cases of AIL (Medeiros et al 1991). EBV has also been detected in a case of B-cell lymphomatoid granulomatosis associated with AIDS (Mittal et al 1990). EBV latent membrane protein is known to have oncogenic properties and EBV infection may well be a factor in lymphomagenesis.

It seems likely, therefore, that lymphomatoid granulomatosis/polymorphic reticulosis/AIL represents a variety of non-Hodgkin's lymphoma rather than specific primary pulmonary/sinonasal disease (Strickler et al 1994, Myers et al 1995), although it has been suggested that pulmonary lymphomatoid granulomatosis is an EBV-related B-cell proliferation distinguishable from angiocentric T-cell lymphomas at other sites (Guinee et al 1994). However, some cases of pulmonary lymphomatoid granulomatosis have been shown to be T-cell lymphomas (Myers et al 1995). One wonders whether the histological features reflect a particular angiocentric pattern of spread rather than a specific cell type, with the large vascular bed of the lung responsible for it being the commonest site of presentation.

Thus, what was originally classified as lymphomatoid granulomatosis can now be shown to be neoplastic with the aid of molecular investigative techniques in a proportion of cases. They appear to be a heterogenous group of neoplasms, with the characteristic histological features of lymphomatoid granulomatosis/AIL seen in both B-cell and T-cell lymphomas. In the recent Revised European American Lymphoma (REAL) classification, they have been classed as angiocentric T-cell lymphomas, but with a reference to cases with a B-cell phenotype (Chan et al 1994). In order to ensure that the correct treatment is instigated, every effort should be made to document the presence of lymphoma and its correct phenotype, perhaps with the term angiocentric immunoproliferative lesion reserved for those cases where proof remains elusive.

Clinical

Most recent series report that patients have an average age of about 50 years (range:4–80) and there is a male preponderance. Cough, dyspnoea, haemoptysis and chest pain may be presenting features and some patients have 'B' symptoms (Medeiros et al 1991, Guinee et al 1994, Myers et al 1995).

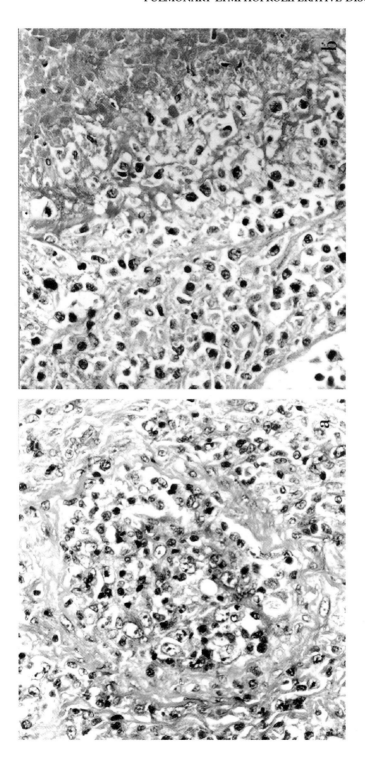

Fig. 3.4 (**a**) Lymphomatoid granulomatosis, classified as AIL grade 2, showing a polymorphic and angiocentric infiltrate including atypical lymphoid cells. H&E × 320. (**b**) Angiocentric lymphoma, classified as AIL grade 3, showing a monomorphic population of atypical lymphoid cells with extensive necrosis. In both cases, the atypical cells were B-cells. H&E × 320.

Imaging generally shows multiple bilateral nodules, but unilateral disease is also described. Although lymphomatoid granulomatosis typically presents in the lung or the skin (Katzenstein et al 1979, Angel et al 1994), it may also primarily affect the gastrointestinal tract (Rubin et al 1983), brain (Colby 1989, Kleinschmidt-DeMasters et al 1992), striated muscle (Schmalzl et al 1982) and bladder (Feinberg et al 1987).

Certain associations between these lymphoid proliferations and other disorders are of interest. Patients with AIL may have underlying defects of cell-mediated immunity and these may be congenital, e.g. in association with Wiskott-Aldrich syndrome (Ilowite et al 1986), or acquired as in AIDS (Colby 1989), after treatment for acute lymphoblastic lymphoma (Bekassy et al 1985), in agnogenic myeloid metaplasia (Naschitz et al 1984) and in follicular lymphoma (Imai et al 1992). There is also a similarity between AILs and post-transplant lymphoproliferative disorders: both show angiocentricity when involving the lung, both express EBV antigens and both exhibit a range of monoclonality, oligoclonality and polyclonality (Swerdlow 1992, Burke 1994, Myers et al 1995). Thus, there is an association between AIL and immunosuppressive states, but whether the risk is greater than for lymphomas in general is unknown.

Pathology

Typically, there is a polymorphous, angiocentric and angiodestructive lymphoid infiltrate consisting of lymphocytes, plasma cells, histiocytes and sometimes eosinophils. Some of the lymphoid cells are atypical, the degree of atypia being the principal variable when grading these lesions. Necrosis and granuloma formation are additional features (Fig. 3.4).

Treatment and survival

Information on treatment is scarce: in one series, 7 of 8 patients with grade 3 AIL went into remission on chemotherapy but, of 7 others that eventually progressed to frank lymphoma and subsequently received chemotherapy, only one responded, suggesting that conservative treatment may compromise the ability to achieve complete remission later (Lipford et al 1988). Lymphomatoid granulomatosis may respond to CHOP combination chemotherapy (Drasga et al 1984) and to bone marrow transplantation (Bernstein et al 1986). In a report of 6 patients undergoing combination chemotherapy, 4 went into remission and 2 failed to respond (Myers et al 1995). It is clear, therefore, that AIL is aggressive and associated with a high mortality rate if untreated.

REACTIVE PULMONARY LYMPHOID DISORDERS

There are numerous reactive pulmonary disorders that contain a prominent lymphoid component, for example extrinsic allergic alveolitis, cryptogenic

fibrosing alveolitis and sarcoidosis, but most of these are clinically and histologically distinct entities that are easily differentiated from malignant lymphoproliferative disorders. However some, such as lymphoid interstitial
pneumonitis and follicular bronchitis/bronchiolitis, have features in common
with pulmonary lymphomas and must be considered in the differential diagnosis of a predominantly lymphoid pulmonary infiltrate.

Lymphoid interstitial pneumonitis

The term lymphoid interstitial pneumonitis (LIP) was introduced to describe
a diffuse lymphocytic interstitial infiltrate that could be distinguished from
the usual form of interstitial pneumonitis (UIP) (Liebow & Carrington
1969), though some patients with LIP have been shown to develop progressive interstitial fibrosis, as did those with UIP (Strimlan et al 1978).

Clinical findings

The disease is commoner in females and the average age at presentation is
about 50 years. The usual presenting symptoms are dyspnoea, cough and
chest pain. Haemoptysis has occasionally been described. Patients tend to
have a restrictive ventilatory defect. Imaging is characteristically described as
showing reticular, coarse reticulonodular or fine reticulonodular shadowing
(Liebow & Carrington 1973, Strimlan et al 1978, Koss et al 1987, Nicholson
et al 1995b).

There are clinical associations with Sjögren's syndrome (Liebow &
Carrington 1973, Strimlan et al 1976), Hashimoto's thyroiditis (Julsrud et al
1978), pernicious anaemia (Levinson et al 1976), chronic autoimmune hepatitis (Helman et al 1977), autoimmune haemolytic anaemia (Liebow &
Carrington 1973, DeCoteau et al 1974), primary biliary cirrhosis (Koss et al
1987), myasthenia gravis (Liebow Carrington 1973), and AIDS, particularly
in children (Grieco & Chinoy-Acharya 1985, Solal-Celigny et al 1985,
Morris et al 1987). Many patients with LIP show abnormalities of
immunoglobulin production, typically hyper- or hypo-gammaglobulinaemia,
or a monoclonal gammopathy (Montes et al 1968, Liebow & Carrington
1973, Church et al 1981).

Pathology

The dominant feature is an interstitial infiltrate of small lymphocytes, plasma
cells and histiocytes, with granuloma formation and germinal centres (Fig.
3.5) (Strimlan et al 1978, Koss et al 1987, Nicholson et al 1995b).
Immunohistochemistry shows that B-cells are mainly limited to the germinal
centres, often highlighting more follicles than are seen on routine sections.
The interstitial lymphocytes are predominantly T-cells mixed with scattered
B-cells (Fig. 3.6) (Nicholson et al 1995b).

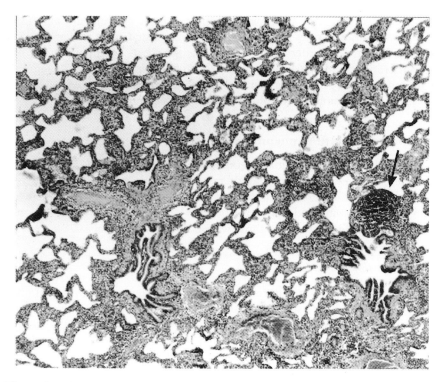

Fig. 3.5 Lymphoid interstitial pneumonitis showing expansion of the interstitium by a lymphoid infiltrate that is less marked than in the lymphoma in Figure 3.1. Note the peribronchiolar lymphoid follicle (arrow). H&E × 50.

Follicular bronchiolitis

This term has been used to describe pathological features associated with various systemic disorders. When there is airway dilatation associated with prominent lymphoid hyperplasia, for example in cystic fibrosis, the term follicular bronchiectasis is sometimes used.

Clinical findings

Follicular bronchiolitis commonly affects people in middle age but there is a wide age range and, in the group with connective tissue disorders, females predominate. They present with progressive shortness of breath, fever, cough and recurrent upper respiratory tract infections, together with bilateral reticulonodular or reticular shadowing on chest X-ray. They fall into three groups: those with connective tissue disorders, those with immune deficiency syndromes, and those of uncertain aetiology. This last group is possibly related to hypersensitivity states (Fortoul et al 1985, Yousem et al 1985).

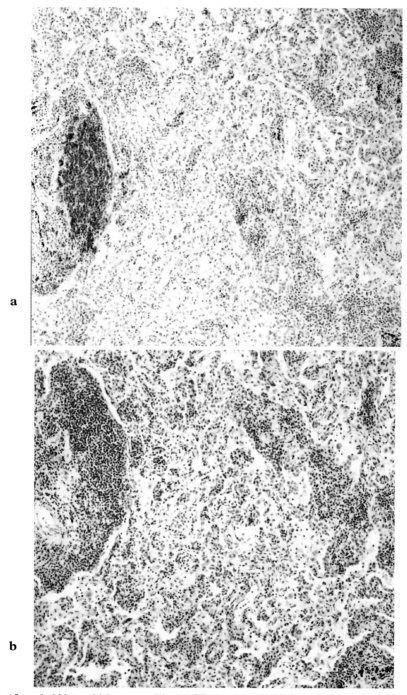

Fig. 3. 6 Lymphoid interstitial pneumonitis. (**a**) CD20 staining highlights a B-cell aggregate: (**b**) CD3 staining shows that the neighbouring interstitial infiltrate consists predominantly of T-cells. Both immunoperoxidase × 45.

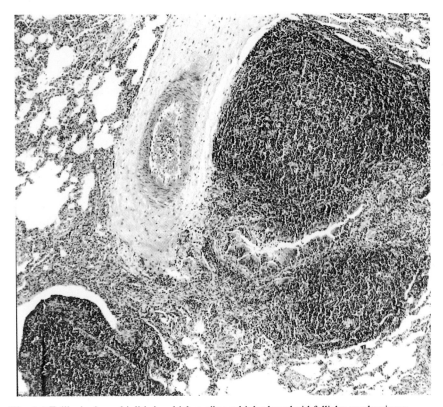

Fig. 3.7 Follicular bronchiolitis in which peribronchiolar lymphoid follicles predominate, although a mild interstitial infiltrate is also seen. H&E × 50.

Pathology

There is abundant peribronchiolar germinal centre formation with lymphocytes infiltrating the overlying epithelium. The airways are often compressed. Some cases show extension of a mixed lymphoid infiltrate into the interstitium, along interlobular septa or beneath the pleura (Fig. 3.7) (Fortoul et al 1985, Yousem et al 1985, Nicholson et al 1995b).

Aetiology

Since their initial descriptions, there has been debate about whether lymphoid interstitial pneumonitis and follicular bronchiolitis represent distinct pathological entities or non-specific responses to injury (Liebow & Carrington 1973, Yousem et al 1985, Koss et al 1987). A review of benign pulmonary lymphoid disorders suggested that lymphoid hyperplasia is the basic underlying pathogenetic mechanism (Kradin & Mark 1983), and the histological features support this view. Follicular bronchiolitis and lymphoid interstitial pneumonitis appear to represent different ends of the spectrum of hyperplasia within the pulmonary immune system, the former being characterised by the predominance of lymphoid follicles with a minor alveolar interstitial inflammatory component, and the latter by a heavy lymphoid infiltrate of the alveolar interstitium but with lymphoid follicles generally located around airways. These infiltrates show a polyclonal pattern after amplification of the heavy chain gene by PCR (Nicholson et al 1995b). Clinically, they are also similar: both disorders are commonest in middle age, and are associated with gammopathies, connective tissue disorders and immunodeficiency (Strimlan et al 1978, Fortoul et al 1985, Yousem et al 1985, Koss et al 1987, Nicholson et al 1995b).

However, only LIP seems to carry a risk of progression to lymphoma, though this is extremely rare (Kradin et al 1982, Teruya-Feldstein et al 1995). Some cases described as lymphomatous transformation may well have been neoplastic from the outset, as the histological features of lymphoma and lymphoid interstitial pneumonitis can be indistinguishable on routine histology. Furthermore, the histology of LIP can be difficult to distinguish from that of extrinsic allergic alveolitis and the final diagnosis depends on clinical correlation (Colby 1988).

Treatment and survival

Most patients are treated with steroids, cytotoxic therapy being an additional option. Responses are variable: some patients show radiological resolution, some remain stable and some progress. In occasional cases, death has been attributed to LIP (Strimlan et al 1978, Koss et al 1987, Nicholson et al 1995b).

DIFFERENTIAL DIAGNOSIS OF PULMONARY LYMPHOID LESIONS

MALT lymphoma vs reactive infiltrates

There are few problems in identifying the confluent sheets of blast cells of a high grade lymphoma, other than distinguishing the tumour from anaplastic large cell carcinoma. The main problem lies in the distinction between low-grade lymphomas of MALT origin and lymphoid interstitial pneumonitis. The clinical history may provide information favouring one diagnosis or the other, but there are no absolute differences. If one is dealing with a resection specimen, the histological features of a lymphoma are characteristic, showing a destructive mass. Lymphoid interstitial pneumonitis does not infiltrate and destroy the alveolar architecture though it may progress to interstitial fibrosis. Thickening of the alveolar septa by the lymphoid infiltrate is less marked in lymphoid interstitial pneumonitis. Vascular infiltration and lymphoepithelial lesions are more common in lymphoma than in reactive lymphoid infiltrates, but neither is a specific marker of malignancy.

The immunohistochemical findings in a reactive infiltrate are of aggregated B-cells which are usually peribronchial or septal in distribution, whilst a predominantly T-cell infiltrate and only scattered B-cells are seen in the alveolar interstitium. In lymphomas of MALT origin, B-cells infiltrate widely throughout the parenchyma and this is a useful distinguishing feature. However, one has to be wary of occasional cases with a predominant reactive T-cell population which may mask lymphoma, and also be aware of extrapulmonary T-cell lymphomas/leukaemias infiltrating the interstitium. Confirmation of lymphoma can be provided by demonstrating light chain restriction or monoclonality by PCR. In our series, one case previously diagnosed as LIP was shown to have a monoclonal band and was re-classified as a low grade B-cell lymphoma (Nicholson et al 1995b).

In practice, there is rarely a problem with resection specimens; the difficulties arise in the assessment of biopsies. With open lung biopsies, a lymphomatous infiltrate may be indistinguishable from a lymphoid interstitial pneumonitis, especially when there is neither architectural destruction nor sclerosis. In these cases, the distribution of B- and T-cells described above is valuable. In transbronchial or percutaneous needle biopsies, high grade lymphoma can be recognised by an infiltrate of blast cells, but the small amount of tissue and crush artefact often preclude adequate assessment of low grade lymphoma. Light chain restriction or the presence of a monoclonal band would support the diagnosis of lymphoma, but often there is insufficient tissue for either of these investigations.

If lymphoma is suspected, judicious sectioning of the tissue is advised, otherwise valuable material which could otherwise have been used for immunohistochemistry and gene rearrangement studies may be lost in the process of initial levelling.

MALT lymphoma vs other lymphoma

With regard to secondary involvement of the lung by lymphomas, there is usually a history of previous disease. If there is doubt in low grade cases, cytogenetic and immunohistochemical profiles may be of help (Wotherspoon et al 1990, Clark et al 1992). Differentiation between lymphomatoid granulomatosis and primary pulmonary high grade B-cell lymphoma rests on the presence or absence of angiocentricity, though this is prone to observer variation. Hodgkin's disease can be primary in the lung, but this is very rare and the characteristic histology is readily distinguishable from MALT lymphoma (Radin 1990). Secondary involvement of the lung by Hodgkin's disease is far more common (Berkman & Breuer 1993).

PLEURAL LYMPHOMAS

Primary pleural lymphomas are extremely rare and appear to be consistently associated with chronic inflammation of the pleura resulting from therapeutic artificial pneumothorax or tuberculous pleuritis (Iuchi et al 1987, Iuchi et al 1989). Most cases have been described in Japan, suggesting the involvement of an environmental factor, although occasional series from Western countries are also on record (Martin et al 1994, Hsu et al 1996). There is a strong association with EBV and localised immunosuppression secondary to chronic inflammation has been suggested as a possible cause of an EBV-driven B-cell proliferation (Fukayama et al 1993, Martin et al 1994, Ohsawa et al 1995). Histologically, these are high grade lymphomas which tend to be immunoblastic and most are of B-cell phenotype. Some are of null-cell phenotype and a single case of T-cell lymphoma has also been described (Nakamura et al 1995, Ohsawa et al 1995). Differentiation from other forms of high grade pulmonary non-Hodgkin's lymphoma rests on localisation to the pleura and a characteristic history of long-standing chronic inflammation. Some patients have gone into remission following chemotherapy, but the majority have died of their disease.

KEY POINTS FOR CLINICAL PRACTICE

1. Most primary pulmonary lymphomas arise from bronchial MALT and show histological features similar to MALT lymphomas arising in other mucosal sites. What was once termed pseudolymphoma is now thought to be lymphoma from the outset.

2. Many cases of lymphomatoid granulomatosis/angiocentric immuno-proliferative lesion have been shown to be neoplastic. They usually represent systemic extranodal B- or T-cell lymphomas, with spread to the lung. Many are associated with Epstein-Barr virus infection.

3. Lymphoid interstitial pneumonitis and follicular bronchiolitis represent overlapping patterns of hyperplasia in the pulmonary immune system.

4. Reactive infiltrates may be indistinguishable from low grade lymphoma on routine histology, but immunohistochemistry and gene analysis can provide useful additional diagnostic information.

5. Pleural lymphomas are extremely rare. They are associated with long-standing chronic inflammation of the pleura, have a B-cell phenotype and are strongly associated with EBV infection.

REFERENCES

Addis B J, Hyjek E, Isaacson P G 1988 Primary pulmonary lymphoma: a re-appraisal of its histogenesis and its relationship to pseudolymphoma and lymphoid interstitial pneumonia.

Histopathology 13: 1–17

Angel C A, Slater D N, Royds J A et al 1994 Epstein-Barr virus in cutaneous lymphomatoid granulomatosis. Histopathology 25: 545–548

Bekassy A N, Cameron R, Garwicz S et al 1985 Lymphomatoid granulomatosis during treatment of acute lymphoblastic lymphoma in a 6 year old girl. Am J Paediatr Hematol Oncol 7: 377–380

Berkman N, Breuer R 1993 Pulmonary involvement in lymphoma. Respiratory Medicine 87: 85–92

Bernstein M L, Reece E, De Chadarevian J P et al 1986 Bone marrow transplantation in lymphomatoid granulomatosis. Report of a case. Cancer 58: 969–972

Bienenstock J, Johnston N, Perey D Y 1973a Bronchial lymphoid tissue. II Functional characteristics. Lab Invest 28, 693–698

Bienenstock J, Johnston N, Perey D Y 1973b Bronchial lymphoid tissue. I. Morphologic characteristics. Lab Invest 28: 686-692

Burke M M 1994 Complications of heart and lung transplantation and of cardiac surgery. In: Anthony P P, MacSween R N M (eds) Recent Advances in Histopathology, No. 16. London, Churchill Livingstone, pp. 95–122

Chan J K, Banks P M, Cleary M L et al 1994 A proposal for classification of lymphoid neoplasms (by the International Lymphoma Study Group). Histopathology 25: 517–536

Church J A, Isaacs H, Saxon A et al 1981 Lymphoid interstitial pneumonitis and hypogammoglobulinaemia in children. Am Rev Resp Dis 124: 491–496

Clark H M, Jones D B, Wright DH 1992 Cytogenetic and molecular studies of t(14;18) and t(14;19) in nodal and extranodal B-cell lymphoma. J Pathol 166: 129–137

Colby T V 1988 Lymphoproliferative diseases. In: Dail D H, Hammar S P (eds) Pulmonary Pathology. New York Springer-Verlag pp. 713

Colby T V 1989 Central nervous system lymphomatoid granulomatosis in AIDS? Hum Pathol 20: 301–302

Colby T V, Carrington C B 1982 Malignant lymphoma simulating lymphomatoid granulomatosis. Am J Surg Pathol 6: 19–32

Cordier J F, Chailleux E, Lauque D et al 1993 Primary pulmonary lymphomas. A clinical study of 70 cases in nonimmunocompromised patients. Chest 103: 201–208

Davis W B, Gadek J E 1987 Detection of pulmonary lymphoma by bronchoalveolar lavage. Chest 91: 787–790

Decoteau W E, Tourville D, Ambrus J L et al 1974 Lymphoid interstitial pneumonia and autoerythrocyte sensitization syndrome. A case with deposition of immunoglobulins on the alveolar basement membrane. Arch Intern Med 134: 519–522

Drasga R E, Williams S D, Wills E R et al 1984 Lymphomatoid granulomatosis. Successful treatment with CHOP combination chemotherapy. Am J Clin Oncol 7: 75–80

Feinberg S M, Leslie K O, Colby T V 1987 Bladder outlet obstruction by so-called lymphomatoid granulomatosis (angiocentric lymphoma). J Urol 137: 989–990

Fiche M, Capron F, Berger F et al 1995 Primary pulmonary non-Hodgkin's lymphomas. Histopathology 26: 529–537

Fortoul T I, Cano-Valle F, Oliva E et al 1985 Follicular bronchiolitis in association with connective tissue diseases. Lung 163: 305–314

Frizzera G 1994 Immunosuppression, autoimmunity and lymphoproliferative disorders. Hum Pathol 25: 627–629

Fukayama M, Ibuka T, Hayashi Y 1993 Epstein-Barr virus in pyothorax-associated pleural lymphoma. Am J Pathol 143: 1044–1049.

Gould S J, Isaacson P G 1993 Bronchus-associated lymphoid tissue (BALT) in human fetal and infant lung. J Pathol 169: 229–234

Grieco M H, Chinoy-Acharya P 1985 Lymphocytic interstitial pneumonia associated with the acquired immune deficiency syndrome. Am Rev Resp Dis 131; 952–955

Guinee Jr D, Jaffe E, Kingma D et al 1994 Pulmonary lymphomatoid granulomatosis. Evidence for a proliferation of Epstein-Barr virus infected B-lymphocytes with a predominant T-cell component and vasculitis. Am J Surg Pathol 18: 753–764

Helman C A, Keeton G R, Benatar S R 1977 Lymphoid interstitial pneumonia with associated chronic active hepatitis and renal tubular acidosis. Am Rev Resp Dis 115: 161–164

Holt P G 1993 Development of bronchus associated lymphoid tissue (BALT) in human lung disease: a normal host defence mechanism awaiting therapeutic exploitation? Thorax 48: 1097–1098

Horning S J, Rosenberg S A 1984 The natural history of initially untreated low-grade non-Hodgkin's lymphomas. N Engl J Med 311: 1471–1475

Hsu N Y, Chen C Y, Pan S T et al 1996 Pleural non-Hodgin's lymphoma arising in a patient with a chronic pyothorax. Thorax 51: 103–104

Ilowite N T, Fligner C L, Ochs H D et al 1986 Pulmonary angiitis with atypical lymphoreticular infiltrates in Wiskott-Aldrich syndrome: possible relationship to lymphomatoid granulomatosis and EBV infection. Clin Immunol Immunopathol 41: 479–484

Imai Y, Yamamoto K, Suzuki K et al 1992 Lymphomatoid granulomatosis (LYG) occurring in a patient with follicular lymphoma during remission. Jpn J Clin Hematol 33: 507–513

Isaacson P G 1990 Lymphomas of mucosa-associated lymphoid tissue (MALT). Histopathology 16: 617–619

Iseman M D, Schwarz M I, Stanford R E 1976 Interstitial pneumonia in angioimmunoblastic lymphadenopathy with dysproteinaemia. Ann Intern Med 85: 752–755

Iuchi K, Aozasa K, Yamato S 1989 Non-Hodgkin's lymphomas of the pleural cavity developing from long-standing pyothorax. Summary of clinical and pathological findings in thirty-seven cases. Jpn J Clin Oncol 19: 249–257

Iuchi K, Ichimiya A, Akashi A et al 1987 Non-Hodgkin's lymphoma of the pleural cavity developing from long standing pyothorax. Cancer 60: 1771–1775

Jaffe E S 1984 Pathologic and clinical spectrum of post-thymic T-cell malignancies. Cancer Invest 3: 413–426

Jones S E, Fuks Z, Kaplan H S et al 1973 Non-Hodgkin's lymphomas. V. Results of radiotherapy. Cancer 32: 682–691

Joseph G, Pandit M., Korfhage L 1993 Primary pulmonary plasmacytoma. Cancer 71: 721–724

Julsrud P R, Brown L R, Li C Y et al 1978 Pulmonary processes of mature-appearing lymphocytes: pseudolymphoma, well-differentiated lymphocytic lymphoma and lymphocytic interstitial pneumonitis. Radiology 127: 289–296

Kamel O W, Van De Rijn M, Le Brun D P et al 1994 Lymphoid neoplasms in patients with rheumatoid arthritis and dermatomyositis; frequency of Epstein-Barr virus and other features associated with immunosuppression. Hum Pathol 25: 638–643

Katzenstein A L, Peiper S C 1990 Detection of Epstein-Barr virus genomes in lymphomatoid granulomatosis: analysis of 29 cases by the polymerase chain reaction technique. Mod Pathol 3: 435–441

Katzenstein A L, Carrington C B, Leibow A A 1979 Lymphomatoid granulomatosis: a clinicopathologic study of 152 cases. Cancer 43: 360–373

Kennedy J L, Nathwani B N, Burke J S et al 1985 Pulmonary lymphomas and other pulmonary lymphoid lesions. A clinicopathologic and immunologic study of 64 patients. Cancer 56: 539–552

Kleinschmidt-Demasters B K, Filley C M, Bitter M A 1992 Central nervous system angiocentric, angiodestructive T-cell lymphoma (lymphomatoid granulomatosis). Surg Neurol 37: 130–137

Koss M N 1995 Pulmonary lymphoid disorders. Semin Diagn Pathol 12: 158–171

Koss M N, Hochholzer L, Nichols P W et al 1983 Primary non-Hodgkin's lymphoma and pseudolymphoma of lung: a study of 161 patients. Hum Pathol 14: 1024–1038

Koss M N, Hochholzer L, Langloss J M et al 1987 Lymphoid interstitial pneumonia: clinicopathological and immunopathological findings in 18 cases. Pathology 19: 178–185

Kradin R L, Mark E J 1983 Benign lymphoid disorders of the lung, with a theory regarding their development. Hum Pathol 14: 857–867

Kradin R L, Young R H, Kradin L A et al 1982 Immunoblastic lymphoma arising in chronic lymphoid hyperplasia of the pulmonary interstitium. Cancer 50: 1339–1343

L'Hoste R J, Filippa D A, Lieberman P H et al 1984 Primary pulmonary lymphomas. A clinicopathological analysis of 36 cases. Cancer 54: 1397–1406

Levinson A I, Hopewell P C, Stites D P et al 1976 Coexistent lymphoid interstitial pneumonia, pernicious anaemia and agammaglobulinaemia. Arch Inter Med 136: 213–216

Li G, Hansmann M L, Zwingers T et al 1990 Primary lymphomas of the lung: morphological, immunohistochemical and clinical features. Histopathology 16: 519–531

Liebow A A, Carrington C B 1969 The interstitial pneumonias. In: Simon M (ed) Frontiers in pulmonary radiology. New York, Grune and Stratton, pp. 102–141

Liebow A A, Carrington C B 1973 Diffuse pulmonary lymphoreticular infiltrations associated with dysproteinaemia. Med Clin North Am 57: 809–843

Liebow A A, Carrington C R, Friedman P J 1972 Lymphomatoid granulomatosis. Hum Pathol 3: 457–458

Lipford E H, Margolick J B, Longo D L et al 1988 Angiocentric immunoproliferative lesions: a clinicopathologic spectrum of post-thymic T-cell proliferations. Blood 72: 1674–1681

Longo D L, Glatstein E, Duffey P L et al 1989 Treatment of localized aggressive lymphomas with combination chemotherapy followed by involved-field radiation therapy. J Clin Oncol 7: 1295–1302

Martin A, Capron F, Liguory-Brunard M et al 1994 Epstein-Barr virus-associated primary malignant lymphomas of the pleural cavity occurring in longstanding pleural chronic inflammation. Hum Pathol 25: 1314–1318

McDermott M R, Bienenstock J 1979 Evidence for a common mucosal immunologic system. Migration of B immunoblasts into intestinal, respiratory, and genital tissues. J Immunol 122: 1892–1898

Medeiros L J, Peiper S C, Elwood L et al 1991 Angiocentric immunoproliferative lesions: a molecular analysis of eight cases. Hum Pathol 22: 1150–1157

Medeiros L J, Jaffe E S, Chen Yet al 1992 Localisation of Epstein-Barr viral genomes in angiocentric immunoproliferative lesions. Am J Surg Pathol 16: 439-447.

Miller T P, Jones S E 1983 Initial chemotherapy for clinically localized lymphomas of unfavorable histology. Blood 62: 413–418

Mittal K, Neri A, Feiner H et al 1990 Lymphomatoid granulomatosis in the acquired immunodeficiency syndrome. Evidence of Epstein-Barr virus infection and B-cell clonal selection without myc rearrangement. Cancer 65: 1345–1349

Mohamedani A A, Bennett M K 1985 Angiofollicular lymphoid hyperplasia in a pulmonary fissure. Thorax 40: 686–687

Montes M, Tomasi Jr T B, Noehreun T H et al 1968 Lymphoid interstitial pneumonia with monoclonal gammopathy. Am Rev Resp Dis 98: 277–280

Morris J C, Rosen M J, Marchevsky A et al 1987 Lymphocytic interstitial pneumonia in patients at risk from the acquired immune deficiency syndrome. Chest 91: 63–67

Myers J L, Kurtin P J, Katzenstein A A et al 1995 Lymphomatoid granulomatosis. Evidence of immunophenotypic diversity and relationship to Epstein-Barr virus infection. Am J Surg Pathol 19: 1300–1312

Nakamura S, Sasajima Y, Koshikawa T et al 1995 Ki-1 (CD30) positive anaplastic large cell lymphomas of T-cell phenotype developing in association with long-standing tuberculous pyothorax: report of a case with detection of Epstein-Barr genome in the tumour cells. Hum Pathol 26: 1382–1385

Naschitz J E, Yeshurun D, Grishkan A et al 1984 Lymphomatoid granulomatosis of the lung in a patient with agnogenic myeloid metaplasia. Respiration 45: 316–320

Ngan B Y, Warnke R A, Wilson M et al 1991 Monocytoid B-cell lymphoma: a study of 36 cases. Hum Pathol 22: 409–421

Nicholson A G, Wotherspoon A C, Diss T C et al 1995a Pulmonary B-cell non-Hodgkin's lymphomas. The value of immunohistochemistry and gene analysis in diagnosis.

Histopathology 26: 395–404

Nicholson A G, Wotherspoon A C, Diss T C et al 1995b Reactive pulmonary lymphoid disorders. Histopathology 26: 405–412

Ohsawa M, Tomita Y, Kanno H et al 1995 Role of Epstein-Barr virus in pleural lymphomagenesis. Mod Pathol 8: 848–853

Ortiz-Hidalgo C, Wright D H 1992 The morphological spectrum of monocytoid B-cell lymphoma and its relationship to lymphomas of mucosa-associated lymphoid tissue. Histopathology 21: 555–561

Pabst R 1992 Is BALT a major component of the human lung immune system? Immunology Today 13: 119–122

Pabst R, Gehrke I 1990 Is the bronchus-associated lymphoid tissue (BALT) an integral structure of the lung in normal mammals, including humans? Am J Resp Cell Mol Biol 3: 131–135

Pisani R J, Deremee R A 1990 Clinical implications of the histopathologic diagnosis of pulmonary lymphomatoid granulomatosis. Mayo Clin Proc 65: 151–163

Portlock C S 1982 Deferral of initial therapy for advanced indolent lymphomas. Cancer Treatment Rep 66: 417–419

Radin A I 1990 Primary pulmonary Hodgkin's disease. Cancer 65: 550–563

Richmond I, Pritchard G E, Ashcroft T et al 1993 Bronchus associated lymphoid tissue (BALT) in human lung: its distribution in smokers and non-smokers. Thorax 48: 1130–1134

Rubin L A, Little A H, Kolin A et al 1983 Lymphomatoid granulomatosis involving the gastrointestinal tract. Two case reports and a review of the literature. Gastroenterology 84: 829–833

Rudzik R, Clancy R L, Perey D Y et al 1975 Repopulation with IgA-containing cells of bronchial and intestinal lamina propria after transfer of homologous Peyer's patch and bronchial lymphocytes. J Immunol 114: 1599–1604

Saldana M J, Patchefsky A S, Israel H I et al 1977 Pulmonary angiitis and granulomatosis. The relationship between histological features, organ involvement and response to treatment. Hum Pathol 8: 391–409

Saltzstein S L 1963 Pulmonary malignant lymphomas and pseudolymphomas: classification, therapy and prognosis. Cancer 1: 928–955

Schmalzl F, Gasser R W, Weiser G et al 1982 Lymphomatoid granulomatosis with primary manifestation in the skeletal muscular system. Klin Wochensch 60: 311–316

Shiota T, Chiba W, Ikeda S et al 1993 Gene analysis of pulmonary pseudolymphoma. Chest 103: 335–338

Solal-Celigny P, Couderc L J, Herman D et al 1985 Lymphoid interstitial pneumonitis in acquired immunodeficiency syndrome-related complex. Am Rev Resp Dis 131: 956–960

Sprague R I, Deblois G G 1989 Small lymphocytic pulmonary lymphoma. Diagnosis by transthoracic fine needle aspiration. Chest 96: 929–930

Strickler J G, Meneses M F, Haberman T M et al 1994 Polymorphic reticulosis: a reappraisal. Hum Pathol 25: 659–665

Strimlan C V, Rosenov E C, Divertie M B et al 1976 Pulmonary manifestations of Sjögren's syndrome. Chest 70: 354–361

Strimlan C V, Rosenow E C, Weiland L H et al 1978 Lymphocytic interstitial pneumonitis. Review of 13 cases. Ann Intern Med 88: 616–621

Swerdlow S H 1992 Post-transplant lymphoproliferative disorders: a morphologic, phenotypic and genotypic spectrum of disease. Histopathology 20: 373–385

Symmons D P 1985 Neoplasms of the immune system in rheumatoid arthritis. Am J Med 78(1A): 22–28

Tanaka Y, Sasaki Y, Kurozumi H et al 1994 Angiocentric immunoproliferative lesion associated with chronic active Epstein-Barr virus infection in an 11 year old boy. Clonotropic proliferation of Epstein-Barr virus-bearing CD4+ T lymphocytes. Am J Surg Pathol 18: 623–631

Teruya-Feldstein J, Temeck B K, Sloas M M et al 1995 Pulmonary malignant lymphoma of mucosa-associated lymphoid tissue (MALT) arising in a pediatric HIV-positive patient. Am J Surg Pathol 19: 357–363

Turner R R, Colby T V, Dogget R S 1984 Well-differentiated lymphocytic lymphoma. A study of 47 patients with primary manifestation in the lung. Cancer 54: 2088–2096

Uppal R, Goldstraw P 1992 Primary pulmonary lymphoma. Lung Cancer 8: 95–100

Veltri R W, Raich P C, McClung J E et al 1982 Lymphomatoid granulomatosis and Epstein-Barr virus. Cancer 50: 1513–1517

Weiss L M, Yousem S A, Warnke R A 1985 Non-Hodgkin's lymphoma of the lung. A study of 19 cases emphasizing the utility of frozen section immunologic studies in differential diagnosis. Am J Surg Pathol 9: 480–490

Wong K F, Chan J K, Ng C G et al 1992 CD56 (NKH1)-positive hematolymphoid malignancies: an aggressive neoplasm featuring frequent cutaneous/mucosal involvement, cytoplasmic azurophilic granules, and angiocentricity. Hum Pathol 23: 798–804

Wotherspoon A C, Finn T M, Isaacson P G 1995 Trisomy 3 in low-grade B-cell lymphomas of mucosa-associated lymphoid tissue. Blood 85: 2000–2004

Wotherspoon A C, Pan L, Diss T C et al 1990 A genotypic study of low-grade B-cell lymphomas, including lymphomas of mucosa-associated lymphoid tissue (MALT). J Pathol 162: 135–140

Wotherspoon A C, Soosay G N, Diss T C et al 1990 Low grade primary B-cell lymphoma of the lung. An immunohistochemical, molecular and cytogenetic study of a single case. Am J Clin Pathol 94: 655–660

Wotherspoon A C, Ortiz-Hidalgo C, Falzon M R et al 1991 *Helicobacter pylori*-associated gastritis and primary B-cell gastric lymphoma. Lancet 338: 1175–1176

Wotherspoon A C, Pan L, Diss T C et al 1992 Cytogenetic study of B-cell lymphoma of mucosa-associated lymphoid tissue. Cancer Genet Cytogenet 58: 35–38

Yousem S A, Colby T V, Carrington C B 1985 Follicular bronchitis/bronchiolitis. Hum Pathol 16: 700–706

Zylak C J, Banerjee R, Galbraith P A et al 1976 Lung involvement in angioimmunoblastic lymphadenopathy. Radiology 121: 513–519

4

Risk assessment in breast cancer

T. J. Anderson   D. L. Page

In the past decade there has been a major international effort to improve the histopathological assessment of breast tissue specimens so that a report, as complete as possible, can be routinely constructed. Several recommendations have been published (Connolly & Schnitt 1988, Connolly et al 1995, NHSBSP Pathology Reporting 1995) to encourage a uniform approach to the handling, processing and reporting of specimens. The introduction of a national programme of breast cancer screening in the UK, and other, more limited schemes in Europe and North America have led to a broader experience of lesions and a need for wider appreciation of how best to approach some of the more contentious or borderline aspects of breast histopathology.

This contribution attempts to assess the current status of breast cancer evaluation and define information on breast cancer risk that can be obtained from histopathology. Three major areas are reviewed: potentially premalignant lesions, carcinoma *in situ*, and prognostic indicators in invasive breast cancer.

POTENTIALLY PREMALIGNANT LESIONS

Histological indicators of increased risk

Lesions of premalignant potential are the atypical hyperplasias which have specific histopathological definitions (Page et al 1987a, Page & Rogers 1992) and have been shown in several follow-up studies to indicate an increased risk of cancer development in the range of 4–5 times that of women of the same age. This information has been available for some time (Dupont & Page 1985), and was confirmed repeatedly (London et al 1992, Dupont et al 1993). The importance of recognising these atypical hyperplastic lesions (Fig. 4.1) is that they can easily be over-diagnosed as carcinoma *in situ* and so result in a much greater level of concern for the patient's well-being than is appropriate. It is important to recognize that these changes are indicators or markers of an increased cancer risk that applies to all parts of both breasts, but they are not obligate (Gallager 1980). In contrast, there are obligate lesions that are committed, in a large percentage of cases, to progress to invasion and metastasis if not completely removed, e.g. non-comedo or low grade ductal carcinoma *in situ*.

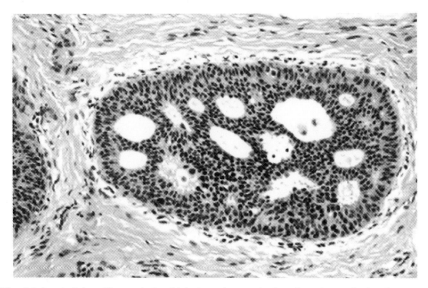

Fig. 4.1 Atypical ductal hyperplasia which shows low grade ductal carcinoma *in situ* of cribriform type centrally, but the cells on the outer aspect, adjacent to the surrounding connective tissue are normally polarised, and have an increased amount of cytoplasm. Therefore, the apparently neoplastic cell population does not involve the entire space. HE x40

Definition and implications of atypical hyperplasia

The histopathological criteria for recognition of the atypical hyperplasias have been well presented in several publications (see comment in NHSBSP Pathology Reporting 1995) and are reproduced here for completeness (Table 4.1). There are both age- and time-dependent factors with regard to the atypical hyperplasias. These lesions are uncommon under the age of 35 years and

Table 4.1

Florid hyperplasia without atypia	Atypical hyperplasia ductal pattern	Non-comedo duct carcinoma *in situ* (DCIS)
Streaming or swirling	Groups of uniform cells lacking crisp pattern definitions of DCIS	Uniform population of evenly spaced cells
Variability of nuclear size and shape		Geometric or papillary patterns of characteristic form
Variability of cell placement	Limited extent of lesion	
	Not completely involving two basement membrane-bound spaces	
Irregular intercellular spaces (particularly slit-like)		More extensive, or larger than atypical hyperplasia
	Less than 2–3 mm in size	

the implications for this age group are unproven largely because of their rarity. They are commonest in the age group of 45–55 years in which their malignant potential is well-proven (Page & Dupont 1990, McDivitt et al 1992). After the age of 55 years atypical lobular hyperplasia (ALH) may have less importance because these lesions tend to disappear after the menopause and few women have been studied for the consequent risk of cancer in this age group. For example, no woman over 55 years diagnosed as having ALH developed invasive carcinoma on follow-up (Page et al 1985). It is equally important to be aware that the relative risk from these lesions decreases with time. That is to say, 10 years after a diagnosis of atypical hyperplasia the risk of carcinoma will be more like that for ordinary hyperplasia, which is about twice that in women of the same age (Dupont & Page 1989). The reason for this is unknown but the finding strongly suggests that the risk is small beyond 10–15 years (Page & Dupont 1993, Page et al 1995b).

The differences between relative risk, which indicates the importance of a lesion in a population, and absolute risk, which applies to an individual patient, can be both mathematically and judgmentally difficult. It is also important to be aware of the adverse interplay of a 'first degree' family history. The currently accepted view is that these atypical hyperplastic lesions have a moderately increased relative risk compared to the high relative risk indicated by fully developed lobular carcinoma *in situ* and the lesser (non-comedo) examples of ductal carcinoma *in situ*. The absolute risk of breast cancer development in women with atypical hyperplasia without a family history of breast cancer in a first degree relative is about 8% over 10 years. Furthermore, the risk is equally distributed between either breast for both atypical lobular and atypical ductal hyperplasia (ADH).

A lesion termed 'clinging carcinoma' has been evaluated in two follow-up studies by the same group from northern Italy (Eusebi et al 1989, 1994). On each occasion these changes, which are often histologically similar to those of ADH, have been found to indicate an increased risk of carcinoma development that is analogous to that found for ADH. Thus, the term 'clinging carcinoma' requires the qualification that it is of much less risk to life than most other lesions called carcinoma *in situ*.

Fibroadenoma

A follow-up study over 20 years revealed fibroadenoma as a *long-term* risk factor for invasive breast cancer (Dupont et al 1994). The relative risk was just over twice that of controls, but this increased to more than three times in cases of 'complex' fibroadenoma. The latter are distinguished by having cysts over 3 mm in diameter, sclerosing adenosis, epithelial calcification or papillary apocrine changes, and constitute about one third of all fibroadenomas. Adjacent proliferative disease and family history both increase the risk further to almost four times, but of particular relevance is the absence of any increased risk when these factors and 'complexity' are lacking.

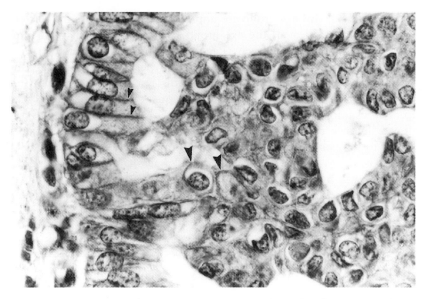

Fig. 4.2 Antibody to fodrin decorates the lateral aspects of the cells adjacent to a capillary and basement membrane complex running vertically at the far left of the photograph. The lateral compartments of the normally polarised cells are darkly stained (small arrows). Cells in an area of hyperplasia are stained all around their membranes (larger arrows). Immunoperoxidase x180

Recent developments

Detection of atypical hyperplasia by fine needle aspiration cytology would be clinically useful but the procedure has been found to be impractical, largely because the cytological features of atypia do not reflect the specific histological features (Sneige & Staerkel 1994, Stanley et al 1993).

Molecular characterisation of these lesions is as yet poorly developed because of their small size and relative rarity. Some ADH lesions are aneuploid (Norris et al 1987, Teplitz et al 1990, Allred et al 1993), or have been found to be monoclonal (Lakhani et al 1995). It is likely that some of the alterations of growth pattern are related to cell adhesion and polarity. The actin- and catenin-related protein 'fodrin' (a non-erythrocyte spectrin) has been shown to decorate the lateral cell membrane of polarized breast epithelial cells, and whilst it is present in florid hyperplasia without atypia (Fig. 4.2), it is absent in atypical hyperplasia (Simpson & Page 1992). Recently, cyclin D has been shown to be over-expressed in low grade ductal carcinoma *in situ*, but not in ADH, another important indication of their fundamentally different biology (Weinstat-Saslow et al 1995). It is also possible that the few ADH lesions that over-express cyclin D may be more aggressive than the others. Cyclin D has a powerful influence in cell cycle control, specifically at the point of exit from G1, and is overexpressed in many neoplasms.

BREAST CARCINOMA *IN SITU*

There are three clinical situations in which breast carcinoma *in situ* (CIS) alone may be diagnosed: serendipitously or as a result of review; by mammographic screening; and at symptomatic presentation. Patients who fall into these categories are not strictly comparable as the selection bias applying to each is different and they may vary in both natural history and outcome.

The historical background that has brought us to today's understanding is described in a review by Fechner (1993). The adoption of 'ductal' and 'lobular' terminologies to distinguish different histological patterns of cancer is also rooted in history and will be retained despite awareness of the imperfections (Page & Anderson, 1993). The term lobular neoplasia is accepted as encompassing the full spectrum of lobular carcinoma *in situ* (LCIS) and ALH. Both carry an increased risk of invasive breast cancer, although the relative risk differs by a factor of 2. This gives added relevance to adhering to criteria to distinguish the poles of the spectrum (Page et al 1985, Page & Dupont 1990). The important features are the character and architecture of the cell population as well as the degree of 'space' filling and distension. The lesser end of the spectrum, ALH, is diagnosed when at least one of the criteria fails to be met in over 50% of the acini within a lobular unit (Page et al 1991). A factor emerging from this last study was that disease extent increased the relative risk, and this has also been confirmed in a report from Denmark (Ottesen et al 1993). Criteria for the diagnosis of lobular pathology were laid down in NHSBSP Pathology Reporting, (1995) which should promote a more uniform recording of its incidence. However, in practice it is the 'ductal' varieties of CIS which command most attention both in terms of classification and their relevance to management and outcome.

Classification of ductal carcinoma *in situ* (DCIS)

It is a matter of current debate whether to retain the traditional method that primarily separated the architectural patterns into comedo and non-comedo sub-groups (Page et al 1987b) or to introduce qualitative aspects such as nuclear grade, differentiation or necrosis (Lagios 1989, Ottesen et al 1992, Poller et al 1994). There are also distinctions to be made on functional, molecular and genetic grounds (Poller et al 1993, Stratton et al 1995). It would seem sensible to take the pragmatic approach of requiring any system to have proven utility as a guide to clinical management or outcome, and to recognize that the latter would be based on probabilities. There are three schools of thought, based on:

(i)   differentiation, mainly based on nuclear morphology, and cell polarisation (Holland et al 1994),

(ii) nuclear grade and necrosis (Silverstein et al 1995),

(iii)   architectural pattern and nuclear grade,
         with separate identification of special types (Scott et al 1996).

It is a essential that any classification should permit consistency in evaluation by the same or different histopathologists.

Several authors (Bobrow et al 1994, Zafrani et al 1994) have attested to the practicality of the European proposal (Holland et al 1994), which divides tumours into high, intermediate and low grades, but there are no studies with sufficient follow-up to determine the clinical importance of this. The second system, now generally referred to as the Van Nuys proposal, also divides these lesions into three groups, with the first comprising DCIS with high nuclear grade and the other two determined solely by the presence or absence of necrosis. It has been demonstrated to have a capacity to discriminate for disease free survival, as well as to identify a particular group of cancers (with high grade nuclei) that benefits from the addition of radiotherapy (Silverstein et al 1995). This experience, however, has not been universal (Arnesson et al 1989). The third system (Table 4.2) is essentially a modification of the original by Lagios (1989) which favoured four categories, but now acknowledges that there is no value in recognising as separate high grade lesions with remnants of cribriform or micropapillary patterns. This system also distinguishes an intermediate grade of DCIS (Fig. 4.3) and has the added virtue of separating out the relatively infrequent micropapillary pattern in pure form (Fig. 4.4) that has been documented in two studies to be associated with extensive disease (Patchefsky et al 1989, Bellamy et al 1993). Furthermore, this classification defines patterns seen less commonly, such as apocrine (Raju et al 1993, O'Malley et al 1994) (Fig. 4.5). Another feature of this system is the incorporation of quantitative criteria to assist appropriate categorisation.

The classification system adopted for the second edition of the NHSBSP Pathology Reporting document (1995) is a hybrid of the first and third, but

Table 4.2 Subclassification of ductal carcinoma *in situ* of the breast. (Adapted from Scott et al 1996)

Histology	Nuclear grade	Necrosis	Grade
Comedo	High	Extensive	High
Intermediate*	Intermediate	Focal and Absent	Intermediate
Non-comedo**	Low	Absent	Low
Special feature cases e.g. apocrine, clear cell, micropapillary (diffuse)	Usually low	Absent***	Usually low

* often a mixture of non-comedo patterns

** solid, cribriform, papillary or focal micropapillary

*** micropapillary is often characterised by the abundance of apoptosis.

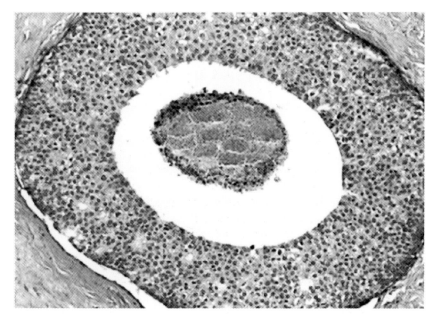

Fig.4.3 This intermediate grade ductal carcinoma *in situ* demonstrates a limited amount of necrosis, present only in 2–3 basement membrane bound spaces and qualifies as an intermediate grade because of some grade two nuclei and the presence focal of necrosis. HE x40

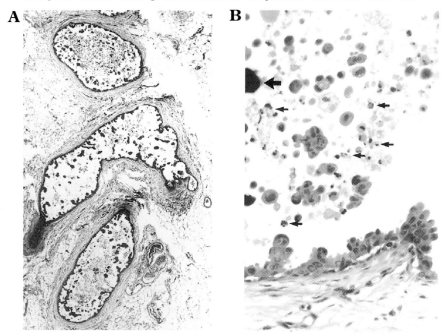

Fig. 4.4 (A) Several adjacent terminal duct-lobular units are expanded with a peripheral rim of uniform cells showing bulbous micropapillary structures and a lumen partially occupied by degenerate material. HE x5. **(B)** Many apoptotic fragments are seen at high magnification (arrows). HE x55

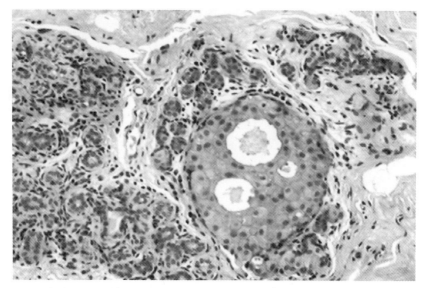

Fig. 4.5 A portion of a low grade apocrine ductal carcinoma is shown in the interlobular terminal duct. There is a suggestion of cribriform pattern here, but not as clearly formed as in most cases of DCIS and there is a large amount of cytoplasm with relatively benign appearing nuclei. This lesion approached 8 mm in greatest extent and in some areas completely involved lobular units. HE x40

lacks any quantitative criteria, and it will be of particular interest to learn the findings of the UK DCIS Trial when these become available in the late 1990's.

Distribution of disease

The extent of disease in the breast is as varied as the histological patterns and is bound to be influenced by the presentation, whether clinical or occult, the former being more likely to be widespread. It is essential also to have an understanding of the micro-anatomy of the breast which is radial, segmental but overlapping (Anderson & Page 1992) and to be aware how imperfectly this can be visualized or surgically defined. Studies by Holland et al (1985), using multiple slices, specimen radiology and multiple blocks, established that there could be foci of DCIS up to 2 cm from the reference lesion, giving a clear signal of the practical implications. Using similar serial techniques (Holland et al 1990) it was also shown that the non-comedo varieties without microcalcification often extended more widely than expected and occupied more than one quadrant in 23% of cases. The same group has recently established that DCIS shows both continuous and interrupted growth, the former usually high grade and the latter mostly low grade (Faverly et al 1994).

Another study identified 27 women with DCIS among 110 symptomatic women with nipple discharge and demonstrated that there was discontinuous intraductal spread of carcinoma in segmental resections performed under nipple duct dye injection control (Ohuchi et al 1994). Residual DCIS was found in 75% of patients with such spread who later had a mastectomy, indicating that, in terms of natural history, the delay inherent in clinical presentation is associated with more disseminated disease. Further data on the spread of DCIS have come from the use of computer aided graphics, with two groups confirming that the distribution is segmental (Ohtake et al 1995, Moffat & Going 1996). The first study concerned intraductal extension at the borders of invasive cancers, but the principle was nevertheless established for the pathways of intraductal spread in three dimensions. The impossibility of defining surgical planes relevant to the involved duct was clear. The exciting and novel discovery in both studies was the identification of anastomoses connecting separate duct-lobular systems (Fig. 4.6). The impracticality of defining each and every excision margin is obvious to histopathologists and will gradually be appreciated by surgeons.

From these descriptions it is evident that the options for therapy will be heavily influenced by the histopathological data, which must therefore contain the essentials for effective communication. Radiologists' opinion on disease distribution will also be relevant (Holland et al 1990, Stomper & Connolly 1992, Evans et al 1994) and both, indeed, must be taken into account in multidisciplinary assessment. It is likely that information on the histological characteristics and extent of DCIS is of more relevance than comments about margins.

Relation to management

Disease margins

From the foregoing sections it is obvious that the histopathologist can provide helpful information as a guide to management. Breast conservation therapy is now more frequently offered than before, but the factors useful for making that choice in relation to DCIS are still debated. We suggest that three factors

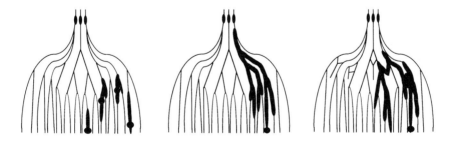

Fig. 4.6 Three possible modes for extension of non-invasive carcinoma. Left, multicentric development. Middle, unicentric development with continuous extension within ducts. Right, unicentric development with continuous extension through anastamoses connecting adjacent duct-lobular systems (after Ohtake et al, 1995).

to consider are a) margins, b) extent of disease and c) biological markers. The assessment of excision margins was described by Anderson (1989) and it is addressed in an appendix to the current NHSBSP Pathology Reporting document (1995). Completeness of excision has been variably regarded as either 'cancer not cut across', or 'only 1 mm, 2 mm, and up to 10 mm from the margin'. The statement, in any case, cannot be absolute (Carter 1986, Connolly & Schnitt 1988), and orientation of the excised specimen to its position in the body is likely to be imperfect. However, this should not be used as an excuse to avoid such assessment when this is of proven value. The approach should be consistent and surgeons should supply specimens according to an agreed protocol (NHSBSP QA Guidelines for Surgeons 1996). Certainly the evidence in cases of invasive disease for reduced recurrence comparing close margins (within 2 mm, 32%) with those not involved (26%) is unimpressive (Frazier et al 1989), and the experience of Solin et al (1991) is similar. Furthermore, numerous studies have reported a much higher incidence of residual DCIS on re-excision or mastectomy than is observed in translation to rates of recurrence (Frykeberg & Bland 1994). This indicates that not all residual disease becomes clinically apparent. It is best therefore to avoid statements that assert clearance, but rather to report the least distance in mm. In addition it is as well to remember that other factors may prevail in deciding further management in any given case (Morrow 1995).

Extent of disease

The extent of DCIS can be evaluated by mammography in many cases but underestimation by at least 20 mm for both comedo (16%) and non comedo (27%) types has been demonstrated (Holland et al 1990). There is also the problem of interrupted growth (Faverly et al 1994). The histopathologist should report the measured extent from the sections taken, ideally mapped in relation to the specimen radiograph for orientation and in three dimensions (sides, roof and floor of biopsies). Common sense must prevail over the extent of tissue sampling, which will be influenced by case presentation and the nature of the lesion (Connolly & Schnitt 1988). Larger lesions (25 mm or greater) are more likely to show microinvasion, and the propensity for micropapillary DCIS to be widespread or of multiquadrant distribution should be remembered. The number of ducts involved, fewer in DCIS identified by chance rather than screening (Patchefsky et al 1989), does not appear to be important.

There is no general agreement on the upper size limit of lesions suitable for conservation therapy. Even the pragmatic approach used in the conservation trial of the Danish Breast Cancer Co-operative Group (Ottesen et al 1992) distinguishing three groups of DCIS as (i) microfocal (5 mm or less), (ii) diffuse, and (iii) tumour forming, had only limited value.

At a median follow-up of almost 5 years there were recurrences in all groups, though these were three and four times more frequent in the diffuse and tumour forming groups, respectively, than in the microfocal group. However, invasive recurrence was seen in all groups and the issue remains one of probabilities that are difficult to determine.

Molecular markers

Attempts to use functional or genetic markers to characterize DCIS have produced varied results that have so far been of no value in prognosis. Immunohistochemical demonstration of steroid receptors has illustrated the heterogeneity of cancer cell populations and positivity rates vary with histological type (Zafrani et al 1994, Bobrow et al 1995, Leal et al 1995). Common findings have been a low frequency of positivity in high grade and a high frequency in low grade DCIS, but there is no correlation with response to Tamoxifen as there is in invasive cancers (Early Breast Cancer Trialists Collaborative Group, 1992). Furthermore, tamoxifen may sometimes act through mechanisms unrelated to steroid receptors.

Interpreting the results of oncogene (p53, c-erbB-2) disregulation has not been helpful, either for management or to interpret biology (Allred et al 1992a, Poller et al 1993). The evidence of variability in bcl-2 positivity between histological patterns of DCIS (Axelsen et al 1994) that may affect responses to radiotherapy is promising. The product of this oncogene inhibits apoptosis and is radioprotective (Hockenbery et al 1993), so the strong positivity for bcl-2 found commonly in the cribriform and low grade DCIS lesions may be highly relevant. Likewise, nm23 expression (Simpson et al 1994) varies in amount in comedo DCIS depending on whether it is associated with invasive carcinoma (less) or not (more). This could have practical relevance in suggesting that a DCIS lesion was unlikely to have invasive foci.

Relation to outcome

While it is clear that DCIS varies in its presentation, nature and biology, as well as in its response to treatment, there are common denominators which help to predict the clinical outcome (Table 4.3). The series are grouped to emphasize characteristics of presentation and management. The following points can be made:

(i) all series show recurrence, usually below the 20% level, with both invasive and non invasive recurrence represented about equally

(ii) all show a strong tendency to recur on the same side and at the same location as the original

(iii) all confirm that comedo DCIS has the highest recurrence rate

(iv) the interval from diagnosis to recurrence varies with type and grade of DCIS.

Table 4.3 Presentation and outcomes of ductal carcinoma *in situ*

Author	Presentation	Radiotherapy	Number of cases	Follow-up	% Recurrence	Significant pathology correlation
Lagios 1990/95	Mammographic	No	79	10y (mean)	16 (31 high grade) (2 low grade)	comedo CIS
Schwartz 1992	Mammographic Incidental	No No	60 12	12y (median 6y)	15 0	comedo CIS
Ottesen 1992	Mammographic Clinical Incidental	No No No	38 50 60	2-8y (median 6y)	22	comedo CIS
Bellamy 1993	Mammographic Clinical Incidental	No No No	58 59 13	2-15y (median 5y)	11	comedo CIS
Solin 1993	Not stated (8 institutions)	Yes	172	16y (median 7y)	9	comedo CIS
Silverstein 1995	Mammographic + clinical (1 institution)	Yes No	139 99	1-12y (median 6y)	13	comedo CIS
Betsill 1978*	Incidental	No	25	22y	28	low grade, non comedo CIS
Page 1982/1995a*	Incidental	No	28	24y	36	low grade, non comedo CIS

*initial surgery was not intended to be excisional

When recurrence takes the form of invasive disease, the prognosis is considerably worse. Poor local control may thus lead to increased mortality.

Three conclusions can be drawn from this appraisal. First, even incidentally detected DCIS cannot be ignored, particularly if it meets established criteria (Page et al 1987b). Second, all treatments carry a probability of failure, but histopathologists can provide useful information that discriminates between those at high and those at low risk. This should include, as a minimum, type, nuclear grade, the measured extent and relation to margins. Third, we must acknowledge that while we do know the likely outcome for groups of women in similar categories, we are unable to predict this for the individual.

PROGNOSIS OF INVASIVE BREAST CANCER

The last few years have produced major changes in the practical approach to prognostication in breast cancer. The hope that molecular or biological indicators or markers would replace classic histopathological features has given way to the realisation that such features are still useful, but only if they are assessed rigorously. It is also clear that clinical practice demands frequent, continual demonstration of such utility and/or large, combined centre clinical trials (Fielding 1992). In such trials negative results may be as meaningful as positive ones and publication of both is important (Page 1994, Pearn 1995).

Definition and implications

The basis of the clinical usefulness of prognostic indicators in breast cancer is experience, which needs to be broad, continuing and consistent. Thus, we must begin with the TNM approach (features of tumour, nodal status, and distant metastasis) and accept the key roles of cancer size and nodal status. The anatomical extent of disease provides the main criterion for selection of therapy and deserves proper emphasis. It integrates these two measures to emphasize the poor prognostic significance of large cancer size and to de-emphasize the importance of very small lymph node metastases. The presence of distant metastases over-rides all other considerations. Further important distinction to be made is between factors that are prognostic and those that are predictive of response to adjuvant treatment (Gasparini et al 1993), though how this might always be accomplished has not been adequately determined.

Prognostic indicators are most useful if they are intuitively understandable from basic concepts of solid tumour pathology. There should be a biological rationale that makes sense of the notion that these indicators are intrinsic components of disease progression. Thus, the presence of nodal metastases is a strong indicator of the capacity for distant metastatic spread, with mass and number probably also reflecting length of time since attainment of this capacity (Tubiana & Koscielny 1991). It has long been known that increasing size

Table 4.4 Prognostic markers for breast cancer: ranking of utility and certainty. (Adapted from Henson et al 1995.)

A.	Well-supported, routinely available and expected
	Pathological TNM staging
	Histological type
	Histological grade
	Combined (differentiation, nuclear and mitotic)
	Nuclear
	Mitotic
	Oestrogen and progestogen receptors: biochemical
B.	Extensively studied
	1. Widely accepted as useful, tested in large trials
	Proliferation markers
	Mitotic count (several methods)
	S-phase(flow cytometry)
	Ki-67 (MIB1)
	Oestrogen/progestogen receptor by immunoassay
	(tissue and cytosol)
	2. Correlative studies done with inconsistent results and varied definitions. Possibly useful to predict responsiveness to therapy
	c-erbB-2
	p53
	Angiogenesis by immunocytochemistry
	Vascular invasion by histology
C.	Currently do not meet degree of acceptance of A or B
	all others = a very long list

of the primary cancer adds poor prognostic implication to any nodal status measured by the number of positive nodes (Fisher 1983). However, this may not be true at the extreme ends of the spectrum (Page 1991). Carter et al (1989), using data from a large group, predominantly of symptomatic women, showed that cancers less than 0.5 cm in diameter with nodal metastases had a worse prognosis than those 1 cm in size with a similar metastatic burden. The practical implications of this observation are not evident.

Several useful reviews on the topic of prognostication are available (Mansour et al 1994, Simpson & Page 1994, Burke et al 1995, Henson et al 1995, Leong & Lee 1995, Pinder et al 1995) and specific recommendations are provided in NHSBSP Pathology Reporting (1995) and by Connolly et al (1995). These address the status at primary diagnosis and prognosis is largely concerned with three events, namely, early death, time to recurrence and long term survival. It is now clear that the same factors may not be useful for each event and the ability of some to discriminate may diminish with time (Page 1991). Breast conservation has led to another prognostic consideration namely, the predictors of local recurrence. The major determinant of the latter is the extent of *in situ* disease and the surgical operation performed (Morrow et al 1995, Page & Johnson 1995, Veronesi et al 1995b, Veronesi et al 1995c) The importance of defining subsets with regard to treatment response is demonstrated even in advanced (Dunphy et al 1994) or locally extensive disease (Gardin et al 1995, Veronesi et al 1995a). The most frequently validated and accepted elements of prognostication are presented in Table 4.4.

Histopathological factors

It is clear that for choice of therapy, lymph node status is of primary concern (Goldhirsch et al 1995). However, some specific questions are unanswered such as microscopic lymph node involvement and extension of tumour from lymph nodes.

Size and lymph node status

Specific recommendation for microscopic measurement of invasive cancers have been made to promote consistency in reporting (NHSBSP Pathology Reporting, 1995). However, some breast cancers are difficult to measure and this needs to be documented in the report as indeterminate. The size of the invasive component is much more important for prognosis than the extent of the *in situ* component. The latter is of separate importance and is undoubtedly the most significant element determining local recurrence. If the extent of *in situ* disease is contained within the original excision and there are negative margins, then recurrence is highly unlikely (Johnson et al 1995, Page & Johnson 1995).

Extensive lymph node involvement is related to poor prognosis (Fisher et al 1983). The importance of minimal involvement of lymph nodes as, for example, one or two microscopically involved lymph nodes (defined by TNM as less than 2 mm), or of even less involvement (by occasional cells determined by immunocytochemistry), is uncertain. A prognostic difference has been demonstrated for micrometastases confined to capsular lymphatics or subcapsular sinus (worse) as distinct from those present only in the lymphoid tissue (better) (Hartveit & Lilleng 1996). The reasons for this apparent paradox are unknown. Sentinel lymphadenectomy may improve matters by focusing on this micrometastasis subset (Guiliano et al 1995). The technique involves selection of lymph nodes after peri-tumoral injection of 3–5 ml iso-sulphan blue vital dye which results in an increased yield of micrometastases. However, 40% were immunodetected by cytokeratins, and since discriminations for recurrence or patient survival between those with such micrometastases and the node negative cases has not been established (Galea et al 1991, deMascarel et al 1992).

It is also debatable whether extension of metastatic carcinoma into perinodal soft tissue has prognostic significance (Donegan et al, 1993). Most studies that have made this contention may not have been controlled for extent of involvement or histological grade.

Grade and type

The method of grading should be documented. A modification of the Scarff, Bloom and Richardson method is now incorporated in the NHSBSP Pathology Reporting document (1995), and is gaining wide acceptance. There may be additional merit in incorporating a proportional mitotic count (Simpson & Page 1994).

Special histological type is of prognostic importance beyond grade in only about 20% of invasive breast cancers (Page 1991) and pure features of a special type must be present. A cut-off point of 90% is a practical recommendation (Anderson et al 1986, 1991; NHSBSP Pathology Reporting 1995). The importance of recognising variants of special type in a consistent manner has still to be determined (Page & Anderson 1993). The use of the term 'invasive lobular' without nuclear grade is probably inappropriate (Ladekarl & Sorensen 1993) The classical type of lobular carcinoma must have low grade nuclei. There are cancers with dominant individual cell infiltration which have high nuclear grade and even a reasonable number of mitoses. Such cases have been called 'infiltrating breast carcinoma with lobular features, intermediate or high grade' or 'pleomorphic lobular carcinoma' and distinction from classical is important as the outcome is worse.

Proliferative activity

An additional measure of proliferation rate besides mitotic count is useful in confirming the growth fraction (Baak 1990, Simpson et al 1992). Exactly what the cut-off points for each of these might be and indeed whether the current cut-off points used for mitotic count should remain at the classic levels is under question. In specific instances, such as the node negative versus node positive breast cancers, different cut-offs may be required. The antibody MIB-I, which recognises the Ki-67 antigen in fixed tissue, may be particularly useful (Keshgegian & Cowan 1995), but mitotic rates probably provide the same information (Simpson et al 1994, Pereira et al 1995). Ploidy by itself does not provide independent information on prognosis in invasive breast cancer (Going et al 1993, Pfistirer et al 1995).

Immunocytochemistry

Immunocytochemical methods are available for the evaluation of oestrogen and progesterone receptors in invasive breast cancers (Barnes & Millis, 1995). Stratification of cases into categories of definitely negative, borderline or probably low, and positive, can be done with a reproducibility that is clinically useful. Immunocytochemical assessment avoids some of the pitfalls of the biochemical method (Parl & Posey 1988, Esteban et al 1994), such as finding oestrogen receptor in normal breast tissue adjacent to an infiltrating carcinoma and thereby assigning oestrogen receptor positive status to it. This may also happen when an *in situ* component expresses receptor and the invasive component does not. This implies the oestrogen receptor status in *in situ* carcinoma is of no value, whether it is associated with invasive carcinoma or not. There is no definite evidence of this either way. The other common pitfall of a biochemical procedure that is avoided by immunocytochemistry is sampling error. Poorly cellular cancers, particularly invasive lobular carcinomas that are regularly oestrogen receptor positive, may appear to be borderline or negative in biochemical evaluation because of the few cells present in the sample.

Other markers which have been widely tested include c-erbB-2 and p53 but there is no consensus on their value (Mansour et al 1994, Page 1994, Dowell & Hall 1995, Pinder et al 1995). Measurement of c-erbB-2 seems most useful in node positive disease, but it may be regarded as superfluous because these patients will be offered further treatment anyway (Muss et al 1995). For node negative cases however, it may well be true that c-erbB2 positivity indicates a greater likelihood of responsiveness to chemotherapy. This possibility has been presented (Allred et al, 1992b), and is under further study. Confirmation that p53 may have similar prognostic significance is not established and studies have been quite conflicting.

Recent developments

Although there have been rapid advances in our understanding of molecular biological associations in breast neoplasia, speed of transfer into clinical practice has not been commensurate. Perhaps the most promising are therapeutic advances related to factors which modulate angiogenesis (Folkman 1995). However, assessment of vascularity by current methods has not proved to be of practical value (Axelsson et al 1995, Costello et al 1995, Goulding et al 1995, Fox et al 1995, Page & Jensen 1995). Determination of vascular density within the tumour by immunocytochemical methodologies using antibodies to factor VIII, CD 31 or CD 34 have shown promise, but further large clinical trials in association with other markers are probably needed.

The importance of peri-tumoral vessel involvement, usually lymphatic, is uncertain because of the problems of its routine identification. This is probably over-cautious and the recommendations in the appendix to the NHSBSP Pathology Reporting document (1995), which encourage identification on ordinary H & E sections, are well supported by two large series (Clemente et al 1992, Pinder et al 1994). We believe that in something between 10% and 20% of large invasive breast cancers peri-tumoral lymphatic invasion is quite evident and should be reported. In cases in which the lymph nodes are histologically negative this information assumes particular significance in determining whether adjuvant chemotherapy or boosted local radiotherapy should be offered to the patient.

There is a special treatment issue relating to node negative tumours less than 2 cm in size traditionally regarded as 'early' or stage I. Most oncologists will not give chemotherapy to young women who have invasive breast cancers of less than 1 cm in size, yet it is important to consider such therapy in situations where those small cancers have a high histological grade. The evidence from studies in which small cancers have been separately evaluated is that treatment failures within five years have been confined to those with high grade lesions (Stierer et al 1992, Rosner 1993).

KEY POINTS FOR CLINICAL PRACTICE

1. Atypical hyperplasia is uncommon but recognition according to specific criteria identifies a group of women who are at a significantly increased risk of breast cancer.

2. Better molecular biological definition of such histologically well characterised lesions will help to clarify the likelihood of progression to invasive breast cancer.

3. Ductal carcinoma *in situ* (DCIS) varies in its distribution in the breast, histological architecture and grade, and there is good evidence that all three features should be considered when deciding upon treatment.

4. There is growing evidence that distinctions can be made between DCIS with high and low likelihood of local recurrence, but further studies are required for validation.

5. The long list of prognostic factors for invasive breast cancer can be divided into two: those routinely available from histopathology (size, nodal status, type, grade and steroid receptor status); and biological indicators (proliferation markers, oncogene disregulation, vascular factors).

6. The aim must be to achieve consistent evaluation of established prognostic factors and to develop facilities to test and then implement the supplementary evaluations which prove to be of value.

REFERENCES

Allred DC, Clark GM, Molina R et al 1992a Overexpression of HER-2/neu and its relationship with other prognostic factors change during the progression of *in situ* to invasive breast cancer. Hum Pathol 23: 974-979
Allred DC, Clark GM, Tandon AK et al 1992b Her-2/neu in node-negative breast cancer: prognostic significance of overexpression influenced by the presence of *in situ* carcinoma. J Clin Oncol 10: 599-605
Allred DC, O'Connell P, Fuqua S 1993 Biomarkers in early breast neoplasia. J Cell Biochem 53: 125-131
Anderson TJ 1989 Breast cancer screening: principles and practicalities for histopathologists. In: Anthony PP, MacSween RNM (eds) Recent advances in histopathology, No.14,

Churchill Livingston, Edinburgh, pp 43-61

Anderson TJ, Page DL 1992 Breast: structure, biology and pathology. In: McGee JOD, Wright NA, Isaacson PG (eds) Oxford Textbook of Pathology, Oxford University Press, Oxford, pp 1643-1670

Anderson TJ, Lamb J, Alexander F et al 1986 Comparative pathology of prevalent and incident cancers detected by breast screening. Lancet 1: 519-523

Anderson TJ, Lamb J, Doonan P et al 1991 Comparative pathology of breast cancer in a randomised trial of screening. Br J Cancer 64: 108-113

Arnesson LG, Smeds S, Fagerberg G et al 1989 Follow-up of two treatment modalities for ductal cancer *in situ* of the breast. Br J Surg 76: 672-675

Axelsen RA, Bellamy COC, Anderson TJ 1994 Bcl-2 expression and cell death in non-invasive breast carcinoma. J Pathol 173: 192

Axelsson K, Ljung BM, Moore DH et al 1995 Tumor angiogenesis as a prognostic assay for invasive ductal breast carcinoma. J Natl Cancer Inst 87: 997-1008

Baak JPA 1990 Mitosis counting in tumours. Hum Pathol 21: 683-685

Barnes DM, Millis RR 1995 Oestrogen receptors: the history, the relevance and the methods of evaluation. In: Kirkham N, Lemoine N (eds). Progress in Pathology Vol 2, Churchill Livingstone, Edinburgh pp 89-114

Bellamy COC, McDonald C, Salter DM et al 1993 Non invasive ductal carcinoma of the breast: the relevance of histological categorization. Hum Pathol 24: 16-23

Bobrow LG, Happerfield LC, Gregory WM et al 1994 The classification of ductal carcinoma *in situ* and its association with biological markers. Semin Diagn Pathol 11: 199-207

Bobrow LG, Happerfield LC, Gregory WM et al 1995 Ductal carcinoma *in situ*: assessment of necrosis and nuclear morphology and their association with biological markers. J Pathol 176: 333-341

Burke HB, Hutter RVP, Henson DE 1995 Breast carcinoma. In: Hermanek P, Gospodarowicz MK, Henson DE, Hutter RVP, Sobin LH (eds). Prognostic factors in cancer. UICC, Springer-Verlag, Berlin pp 165-176

Carter CL, Allen C, Henson DE 1989 Relation of tumor size, lymph node status and survival in 24,740 breast cancer cases. Cancer 63: 181-187

Carter D 1986 Margins of "lumpectomy" for breast cancer. Hum Pathol 17: 330-332

Clemente CG, Boracchi P, Andreola S et al 1992 Peritumoral lymphatic invasion in patients with node-negative mammary duct carcinoma. Cancer 69: 1396-1403

Connolly JL, Schnitt SJ 1988 Evaluation of breast biopsy specimens, patients considered for treatment conservative surgery and radiation therapy for early breast cancer. In: Pathology Annual. Rosen PP, Fechner RE (eds). Appleton and Lange, Connecticut, pp 1-24

Connolly JL, Fechner RE, Kempson RL et al 1995 Recommendations for the reporting of breast carcinoma. From the Association of Directors of Anatomic and Surgical Pathology. Am J Clin Pathol 104: 614-619

Costello P, McCann A, Carney DN et al 1995 Prognostic significance of microvessel density in lymph node negative breast cancer. Hum Pathol 26: 1181-1184

Donegan WL, Stine SB, Samter TG 1993 Implications of extracapsular nodal metastases for treatment and prognosis of breast cancer. Cancer 72: 778-782

Dowell SP, Hall PA 1995 The p53 tumour suppressor gene and tumour prognosis: is there a relationship. J Pathol 177: 221-224

Dunphy FR, Spitzer G, Rossiter FJ et al 1994 Factors predicting long-term survival for metastatic breast cancer patients treated with high-dose chemotherapy and bone marrow support. Cancer 73: 2157-2167

Dupont WD, Page DL 1985 Risk factors for breast cancer in women with proliferative breast disease. N Engl J Med 312: 146-151

Dupont WD, Page DL 1989 Relative risk of breast cancer varies with time since diagnosis of atypical hyperplasia. Hum Pathol 20: 723-725

Dupont WD, Parl FF, Hartmann WH et al 1993 Breast cancer risk associated with proliferative breast disease and atypical hyperplasia. Cancer 71: 1258-1265

Dupont WD, Page DL, Parl FF et al 1994 Long-term risk of breast cancer in women with fibroadenoma. N Engl J Med 331: 10-15

Early Breast Cancer Trialists' Collaborative Group 1992 Systemic treatment of early breast cancer by hormonal, cytotoxic, or immune therapy. 133 randomised trials involving 31,000 recurrences and 24,000 deaths among 75,000 women. Lancet 339: 71-85

Esteban JM, Ahn C, Battifora H et al 1994 Predictive value of estrogen receptors evaluated by quantitative immunohistochemical analysis in breast cancer. Am J Clin Pathol 102(4): S9-S12

Eusebi V, Foschini MA, Cook MG et al 1989 Long-term follow-up of *in situ* carcinoma of the breast with special emphasis on clinging carcinoma. Semin Diagn Pathol 6: 165-173

Eusebi V, Feudale E, Foschini MP et al 1994 Long-term follow-up of *in situ* carcinoma of the breast. Semin Diagn Pathol 11: 223-235

Evans A, Pinder S, Wilson R et al. 1994 Ductal carcinoma *in situ* of the breast: correlation between mammographic and pathologic findings. AJR 162: 1307-1311

Faverly DRG, Burgress L, Bult P et al 1994 Three dimensional imaging of mammary ductal carcinoma *in situ*: clinical implications. Semin Diagn Pathol 11: 193-198

Fechner RE 1993 One century of mammary carcinoma is situ: what have we learned? Am J Clin Pathol 100: 654-661

Fielding LP 1992 The future of prognostic factors in outcome prediction for patients with cancer. Cancer 70: 2367-2377

Fisher B, Bauer M, Wickerham L et al 1983 Relation of number of positive axillary nodes to the prognosis of patients with primary breast cancer. Cancer 52: 1551-1557

Folkman J 1995 Clinical applications of research on angiogenesis. N Engl J Med 333: 1757-1763

Fox SB, Turner GDH, Leek RD et al 1995 The prognostic value of quantitative angiogenesis in breast cancer and role of adhesion molecule expression in tumor endothelium. Breast Cancer Res Treat 36: 219-226

Frazier TG, Wong RW, Rose D 1989 Implications of accurate pathologic margins in the treatment of primary breast cancer. Arch Surg 124: 37-38

Frykberg ER, Bland KI 1994 Overview of the biology and management of ductal carcinoma *in situ* of the breast. Cancer 74: 350-361

Galea M, Athanassiou E, Bell J et al 1991 Occult regional lymph node metastases from breast carcinoma: immunohistochemical detection with antibodies CAM 5.2 and NCR 11. J Pathol 165: 221-227

Gallager HS 1980 The developmental pathology of breast cancer. Cancer 46: 905-907

Gardin G, Rosso R, Campora E et al 1995 Locally advanced non-metastatic breast cancer: Analysis of prognostic factors in 125 patients homogeneously treated with a combined modality approach. Eur J Cancer [A] 9: 1428-1433

Gasparini IG, Pozza F, Harris AL 1993 Evaluating the potential usefulness of new prognostic and predictive indicators in node negative breast cancer patients. J Natl Cancer Inst 85: 1206-1219

Giuliano AE, Dale PS, Turner RR et al 1995 Improved axillary staging of breast cancer with sentinel lymphadenectomy. Ann Surg 222 (3): 394-401

Going JJ, Stanton PD, Cooke TG. 1993 Influence on measurement of cellular proliferation by histology and flow cytometry in mammary carcinomas labelled in vivo with bromodeoxyuridine. Am J Clin Pathol 100: 218-222

Goldhirsch A, Wood WC, Senn HJ et al 1995 International consensus panel on the treatment of primary breast cancer. Eur J Cancer 31A: 1754-1759

Goulding H, Rashid NA, Robertson JF et al 1995 Assessment of angiogenesis in breast carcinoma: An important factor in prognosis? Hum Pathol 26: 1196-1200

Hartveit F, Lilleng PK 1996 Breast cancer: two micrometastatic variants in the axilla that differ in prognosis. Histopathology 28: 241-246

Henson DE, Fielding P, Grignon DJ et al 1995 College of American Pathologists Conference XXVI on clinical relevance of prognostic markers in solid tumors. Arch Pathol Lab Med 119: 1109-1112

Hockenbery DM, Oltvai ZN, Yin X et al 1993 Bcl-2 functions in antioxidant pathway to prevent apoptosis. Cell 75: 1-20

Holland R, Veling SH, Mravunac M et al 1985 Histologic multifocality of Tis, T1-2 breast carcinomas: implications for clinical trials of breast-conserving surgery. Cancer 56: 979-990

Holland R, Hendricks JHCL, Verbeek ALM et al 1990 Extent, distribution, and mammographic/histologic correlations of breast carcinoma *in situ*. Lancet 335: 519-522

Holland R, Peterse JL, Millis RR et al 1994 Ductal carcinoma *in situ*: a proposal for a new classification. Semin Diagn Pathol 11: 167-180

Johnson JE, Page DL, Winfield AC et al 1995 Recurrent mammary carcinoma after local excision: A segmental problem. Cancer 75: 1612-1618

Keshgegian AA, Cnaan A 1995 Proliferation markers in breast carcinoma: mitotic figure count,

S-phase fraction, proliferating cell nuclear antigen, Ki-67 and MIB-1. Am J Clin Pathol 104: 42-49

Ladekarl M, Sorensen FB 1993 Prognostic, quantitative histopathologic variables in lobular carcinoma of the breast. Cancer 72: 2602-11

Lagios MD. 1990 Duct carcinoma *in situ*: pathology and treatment. Surg Clin North Am 70: 853-871

Lagios MD 1995 Heterogeneity of duct carcinoma *in situ* (DCIS): relationship of grade and subtype analysis to local recurrence and risk of invasive transformation. Cancer Lett 90: 97-102

Lagios MD, Margolin FR, Westdahl PR et al 1989 Mammographically detected duct carcinoma *in situ*. Frequency of local recurrence following tylectomy and prognostic effect of nuclear grade on local recurrence. Cancer 63: 618-624

Lakhani SR, Collins N, Stratton MR et al 1995 Atypical ductal hyperplasia of the breast: clonal proliferation with loss of heterozygosity in chromosomes 16q and 17p. J Clin Pathol 48: 611-615

Leal CB, Fernando Schmitt FC, Bento MJ et al 1995 Ductal carcinoma *in situ* of the breast: histologic categorization and its relationship to ploidy and immunohistochemical expression of hormone receptors, p53 and c-erbB-2 protein. Cancer 75: 2123-2131

Leong AS-Y, Lee AKC 1995 Biological indices in the assessment of breast cancer. J Clin Pathol: Clin Mol Pathol 48 M221-M238

London SJ, Connolly JL, Schnitt SJ et al 1992 A prospective study of benign breast disease and the risk of breast cancer. JAMA 267: 941-944

Mansour EG, Ravdin PM, Dressler L 1994 Prognostic factors in early breast carcinoma. Cancer 74: 381-400

deMascarel I, Bonichon F, Coindre JM et al 1992 Prognostic significance of breast cancer axillary lymph node micrometastases assessed by two special techniques: re-evaluation with longer follow-up. Br J Cancer 66: 523-527

McDivitt RW, Stevens JA, Lee NC et al 1992 Histologic types of benign breast disease and the risk for breast cancer. Cancer 69: 1408-1414

Moffat DR, Going JJ 1996 Three dimensional anatomy of complete duct systems in human breast: pathological and developmental implications. J Clin Pathol 49: 48-52

Morrow M. 1995 The natural history of ductal carcinoma *in situ*: implications for clinical decision making. Cancer 76: 113-115

Morrow M, Harris JR, Schnitt SJ 1995 Local control following breast conserving surgery for invasive cancer: results of clinical trials. J Natl Cancer Inst 87: 1669-1673

Muss HB, Thor AD, Berry DA et al 1995 C-erB-2 expression and response to adjuvant therapy in women with node-positive early breast cancer. N Engl J Med 330: 1260-1266

National Health Service Breast Screening Programme (NHSBSP) 1995 Pathology reporting in breast cancer screening (2nd ed) NHSBSP Publication No. 3

National Health Services Breast Screening Programme (NHSBSP) 1996 Quality assurance guidelines for surgeons in breast cancer screening (2nd ed) NHSBSP Publication No. 20

Norris HJ, Bahr GF, Mikel UV 1987 A comparative morphometric and cytophotometric study of intraductal hyperplasia and intraductal carcinoma of the breast. Anal Quant Cytol Histol 10: 1-9

O'Malley F, Page DL, Nelsen E et al 1994 Ductal carcinoma *in situ* of the breast and apocrine cytology: definition of borderline category. Hum Pathol 25: 164-168

Ohtake T, Rikiya A, Kimijima I et al 1995 Intraductal extension of primary invasive breast carcinoma treated by breast conservative surgery: computer graphic three-dimensional reconstruction of the mammary duct-lobular systems. Cancer 76: 32-45

Ohuchi N, Furuta A, Mori S 1994 Management of ductal carcinoma *in situ* with nipple discharge: intraductal spreading of carcinoma is an unfavourable pathologic factor for breast-conserving surgery. Cancer 74: 1294-1302

Ottesen GL, Graversen HP, Blichert-Toft M et al 1992 Ductal carcinoma *in situ* of the female breast: short-term results of a prospective nationwide study. Am J Surg Pathol 16: 1183-1196

Ottesen GL, Graversen HP, Blichert-Toft M et al 1993 Lobular carcinoma *in situ* of the female breast. Short term results of a prospective nationwide study. Am J Surg Pathol 17: 14-21

Page D 1994 The epidemiology of tumor markers in breast cancer management: prognostic markers. Cancer Epidemiology, Biomarkers & Prevention, 3: 101-104

Page D, Johnson J 1995 Controversies in the local management of invasive and non-invasive breast cancer. Cancer Lett 90: 91-96

Page DL 1991 Prognosis and breast cancer-recognition of lethal and favorable prognostic types. Am J Surg Pathol 15: 334-349

Page DL, Dupont WD 1990 Anatomic markers of human premalignancy and risk of breast cancer. Cancer 66: 1326-1335

Page DL, Rogers LW 1992 Combined histologic and cytologic criteria for the diagnosis of mammary atypical ductal hyperplasia. Hum Pathol 23: 1095-1097

Page DL, Anderson TJ 1993 How should we categorise breast cancer. Breast 2: 217-219

Page DL, Dupont WD 1993 Anatomic indicators (histologic and cytologic) of increased cancer risk. Breast Cancer Res Treat 28: 157-166

Page DL, Lagios MD 1994 Pathology and clinical evolution of ductal carcinoma *in situ* (DCIS) of the breast. Cancer Lett 86: 1-4

Page DL, Jensen RA 1995 Angiogenesis in human breast carcinoma: what is the question? Hum Pathol 26: 1173-1174

Page DL, Steel CM, Dixon JM 1995 ABC of breast diseases: Carcinoma *in situ* and patients at high risk of breast cancer. Br Med J 310: 39-41

Page DL, Anderson TJ, Rogers LW 1987a Epithelial hyperplasia. In: Page DL, Anderson TJ (eds) Diagnostic histopathology of the breast, Churchill Livingstone, Edinburgh, pp 120-156

Page DL, Anderson TJ, Rogers LW 1987b Carcinoma *in situ* (CIS). In: Page DL, Anderson TJ. (eds) Diagnostic histopathology of the breast, Churchill Livingstone, Edinburgh, pp 157-192

Page DL, Dupont WD, Rogers LW et al 1985 Atypical hyperplastic lesions of the female breast. A long follow-up study. Cancer 55: 2698-2708

Page DL, Kidd TE, Dupont WD et al 1991 Lobular neoplasia of the breast: higher risk of subsequent invasive cancer predicted by more extensive disease. Hum Pathol 22: 1232-1239

Page DL, Dupont WD, Rogers LW et al 1995 Continued local recurrence of carcinoma 15-25 years after a diagnosis of low grade ductal carcinoma *in situ* of the breast treated by biopsy only. Cancer 76: 1197-1200

Parl FF, Posey YF 1988 Discrepancies of the biochemical and immunohistochemical estrogen receptor assays in breast cancer. Hum Pathol 19: 960-966

Patchefsky AS, Schwartz GF, Finkelstein et al 1989 Heterogeneity of intraductal carcinoma of the breast. Cancer 63: 731-741

Pearn J 1995 Publication: an ethical imperative. Br Med J 310: 1313-1315

Pereira H, Pinder SE, Sibbering DM et al 1995 Pathological prognostic factors in breast cancer. IV: Should you be a typer or a grader? A comparative study of two histological prognostic features in operable breast carcinoma. Histopathology 27: 219-226

Pfisterer J, Kommoss F, Sauerbrei W et al 1995 DNA flow cytometry in node-positive breast cancer — Prognostic value and correlation with morphologic and clinical factors. Anal Quant Cytol Histol 17: 406-412

Pinder SE, Ellis IO, Elston CW 1995 Prognostic factors in primary breast carcinoma. J Clin Pathol 48: 981-983

Pinder SE, Ellis IO, Galea et al. 1994 Pathology prognostic factors in breast cancer. III. Vascular invasion: relationship with recurrence and survival in a large study with long-tem follow-up. Histopathology 24: 41-47

Poller DN, Ellis IO 1995 Ductal carcinoma *in situ* (DCIS) of the breast. In: Kirkham NI, Lemoine NR (eds) Progress in pathology,Vol 1, Churchill Livingstone, Edinburgh, pp 47-87

Poller DN, Roberts EC, Bell JA et al 1993 p53 protein expression in mammary ductal carcinoma *in situ*: relationship to immunohistochemical expression of estrogen receptor and c-erbB-2 protein. Hum Pathol 24: 463-468

Poller DN, Silverstein MJ, Galea M et al 1994 Duct carcinoma *in situ* of the breast: a proposal for a new simplified histology classification association between cellular proliferation and c-erbB-2 protein expression. Mod Pathol 7: 257-262

Raju U, Zarbo RJ, Kubus J et al 1993 The histologic spectrum of apocrine breast proliferations: analysis. Hum Pathol 24: 173-181

Rosner D, Lane WW 1993 Predicting recurrence in axillary-node negative breast cancer patients. Breast Cancer Res & Treat 25: 127-139

Scott MA, Lagios MD, Axelsson K et al 1995 Ductal carcinoma *in situ* of the breast, reproducibility of histologic subtype analysis. Lab Invest 72: 25A

Silverstein MJ, Poller DN, Waisman JR et al 1995 Prognostic classification of breast ductal carcinoma-in-situ. Lancet 345: 1154-1157

Simpson JF, Page DL 1992 Altered expression of a structual protein (Fodrin) within epithelial proliferative disease of the breast. Am J Pathol 141: 285-289

Simpson JF, Page DL 1994 Status of breast cancer prognostication based on histopathologic data. Am J Clin Pathol 102: S3-S8

Simpson JF, Dutt PL, Page DL 1992 Expression of mitoses per thousand cells and cell density in breast carcinoma: a proposal. Hum Pathol 23: 608- 611

Simpson JF, O'Malley F, Dupont WD et al 1994 Heterogeneous expression of nm23 gene product in non invasive breast carcinoma. Cancer 73: 2352-2358

Sneige N, Staerkel GA 1994 Fine-needle aspiration cytology of ductal hyperplasia with and without atypia and ductal carcinoma *in situ*. Hum Pathol 25: 485-492

Solin LJ, Fowble BL, Schultz DJ et al 1991 The significance of the pathology margins of the tumour excision on the outcome of patients treated with definitive irradiation for early stage breast cancer. Int J Radiat Oncol Biol Phys 21: 279-287

Solin LJ, Yeh I, Kurtz J et al 1993 Ductal carcinoma *in situ* (intraductal carcinoma) of the breast treated with breast-conserving surgery and definitive irradiation. Cancer 71: 2532-42

Stanley MW, Henry SM, Zera R 1993 Atypia in breast fine-needle aspiration smears correlates poorly with the presence of a prognostically significant proliferative lesion of ductal epithelium. Hum Pathol 24: 630-635

Stierer M, Rosen HR, Weber R et al 1992 Long term analysis of factors influencing the outcome in carcinoma of the breast smaller than one centimetre. Surg Gynecol Obstet 175: 151-160

Stomper PC, Connolly JL 1992 Ductal carcinoma *in situ* of the breast: correlation between mammographic calcification and tumor sub-type. AJR 159: 483-485

Stratton MR, Collins N, Lakhani SR et al 1995 Loss of heterozygosity in ductal carcinoma *in situ* of the breast. J Pathol 175: 195-201

Teplitz RL, Butler BB, Tesluk H et al 1990 Quantitative DNA patterns in human preneoplastic breast lesions. Anal Quant Cytol Histol 12: 98-102

Tubiana M, Koscielny S 1991 Natural history of human breast cancer: Recent data and clinical implications. Breast Cancer Res Treat 18: 125-140

Veronesi U, Bonadonna G, Zurrida S et al 1995a Conservation surgery after primary chemotherapy in large carcinomas of the breast. Ann Surg 222: 612-618

Veronesi U, Marubini E, Del VM et al 1995b Local recurrences and distant metastases after conservative breast cancer treatments: Partly independent events. J Natl Cancer Inst 87: 19-27

Veronesi U, Salvadori B, Luini A et al 1995c Breast conservation is a safe method in patients with small cancer of the breast. Long-term results of three randomised trials on 1,973 patients. Eur J Cancer [A] 10: 1574-1579

Weinstat-Saslow D, Merino MJ, Manrow RE et al 1995 Overexpression of cyclin D mRNA distinguishes invasive and *in situ* breast carcinomas from non-malignant lesions. Nature Med 1: 1257-1260

Zafrani B, Leroyer A, Forquet A et al 1994 Mammographically detected ductal *in situ* carcinoma of the breast analysed with a new classification: a study of 127 cases: Correlation with estrogen and progesterone receptors, p53 and c-erbB-2 proteins and proliferative activity. Semin Diagn Pathol 11: 208-214

5

Criteria for malignancy in endocrine tumours

T. J. Stephenson

GENERAL CONSIDERATIONS

In the absence of frank invasion or metastasis at the time of presentation, identification of malignancy in certain endocrine neoplasms presents a significant problem for the diagnostic histopathologist. This is because some of the conventional criteria likely to be associated with malignancy in tumours of other tissues – such as elevated mitotic count, hypercellularity, nuclear hyperchromasia and pleomorphism – are commonly seen in benign endocrine tissues as part of their functional state (Carniero & Sobrinho-Simões 1995, Chan & Tsang 1995).

Currently, five principal approaches are being used to enhance prediction of malignancy in endocrine neoplasms.

The first is the careful evaluation of conventional histological features which are then subjected to multi-parameter statistical analysis to determine which constellations of features corrclate most strongly with malignancy. This approach has been successfully applied to adrenal cortical neoplasms (Hough et al 1979, Weiss 1984, van Slooten et al 1985).

The second is correlation between hormones produced and malignant potential. Thus, clinical feminisation or virilisation (Lack et al 1992), and immunohistochemical identification of neuroendocrine differentiation (Haak & Fleuren 1995) point to malignancy in adrenal cortical neoplasms. Similarly, in pancreatic endocrine tumours, expression of gastrin or somatostatin (Heitz 1984) and particularly adrenocorticotrophic hormone (ACTH) (Doppman et al 1994), rather than insulin, are likely to be associated with malignancy.

The third is estimation of proliferative activity (reviewed in this context by DeLellis 1995), either by DNA flow cytometry or immunohistochemical techniques using recently developed antibodies to various components of proliferating cells (McCormick et al 1993, Hall & Coates 1995). Abbona et al (1995) reported significantly higher proliferative activity in aggressive parathyroid carcinomas than in non-aggressive carcinomas and benign lesions. In the thyroid, Katoh et al (1995) found significantly higher proliferative activity in widely, rather than minimally, invasive follicular carcinomas. However, no significant difference was found between the former and follicular adenoma.

The fourth approach, sometimes combined with studies of cell proliferation as above, is the analysis of DNA ploidy. This has so far been disappointing in the prediction of malignancy – not all carcinomas are DNA aneuploid, and DNA aneuploidy is encountered in some benign endocrine neoplasms (reviewed by Sobrinho-Simões 1991). This is particularly true of neuro-endocrine neoplasms (Falkmer & Falkmer 1995).

The fifth approach is the application of molecular biology to the prediction of malignancy (reviewed by Soares & Sobrinho-Simões 1995). For example, loss of retinoblastoma (Rb) gene protein has been reported in some parathyroid carcinomas while adenomas appear to be Rb positive (Cryns et al 1994a). p53 allelic loss and abnormal protein expression have been reported in some parathyroid carcinomas (Cryns et al 1994b). p53 protein accumulation is more common in aggressive than indolent variants of thyroid carcinomas, but there is no clear-cut correlation with histological tumour type (Carr et al 1993, Soares et al 1994). Expression of various oncogenes and growth factors in thyroid neoplasms has been reviewed (Frauman & Moses 1990). However, overlap in the expression pattern between benign and malignant lesions may limit their diagnostic utility (Sobrinho-Simões 1991). In papillary thyroid carcinomas, a novel rearranged form of the ret proto-oncogene designated ptc (Grieco et al 1990) has been detected in a high proportion of cases (Tong et al 1995). It remains to be determined whether this will prove valuable in the differentiation of papillary carcinomas from non-neoplastic papillary lesions. Different splice variants of CD44 are expressed in gastrinomas (which are likely to be malignant), but not in other subtypes of endocrine pancreatic tumours (Chaudhry et al 1994).

Space dictates that this review cannot be comprehensive. Key examples of problems in the prediction of malignancy after recognising that the lesion is a neoplasm will be emphasised. Prior to this, papillary carcinoma of the thyroid will be used to illustrate an even more fundamental problem: the distinction between neoplasia and benign lesions which may mimic it (Rosai 1993a).

Problems in papillary thyroid neoplasia

Failure to identify a papillary neoplasm in the thyroid will result in a lesion with metastatic potential being overlooked (Chan & Tsang 1995). While classical papillary carcinoma (LiVolsi 1992) is unlikely to be missed, variants such as the follicular variant (Tielens et al 1994) may masquerade as benign follicular lesions. Further distinction of hyperplastic epithelial pseudopapillae (Damiani et al 1991) from true papillary neoplasia can present a significant diagnostic problem.

Hyperplastic thyroid epithelial pseudopapillae

These are common and may be seen in association with dyshormonogenetic goitre (Kennedy 1969), multinodular goitre and Graves' thyroiditis. Characteristic features include nuclear enlargement and pleomorphism and columnar

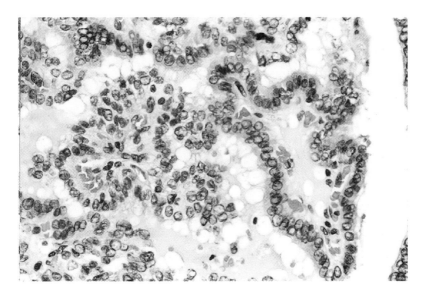

Fig. 5.1 Papillary carcinoma. The papillae have central fibrovascular cores and their epithelium is single-layered. H&E × 190.

change in the epithelial cells. Crucially, the pseudopapillae of hyperplastic states are formed by epithelial multilayering and its infolding into follicles. One variant of this theme, the heaping up of microfollicles within one pole of a larger follicle, is sometimes given the term 'Sanderson polsters' (Rosai et al 1992).

In contrast to this, papillary carcinoma has **true** papillae (Vickery 1981). These have fibrovascular cores (Fig. 5.1) and their epithelium is usually tall with the nuclei near the basement membrane. Papillary carcinoma cells usually have ground glass (DeLellis 1993a), or grooved (Chan & Saw 1986), nuclei. Psammoma bodies, a desmoplastic stroma and lymphocytic infiltration are common (Rosai 1993b). While the presence of psammoma bodies points strongly to a diagnosis of papillary carcinoma, the finding is not absolutely specific (Riazmontazer & Bedayat 1991). In an interesting immunohistochemical study, Damiani et al (1991) have found that the tips of pseudopapillae in hyperplasia fail to stain or do so only weakly with alcian blue and epithelial membrane antigen, while those of the papillae of papillary carcinoma stain strongly.

Follicular variant of papillary carcinoma

The follicular variant of papillary thyroid carcinoma is a distinct histopathological entity (Tielens et al 1994), recognition of which evolved after it had been realised that a mixed follicular-papillary carcinoma of the thyroid does

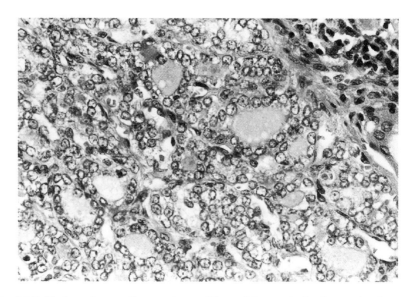

Fig. 5.2 Follicular variant papillary carcinoma. The nuclei are optically-clear, oval and grooved. The change is uniform and sharply distinguished from surrounding thyroid. H&E × 190.

not exist (Sobrinho-Simões 1991). There is controversy as to whether such tumours have a higher propensity to metastasise outside the neck than ordinary papillary carcinoma with some studies (Carcangiu et al 1985) and reviews (Sobrinho-Simões 1991) suggesting that this is so while others point to no difference in metastatic rate (Tielens et al 1994).

It is important to recognise follicular variant papillary thyroid carcinoma because tumours which have the cytological features of papillary carcinoma usually behave as papillary carcinoma even if they lack typical papillary structures (Sobrinho-Simões 1991). Further, a diffuse variant has been described (Sobrinho-Simões et al 1990) which is a diagnostic pitfall due to its lack of encapsulation and has a poor prognosis (Sobrinho-Simões & Fonseca 1994).

Cytological features of follicular lesions, which would not otherwise be important in the identification of follicular carcinoma, thus become important in the identification of follicular variant papillary carcinoma (Fig. 5.2). The nuclear changes which characterise papillary carcinoma have been well described (Rosai 1993 a&b) and include an oval shape associated with pseudo-inclusions or grooves (Chan & Saw 1986) that are parallel to the long axis of the nucleus. These are thought to arise from deep cytoplasmic invaginations into the nucleus (Albores-Saavedra et al 1971). The nuclear chromatin characteristics specific for papillary carcinoma are well known (Kiyoni et al 1994). The features are often given the eponym 'Orphan Annie eye nuclei' (DeLellis 1993a), but descriptive terms – such as pale, clear, optically clear, watery, empty and ground glass (Rosai 1993b) – may be more helpful.

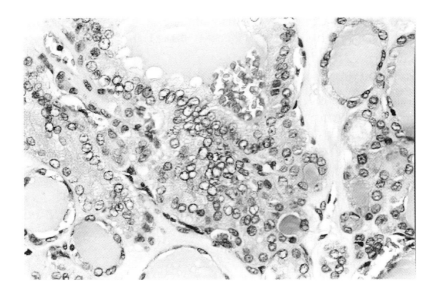

Fig. 5.3 Nuclear clearing in the centre of a hyperplastic nodule in a multinodular goitre. There is a continuum of nuclear appearances from normal to optically clear. The nuclei are mostly round and grooves are not seen. H&E × 190.

These nuclear changes can present a diagnostic problem. Fonseca & Sobrinho-Simões (1995) stress that the nuclei of the cells of some multi-nodular goitres tend to be larger and clearer than those of normal thyroid cells, but without the irregularity of contour associated with papillary neopla-sia. One cause of this clearing might be poor penetration of fixative into the centre of tissues which can lead to loss of nuclear chromatin staining (Baker 1950). This is particularly seen in well encapsulated lesions. The phe-nomenon is not confined to endocrine conditions because it is also seen in poorly fixed lymphocytes (Stansfeld 1992). Such changes in these and other tissues have also been attributed to specific types of tissue processing and the quality of chemical reagents used (Anderson 1988, Slater & Cobb 1988). This artefact occurs chiefly in well encapsulated nodules, either solitary or part of a multinodular goitre, and it is most pronounced in the centre of blocks. Unlike papillary carcinoma nuclei, benign nuclei are the same size as those of ordinary follicular epithelial cells and there is no nuclear grooving. The area affected by artefact has a diffuse border and there are gradations of degree of severity (Fig. 5.3). The ground glass nuclei of papillary carcinoma are abruptly different from surrounding follicular epithelial nuclei with no gradation of the change. They occur anywhere in a block, including the well fixed periphery. Further, thorough sampling sometimes reveals areas of true papillae and/or psammoma bodies in follicular variant papillary carcinoma.

Where diagnostic difficulty still exists after careful consideration of the morphological features, immunohistochemistry for high molecular weight cytokeratins, present in papillary carcinomas including their follicular variant but not in follicular neoplasms (Raphael et al 1994), may be of assistance.

Hürthle cell tumours of the thyroid

Although the oxyphil cell was first described by Askanazy (1898) and the cell described by Hürthle (1894) was in fact the canine C-cell, the eponym 'Hürthle', introduced incorrectly by Ewing (1919), has become entrenched in the literature. For the purposes of this article, the terms oxyphil, Hürthle and Askanazy cell will be treated as synonymous.

Until recently, mystique has surrounded the prediction of behaviour in Hürthle cell tumours, with uncertainty about the histological features and the value of lesion size in predicting malignancy (reviewed by Tallini et al 1992). Fortunately, careful follow-up and correlation with the detailed histological features has clarified the issue (Bruni et al 1987, Bronner & LiVolsi 1988, Gerken et al 1988, Carcangiu et al 1991).

The tinctorial (Chetty 1992), immunohistochemical (Abu-Alfa & Montag 1994) and ultrastructural (Feldman et al 1972) features of thyroid Hürthle cells, thought to be a variant of follicular epithelial cells (Wilensky & Kaufman 1938), are due to the high concentration of mitochondria in the cells (Tremblay & Pearse 1960).

Provided that the specimen has been adequately sampled, morphology adequately predicts behaviour (Bronner & LiVolsi 1988). Capsular (Fig. 5.4) and/or vascular invasion indicate(s) malignancy. In the absence of invasion these neoplasms almost invariably have a benign course (Tallini et al 1992).

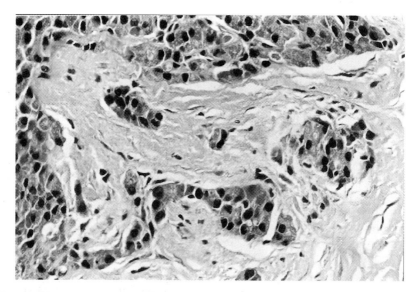

Fig. 5.4 Widespread capsular invasion by Hürthle cell carcinoma. The cells have voluminous granular eosinophilic cytoplasm. H&E × 245.

The majority of carcinomas are solid or trabecular and finding this growth pattern should prompt search for evidence of invasion. A high proportion of cases defined as malignant pursue an aggressive course; the prognosis is similar to that of insular pattern follicular carcinoma. Size alone cannot be used as a criterion of malignancy, although the larger the size, the greater the chance of malignancy (Carcangiu et al 1991).

Less than total thyroidectomy is adequate treatment for histologically benign tumours (Grant 1995). For malignant tumours, aggressive surgical treatment does not diminish the incidence of metastases. Whereas only 2–3% of solitary encapsulated follicular nodules show invasion, this is seen in 30–40% of cases with Hürthle cell cytology. They often show areas of infarction or necrosis – but these do not in themselves indicate malignancy. Nuclear atypia, number of mitoses, cellular pleomorphism and percentage of Hürthle cells are of little prognostic significance.

Unlike 'ordinary' follicular carcinoma, they may metastasise to lymph nodes (Tallini et al 1992). For malignant tumours, no clinical or histological features have been shown to be prognostic. There is some evidence that DNA flow cytometry and immunohistochemical quantification of cell proliferation (Tatayama et al 1994) may identify a group of patients with a particularly poor prognosis. Oncocytic tumours have characteristic mitochondrial and/or nuclear DNA abnormalities. Compared with ordinary follicular carcinomas, a higher proportion of them express Pan-ras, N-myc, TGF-α, TGF-β and IGF-1 (Masood et al 1993).

Parathyroid adenocarcinoma

Parathyroid adenocarcinomas are rare, accounting for only 0.5–6% of cases of primary hyperparathyroidism (DeLellis 1993b, Hakaim & Esselstyn 1993). There are reports suggesting that the condition is both over- (Vetto et al 1993) and under-diagnosed (Sandelin et al 1992). In the latter study, the diagnosis was not appreciated at primary surgery in 19% of 95 patients. Severe recurrent hyperparathyroidism in association with histologically atypical features in the resected gland should alert to the possibility that a diagnosis of parathyroid adenocarcinoma has been overlooked (Fraker et al 1991). LiVolsi & Hamilton (1994) pointed out that these problems arise from the rarity of the tumour and lack of specific histological criteria.

Parathyroid adenocarcinoma has an equal sex incidence, compared with adenoma which is more common in females (Shane & Bilezikian 1982). It presents over a wide age range, reported to be from 28–72 years (mean 45) (Wang & Gaz 1985). Most of the tumours are functional, leading to severe parathyroid bone disease and renal complications of hypercalcaemia at presentation (Shane & Bilezikian 1982). Approximately one-third of patients present with a palpable neck mass due to the relatively large size (mean 6.7 g) of parathyroid adenocarcinomas (Wang & Gaz 1985). At surgery, the diagnosis of malignancy may be suspected if the mass has ill-defined borders with adhesion to soft tissues, thyroid or peri-oesophageal tissues (DeLellis 1993b).

The morphological criteria for the diagnosis of parathyroid adenocarcinoma include: capsular and blood vessel invasion, desmoplastic stroma with fibrous bands (Fig. 5.5), trabecular growth pattern, thickening and hyalinization of the capsule, spindle shaped tumour cells, elevated mitotic count and aberrant mitoses (Schantz & Castleman 1973, Smith & Coombs 1984, Chan & Tsang 1995). Of these features, the presence of fibrous bands stands out as the most helpful for the diagnosis of malignancy, being present in 90% of 67 cases studied (Schantz & Castleman 1973). Caution should be exercised in the interpretation of fibrous bands since these sometimes occur as part of a regressive phenomenon in adenomas, in which case they may be associated with deposition of haemosiderin and surrounded by chronic inflammatory cells (DeLellis 1993b).

Assessment of mitotic activity either by mitotic counts (Schantz & Castleman 1973, Evans 1993), flow cytometry (Harlow et al 1991, Bondeson et al 1993), or immunohistochemistry (Abbona et al 1995) has been proposed as a means of predicting malignancy in parathyroid neoplasia. While there is a statistical tendency for the adenocarcinomas – particularly those with aggressive behaviour – to have higher proliferative activity than adenomas, overlap in the result ranges limits diagnostic utility in the individual case (DeLellis 1995). The main problem appears to be that some parathyroid adenomas, increasingly recognised to be clonal and true neoplasms (Noguchi et al 1994), have high proliferative indices. In one interesting study, nuclear chromatin texture, even when subjected to detailed image analysis, failed to distinguish between benign and malignant parathyroid neoplasms (Einstein et al 1994).

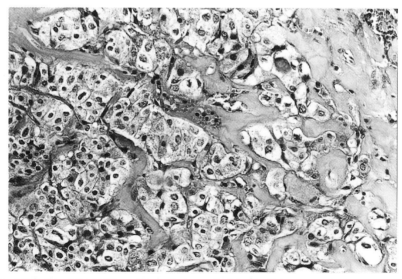

Fig. 5.5 A desmoplastic fibrous stroma between the islands of pleomorphic clear cells is one of the most important defining features of parathyroid adenocarcinoma. H&E × 245.

Capsular invasion is an important distinguishing feature of parathyroid adenocarcinoma, being present in approximately two-thirds of cases, often associated with a capsule which itself is thicker than that encountered in parathyroid adenomas (Schantz & Castleman 1973). However, care should be taken not to confuse occasional entrapped clusters of cells, particularly in the capsules of adenomas which have undergone cystic degeneration, for true invasion (DeLellis 1993b). While clear-cut vascular invasion is only encountered in 10–15% of parathyroid adenocarcinomas, when present it is a useful sign of malignancy (DeLellis 1993).

The growth pattern in parathyroid adenocarcinoma may be trabecular, rosette-like or sheet-like. Nuclear palisading may be present. The tumour cells are generally larger than those in adenomas, but there may be little nuclear pleomorphism (Jacobi et al 1986).

Electron microscopic studies (Altenähr & Saeger 1973, Obara et al 1985) have failed to show any unique features correlating with malignancy in parathyroid neoplasms. Analysis of p53 gene mutation is of uncertain value in the prediction of their malignancy and in one study it was demonstrated in neither adenomas nor carcinomas (Hakim & Levine 1994). In another study, two out of nine carcinomas were p53 immunopositive of which one had p53 allelic loss while the other was genetically non-informative. None of the adenomas had allelic loss (Cryns et al 1994b). Loss of retinoblastoma (Rb) protein has been reported in some parathyroid carcinomas while adenomas appear to be Rb gene positive (Cryns et al 1994a)

A number of benign and malignant lesions can mimic parathyroid adenocarcinoma. The clear cells in the wall of a parathyroid cyst (Calandra et al 1983, Mitmaker et al 1991), atypical oxyphil parathyroid adenoma (Bedetti et al 1984, Wolpert et al 1989) various metastatic tumours (Horwitz 1972, de la Monte 1984) particularly of clear cell type (Underwood 1987), and implantation of parathyroid tissue at previous surgery for benign conditions (Rattner et al 1985, LiVolsi & Hamilton 1994) may mimic parathyroid adenocarcinoma (Smith & Coombs 1984, Cohn 1985). The presence of mitotic figures within a parathyroid adenoma (provided that they are not atypical) is not in itself an indicator of malignancy (DeLellis 1993b). Groups of large atypical cells in parathyroid neoplasms, particularly close to foci of haemorrhage, do not indicate malignancy and are, paradoxically, more common in adenomas (DeLellis 1993b).

When a diagnosis of parathyroid adenocarcinoma is established, the prognosis is poor with an approximate 50% 10 year survival; more patients die from severe hypercalcaemia than the physical effects of metastatic disease (Grimelius & Bondeson 1995).

Adrenal cortical adenocarcinoma

Adenocarcinoma of the adrenal cortex is rare, with an incidence of 1:1 700 000 population or 0.02% of cancers. It has a bimodal age distribution of 10–20

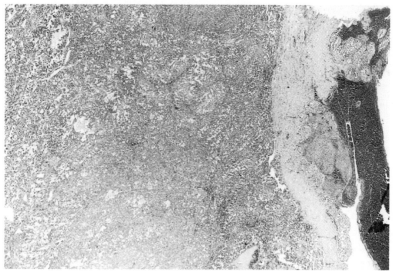

Fig. 5.6 This adrenocortical tumour had invaded through the wall of the inferior vena cava (right) causing considerable difficulty in operative removal and clearly defining itself as malignant. H&E × 65.

and 40–60 years, and the sex incidence is equal (Lack et al 1990). Patients with carcinoma of the adrenal cortex usually have endocrine manifestations – feminisation and masculinisation are pointers to malignancy in adrenal corti-cal neoplasia. Most adrenal carcinomas are large with average weights in reported series being in the range of 750–1500 g, and many tumours are much larger. There is often obvious local spread (Fig. 5.6) or metastasis at operation.

There have been attempts to make the prediction of a malignant course more reliable using multivariate analysis and probability techniques. Hough et al (1979) determined the histological features in adrenal cortical neoplasms associated with the highest Bayesian probabilities of metastasis. These were: broad fibrous bands ($P < 0.0001$), widespread necrosis ($P < 0.0001$), diffuse growth pattern ($P < 0.001$), vascular invasion ($P < 0.001$), cellular pleomor-phism ($P < 0.001$), over 10 mitoses per 10 high power fields (hpf) ($P < 0.02$) and capsular invasion ($P < 0.03$). Weiss (1984) described the histological fea-tures present in more than half of 18 metastasising/recurring adrenal cortical tumours. These included: high nuclear grade (III or IV), mitotic rate over 5 per 50 hpf, compact cells comprising more than 75% of the tumour, diffuse architecture, tumour necrosis and invasion of sinusoidal structures and/or of the capsule.

The problem with these types of study is that they still give no absolute indication of whether an individual adrenal cortical tumour is malignant (Chan & Tsang 1995). In the study by Weiss (1984) the three features found **only** in metastasising or recurring tumours were a mitotic count of over 5 per

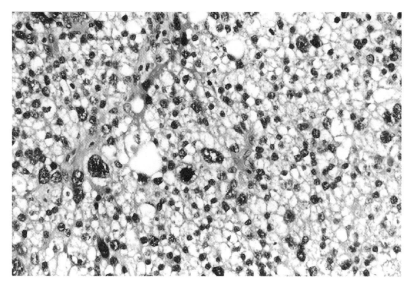

Fig. 5.7 This adrenocortical tumour had no features suggestive of malignancy other than the pronounced nuclear pleomorphism. It had to be described as 'an adrenocortical tumour of uncertain malignant potential'. H&E × 245.

50 hpf, atypical mitoses and invasion of venous structures. These features when present should therefore be regarded as absolute indicators of malignancy. The problem is that not all adrenal cortical adenocarcinomas have one or more of these features. It is inevitable that in a number of cases no firm prediction of behaviour can be made and the term 'adrenal cortical tumour of uncertain malignant potential' may be appropriate (Fig. 5.7). Long term follow up of these is desirable because, although adrenal cortical adenocarcinoma has a reported overall mortality between 70 and 92% (Lack et al 1990), the malignant nature of some tumours can take 10 years to become apparent (King & Lack 1979).

Nuclear DNA content has been advocated as a predictor of malignancy in adrenal cortical neoplasia, but not all adenocarcinomas are aneuploid (Haak et al 1993). In contrast to the findings with many other tumours, Haak et al (1993) found longer survival in patients with aneuploid than with diploid tumours. DNA ploidy combined with morphometric indicators of nuclear pleomorphism and tumor weight have been proposed by Diaz-Cano et al (1993) for prediction of malignancy in discriminant analysis, but they found overlap between benign and malignant tumours. Examination of silver binding nucleolar organiser regions (Ag-NOR) has been advocated for prediction of malignancy, with carcinomas having significantly higher Ag-NOR counts than adenomas in one study (Oz et al 1992).

The differential diagnosis of adrenal cortical adenocarcinoma includes other clear cell tumours such as hepatocellular and renal cell carcinomas – immunohistochemistry for cytokeratin types has been advocated as a means of distinguishing these entities (Gaffey et al 1992). Neuroendocrine differentiation, as evidenced by immunohistochemical detection of synaptophysin and neuron 'specific' enolase (Miettinen 1992, Haak & Fleuren 1995), detection of synaptophysin mRNA (Komminoth et al 1995) and electron microscopy (Miettinen 1992), is encountered in some adrenal cortical tumours including carcinomas. Electron microscopy is valuable in the differential diagnosis of adrenal cortical adenocarcinoma from other similar appearing tumours but there are no specific features indicative of malignancy (Mackay et al 1994).

Pancreatic endocrine tumours

The term 'pancreatic endocrine tumours' has been selected in preference to islet cell tumours since this section would be incomplete without consideration of gastrinomas which are not thought to originate from islets (Capella et al 1995). This is another area where the histopathologist may feel diagnostically impotent since the only unequivocal and universally accepted evidence that they are malignant is the presence of tumour cells in the regional lymph nodes or distant organs where similar endocrine tissues are not normally found (Moffat & Ketcham 1993).

Large size (over 30 mm diameter) and unequivocal angio-invasion are more commonly seen in tumours which prove to be malignant (Moffat & Ketcham 1993), but one of the most consistently prognostic features is the category of the tumour's hormonal product. The most comprehensive data on the relative frequencies of different pancreatic endocrine tumours comes from Ireland (Buchanan et al 1986), where an overall incidence of 3.6 cases per million population per year has been documented (Table 5.1). Insulinomas were as common as non-functional tumours, and were twice as common as

Table 5.1 Prevalence and pathological features of pancreatico-duodenal neuroendocrine tumours (adapted from Buchanan et al 1986)

Tumour type	Incidence	% with metastases
Gastrinoma	2 : 5 million	50
Insulinoma	4 : 5 million	5
VIPoma		40
Glucagonoma		70
Somatostatinoma		70
GRFoma		30
ACTHoma		100
PTH-like-oma		100
Neurotensinoma		> 80
Nonfunctioning	1 : 5 million	60

VIP = vasoactive intestinal peptide
GRF = growth hormone releasing factor
ACTH = adrenocorticotrophic hormone
PTH = parathyroid hormone

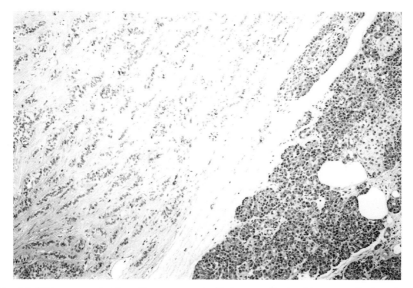

Fig. 5.8 This pancreatic islet cell tumour was well circumscribed, with no vascular invasion and contained insulin. The patient had no evidence of recurrence 10 years after excision. H&E × 55.

gastrinomas, eight times as common as VIPomas and 17 times as common as glucagonomas.

The percentages of cases which Buchanan et al (1986) found to present with or develop metastases are shown in Table 5.1. It can be seen that insulinomas (Fig. 5.8) are the least likely of all the tumour types to metastasise, a finding backed up by all other studies. The expression of gastrin or somatostatin (Heitz 1984) and particularly adrenocorticotrophic hormone (ACTH) (Doppman et al 1994), rather than insulin, are likely to be associated with malignancy. Gastrinomas deserve special mention because they are the second commonest pancreatic endocrine tumour: 60% of them arise in the pancreas. While there is controversy as to whether the extra- or intra-pancreatic primary site affects behaviour, about 50% overall are malignant. It is claimed that metastases confined to lymph nodes correlate with an indolent course while liver metastases predict a very poor prognosis (Moffat & Ketcham 1993). Chaudhry et al (1994) found that different splice variants of CD44 are expressed in gastrinomas but not in other subtypes of endocrine pancreatic tumours. They argue that this difference, with its correlation with malignant behaviour, may relate to CD44 being the principal receptor for hyaluronate which has been implicated in cell-extracellular matrix interactions.

Different metastatic patterns have been reported between the various types of pancreatic endocrine neoplasms (Moffat & Ketcham 1993). Malignant insulinomas favour the regional lymph nodes, while malignant glucagonomas, somatostatinomas and non-functional tumours are much more likely to metastasise to the liver.

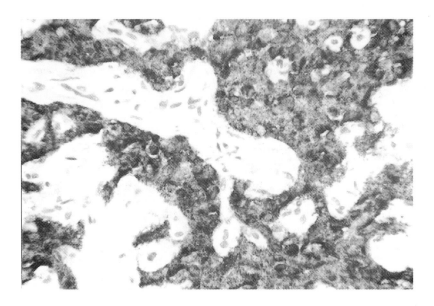

Fig. 5.9 This pancreatic islet cell tumour had no operative or histological evidence of invasion at primary surgery. Immunohistochemistry confirmed that it was producing glucagon. It disseminated to the local lymph nodes within two years of diagnosis. Immunoperoxidase for glucagon × 315.

Although there are theoretical reasons to suspect that non-functional tumours may have a worse prognosis than functional ones because the latter may present at a very small size due to endocrine effects (Norton 1994), a recent study (White et al 1994) indicates no significant prognostic difference. A generally non-functional variant known as poorly differentiated neuroendocrine carcinoma of the pancreas is also recognised. This has the appearance of a 'small blue cell tumour' and is always malignant with a very poor prognosis (Capella et al 1995).

Immunohistochemistry (Fig. 5.9) is generally considered the most convenient method for determining the endocrine content of these tumours (Mukai et al 1982), although differences in endocrine granule morphology at electron microscopy have also been used (Kunz 1986). Where these methodologies are not available, tinctorial methods such as the aldehyde fuschin technique for insulin and the chrome-alum haematoxylin phloxine technique for insulin (blue reaction) and glucagon (red reaction) have been suggested as substitutes (Wilson & Chalk 1996), although they may be less specific.

Techniques such as assessment of DNA ploidy, proliferation indices, Ag-NOR counting, and demonstration of human chorionic gonadotropin (reviewed in Capella et al 1995) have been advocated as aids to prediction of malignancy, but they await clarification and remain at the research stage.

KEY POINTS FOR CLINICAL PRACTICE

1. With endocrine lesions more than with many other areas of tumour pathology, close attention must be paid to the clinical, biochemical and naked eye appearances. The main clues to malignancy may lie outwith the purely histological features.

2. Thorough specimen sampling is essential because the cytological or architectural (invasion) features of malignancy may be focal.

3. DNA ploidy analysis and molecular biological techniques have yielded useful prognostic information, but considerable overlap in findings between benign and malignant lesions means that careful histological evaluation has not been superseded.

4. It is no longer necessary to give non-committal reports on Hürthle cell tumours – histological features can adequately predict malignancy.

5. The features of malignancy in an endocrine tumour can be 'non-conventional'. For example, in the parathyroid, the presence of fibrous bands is a better indicator of malignancy than mitotic count.

6. Good fixation is important to enable nuclear features, including mitotic counts, to be assessed unimpeded by artefacts.

7. In pancreatic endocrine tumours, the identity of any hormonal product is one of the most useful factors in assessing malignant potential.

8. The endocrine system is rich in 'pseudomalignant' conditions and appearances with which it is important to be familiar.

REFERENCES

Abbona GC, Papotti M, Gasparri G et al 1995 Proliferative activity in parathyroid tumours as detected by Ki-67 immunostaining. Hum Pathol 26: 135–138

Abu-Alfa AK, Montag AG 1994 An immunohistochemical study of thyroid Hürthle cells and their neoplasms: the roles of S-100 and HMB-45 proteins. Mod Pathol 7: 529–532

Albores-Saavedra J, Altamirano-Dimas M, Alcorta-Anguizola B et al 1971 Fine structure of human papillary thyroid cancer. Cancer 28: 763–774

Altenähr E, Saeger W 1973 Light and electron microscopy of parathyroid adenocarcinoma. Report of 3 cases. Virchows Archiv [A] 360: 107–122

Anderson G 1988 Enclosed tissue system problem. Institute for Medical Laboratory Sciences Gazette 32, 141–142

Askanazy M 1898 Pathologisch-anatomisch Beitrage zur Kenntniss des Morbus Basedow, insbesondere über die dabei auftretende Muskelerkranking. Dtsch Arch Klin Med 61: 118–186

Baker JR 1950 Cytological technique. Methuen, London. Ch 1, pp 1–21

Bedetti CD, Dekker A, Watson CG 1984 Functioning oxyphil adenoma of the parathyroid gland. A clinicopathological study of ten patients with hyperparathyroidism. Hum Pathol 15: 1121–1126

Bondeson L, Sandelin K, Grimelius L 1993 Histopathological variables and DNA cytometry in parathyroid adenocarcinoma. Am J Surg Pathol 17: 820–829

Bronner MP, LiVolsi VA 1988 Oxyphilic (Askanazy/Hürthle cell) tumors of the thyroid: Microscopic features predict biologic behaviour. Surg Pathol 1: 137–150

Bruni F, Batsakis JG, Luna MA et al 1987 Hürthle cell tumors of the thyroid gland (Abstr). Am J Clin Pathol 88: 528

Buchanan KD, Johnston CF, O'Hare MMT et al 1986 Neuroendocrine tumors: a European view. Am J Med 81(Suppl 68): 14–23

Calandra DB, Shah KH, Prinz RA 1983 Parathyroid cysts: a report of 11 cases including two associated with hyperparathyroid crisis. Surgery 94: 887–892

Capella C, Heitz PU, Hofler H et al 1995 Revised classification of neuroendocrine tumours of the lung, pancreas and gut. Virchows Archiv 425: 547–560

Carcangiu ML, Zampi G, Pupi A et al 1985 Papillary carcinoma of the thyroid. A clinicopathologic study of 241 cases treated at the University of Florence, Italy. Cancer 55: 805–828

Carcangiu ML, Bianchi S, Savino D et al 1991 Follicular Hürthle cell tumors of the thyroid gland. Cancer 68: 1944–1953

Carniero F, Sobrinho-Simões M 1995 Introduction. Pathol Update 2: i–ii

Carr K, Heffess C, Jin L et al 1993 Immunohistochemical analysis of thyroid carcinomas using antibodies to p53 and Ki-67. Appl Immunohistochem 1: 201–207

Chan JKC, Saw D 1986 The grooved nucleus: a useful diagnostic criterion of papillary carcinoma of the thyroid. Am J Surg Pathol 10: 672–679

Chan JKC, Tsang WYW 1995 Endocrine malignancies that may mimic benign lesions. Semin Diagn Pathol 12: 45–63

Chaudhry A, Gobl A, Eriksson B et al 1994 Different splice variants of CD44 are expressed in gastrinomas but not in other subtypes of endocrine pancreatic tumors. Cancer Res 54: 981–986

Chetty R 1992 Hürthle cell neoplasms of the thyroid gland revisited (Review). Austr & New Z J Surg 62: 802–804

Cohn K 1985 Parathyroid carcinoma: the Lahey clinic experience. Surgery 98: 1095–1100

Cryns VL, Thor A, Xu H-J et al 1994a Loss of the retinoblastoma tumor suppressor gene in parathyroid carcinoma. New Engl J Med 330: 757–761

Cryns VL, Rubio MP, Thor AD et al 1994b p53 abnormalities in human parathyroid carcinoma. J Clin Endocrinol Metabolism 78: 1320–1324

Damiani S, Fratamico F, Lapertosa G et al 1991 Alcian blue and epithelial membrane antigen are useful markers in differentiating benign from malignant papillae in thyroid. Virchows Archiv [A] 419: 131–135

de la Monte SM, Hutchins GM, Moore GW 1984 Endocrine organ metastases from breast carcinoma. Am J Pathol 114: 131–136

DeLellis RA 1993a Orphan Annie eye nuclei: a historical note. Am J Surg Pathol 17: 1067–1068

DeLellis RA 1993b Tumors of the parathyroid gland. Atlas of tumor pathology, Third series fascicle 6. Armed Forces Institute of Pathology, Washington pp 25–51 and 93–94

DeLellis RA 1995 Does the evaluation of proliferative activity predict malignancy or prognosis in endocrine tumors? Hum Pathol 26: 131–134

Diaz-Cano S, Gonzalez-Campora R, Rios-martin JJ et al 1993 Nuclear DNA patterns in adrenal cortex proliferative lesions. Virchows Archiv [A] 423: 323–328

Doppman JL, Nieman LK, Cutler GB et al 1994 Adrenocorticotropic hormone-secreting islet cell tumours: are they always malignant? Radiology 190: 59–64

Einstein AJ, Barba J, Unger PD 1994 Nuclear diffuseness as a measure of texture: definition and application to the computer–assisted diagnosis of parathyroid adenoma and carcinoma. J Microsc 176: 158–166

Evans HL 1993 Pathologic diagnosis of parathyroid carcinoma. Int J Surg Pathol 1: 139–142

Ewing J 1919 Neoplastic diseases – a textbook on tumors. 1st edn. Saunders, Philadelphia

Falkmer UG, Falkmer S 1995 The value of cytometric DNA analysis as a prognostic tool in neuroendocrine neoplastic disease. Pathol Update 2: 1–23

Feldman PS, Horvath E, Kovaks K (1972) Ultrastructure of three Hürthle cell tumors of the thyroid. Cancer 30: 1279–1284

Fonseca E, Sobrinho-Simões M 1995 Diagnostic problems in differentiated carcinomas of the thyroid. Pathol Update 2: 1–23

Fraker DL, Travis WD, Merendino JJ et al 1991 Locally recurrent parathyroid neoplasms as a cause for recurrent and persistent primary hyperparathyroidism. Ann Surg 213: 58–65

Fraumann AG, Moses AC 1990 Oncogenes and growth factors in thyroid carcinogenesis. Endocrinol Metabol Clin North Am 19: 479–493

Gaffey MJ, Traweek ST, Mills SE et al 1992 Cytokeratin expression in adrenocortical neoplasia: an immunohistochemical and biochemical study with implications for the differential diagnosis of adrenocortical, hepatocellular and renal cell carcinoma. Hum Pathol 23: 144–153

Gerken K, Nunez C, Broughan T et al 1988 Clinical outcome of Hürthle cell tumors of the thyroid (Abstr). Am J Clin Pathol 90: 498

Grant CS 1995 Operative and postoperative management of the patient with follicular and Hürthle cell carcinoma – do they differ? Endocr Surg 75: 395–403

Grieco M, Santoro M, Berlingieri MT et al 1990 PTC is a novel rearranged form of the ret proto-oncogene and is frequently detected in vivo in human thyroid papillary carcinomas. Cell 60: 557–563

Grimelius L, Bondeson L 1995 Histopathological diagnosis of parathyroid diseases. Pathol Update 2: 73–85

Haak HR, Fleuren GJ 1995 Neuroendocrine differentiation of adrenocortical tumors. Cancer 75: 860–864

Haak HR, Cornelisse CJ, Hermans J et al 1993 Nuclear DNA content and morphological characteristics in the prognosis of adrenocortical carcinoma. Br J Cancer 68: 151–155

Hakaim AG, Esselstyn CB 1993 Parathyroid carcinoma: 50 year experience at the Cleveland Clinic Foundation. Cleveland Clinic J Med 60: 331–335

Hakim JP, Levine MA 1994 Absence of p53 point mutations in parathyroid adenoma and carcinoma. J Endocrinol Metab 78: 103–106

Hall PA, Coates PJ 1995 Assessment of cell proliferation in pathology – what next? Histopathology 26: 105–112

Harlow S, Roth SI, Bauer K et al 1991 Flow cytometric DNA analysis of normal and pathologic parathyroid glands. Mod Pathol 4: 310–315

Heitz PU 1984 Pancreatic endocrine tumors. In: Kloppel G, Heitz PU (eds) Pancreatic pathology. Churchill Livingstone, Edinburgh. pp 206–232

Horwitz CA, Myers WP, Foote FW 1972 Secondary malignant tumours of the parathyroid glands. Report of two cases with associated hypoparathyroidism. Am J Med 52: 797–808

Hough AJ, Hollifield JW, Page DL et al 1979 Prognostic factors in adrenal cortical tumors. A mathematical analysis of clinical and morphologic data. Am J Clin Pathol 72: 390–399

Hürthle K 1894 Beitrage zur Kenntniss der Secretionsonsvorgangs in der Schilddruse. Arch Gesamte Physiol 56: 1–44

Jacobi JM, Lloyd HM, Smith JF 1986 Nuclear diameter in parathyroid carcinomas. J Clin Pathol 39: 1353–1354

Katoh R, Bray CE, Suzuki K et al 1995 Growth activity in hyperplastic and neoplastic human thyroid determined by an immunohistochemical staining procedure using monoclonal antibody MIB-1. Hum Pathol 26: 139–146

Kennedy JS 1969 The pathology of dyshormonogenetic goitre. J Pathol 99: 251–264

King DR, Lack EE 1979 Adrenal cortical carcinoma. A clinical and pathologic study of 49 cases. Cancer 44: 239–245

Kiyono T, Katagiri M, Harada T 1994 The incidence of ground glass nuclei in thyroid diseases. Thyroidology 6: 43–48

Komminoth P, Roth J, Schroder S et al 1995 Overlapping expression of immunohistochemical markers and synaptophysin mRNA in phaeochromocytomas and adrenocortical carcinomas. Implications for the differential diagnosis of adrenal gland tumors. Lab Invest 72: 424–431

Kunz J 1986 Pancreatic endocrine tumours: histological, immunocytochemical and electronmicroscopical investigations. Acta Histochem (Suppl) 33: 233–241

Lack EE, Travis WD, Oertel JE 1990 Adrenal cortical neoplasms. In: Lack EE (ed) Pathology of the adrenal glands. Churchill Livingstone, Edinburgh, pp 115–171

Lack EE, Mulvihill JJ, Travis WD et al 1992 Adrenal cortical neoplasms in the pediatric and adolescent age group: clinicopathologic study of 30 cases with emphasis on epidemiological and prognostic factors. In: Rosen PP, Fechner RE (eds) Pathology Annual 27.1, Appleton & Lange, Norwalk, pp 1–54

LiVolsi VA 1992 Papillary neoplasms of the thyroid: pathologic and prognostic factors. Am J Clin Pathol 97: 426–434

LiVolsi VA, Hamilton R 1994 Intraoperative assessment of parathyroid gland pathology. Am J Clin Pathol 102: 365–373

Mackay B, el-Naggar A, Ordonez NG 1994 Ultrastructure of adrenal cortical carcinoma. Ultrastruct Pathol 18: 181–190

Masood S, Auguste LJ, Westerband A et al 1993 Differential oncogenic expression in thyroid follicular and Hürthle cell carcinomas. Am J Surg 1993: 366–368

McCormick D, Yu C, Hobbs C et al 1993 The relevance of antibody concentration to the immunohistological quantification of cell proliferation-associated antigens. Histopathology 22: 543–547

Miettinen M 1992 Neuroendocrine differentiation in adrenocortical carcinoma. New immunohistochemical findings supported by electron microscopy. Lab Invest 66: 169–174

Mitmaker B, Lerman S, Lamoureux E et al 1991 Parathyroid cyst: diagnosis and treatment of an unusual surgical problem. Can J Surg 34: 59–61

Moffat FL, Ketcham AS 1993 Metastatic proclivities and patterns among APUD cell neoplasms. Semin Surg Oncol 9: 443–452

Mukai K, Greider MH, Grotting JC et al 1982 Retrospective study of 77 pancreatic endocrine tumours using the immunoperoxidase method. Am J Surg Pathol 6: 387–399

Noguchi S, Motomura K, Inaji II et al 1994 Clonal analysis of parathyroid adenomas by means of the polymerase chain reaction. Cancer Lett 78: 93–97

Norton JA 1994 Neuroendocrine tumours of the pancreas and duodenum. Curr Prob Surg 31: 77–156

Obara T, Fujimoto Y, Yamaguchi K et al 1985 Parathyroid carcinoma of the oxyphil cell type. A report of two cases, light and electron microscopic study. Cancer 55: 1482–1489

Oz B, Dervisoglu S, Dervisoglu M et al 1992 Silver binding nucleolar organiser regions in adrenocortical neoplasia. Cytopathology 3: 93–99

Raphael SJ, McKeown-Eyssen G, Asa SL 1994 High-molecular-weight cytokeratin and cytokeratin-19 in the diagnosis of thyroid tumors. Mod Pathol 7: 295–300

Rattner DW, Marrone GC, Kasdon E et al 1985 Recurrent hyperparathyroidism due to implantation of parathyroid tissue. Am J Surg 149: 745–748

Riazmontazer N, Bedayat G 1991 Psammoma bodies in fine needle aspirates from thyroids containing nontoxic hyperplastic nodular goitres. Acta Cytologica 35: 563–566

Rosai J 1993a Papillary carcinoma. In: LiVolsi VD, DeLellis RA (eds) Pathobiology of the parathyroid and thyroid glands. Williams & Wilkins, Baltimore. pp 139–165

Rosai 1993b Papillary carcinoma (Review) Monogr Pathol 35: 138–165

Rosai J, Carcangiu ML, DeLellis RA 1992 Tumors of the thyroid gland. Atlas of tumor pathology, Third series fascicle 5. Armed Forces Institute of Pathology, Washington. pp 297–316

Sandelin K, Auer G, Bondeson L et al 1992 Prognostic factors in parathyroid cancer: a review of 95 cases. World J Surg 16: 724–731

Schantz A, Castleman B 1973 Parathyroid carcinoma. A study of 70 cases. Cancer 31: 600–605

Shane E, Bilezikian JP 1982 Parathyroid carcinoma. A study of 70 cases. Endocr Rev 3: 218–226

Slater DN, Cobb N 1988 Enclosed tissue processors. Institute for Medical Laboratory Sciences Gazette 32, 543–544

Smith JH, Coombs RRH 1984 Histological diagnosis of carcinoma of the parathyroid gland. J Clin Pathol 37: 1370–1378

Soares P, Sobrinho-Simões M 1995 Recent advances in cytometry, cytogenetics and molecular genetics of thyroid tumours and tumour-like conditions. Pathol Update 2: 24–37

Soares P, Cameselle-Teijerio J, Sobrinho-Simões M 1994 Immunohistochemical detection of p53 in differentiated, poorly differentiated and undifferentiated carcinomas of the thyroid. Histopathology 24: 205–210

Sobrinho-Simões M 1991 Thyroid oncology: the end of the dogmas. Endocr Pathol 2: 117–119

Sobrinho-Simões M, Fonseca E 1994 Recently described tumours of the thyroid. In: Anthony PP, MacSween RNM (eds) Recent advances in histopathology volume 16. Churchill

Livingstone, Edinburgh. pp 213–229

Sobrinho-Simões, M, Soares J, Carneiro F et al 1990 Diffuse follicular variant of papillary carcinoma of the thyroid: report of eight cases of a distinct aggressive type of thyroid tumour. Surg Pathol 3: 189–203

Stansfeld AG 1992 An introduction to biopsy interpretation. In: Stansfeld AG, d'Ardenne AJ (eds) Lymph node biopsy interpretation. Churchill Livingstone, Edinburgh. p 50

Tallini G, Carcangiu ML, Rosai J 1992 Oncocytic neoplasms of the thyroid gland. Acta Pathol Jpn 42: 305–315

Tatayama H, Yang YP, Eimoto T et al 1994 Proliferative cell nuclear antigen expression in follicular tumours of the thyroid with special reference to oxyphilic cell lesions. Virchows Archiv 424: 533–537

Tielens ET, Sherman SI, Hruban RH et al 1994 Follicular variant of papillary thyroid carcinoma. Cancer 73: 424–431

Tong Q, Li Y, Smanik PA et al 1995 Characterisation of the promoter region and oligomerization domain of H4 (D10S170), a gene frequently rearranged with the ret proto-oncogene. Oncogene 10: 1781–1787

Tremblay G, Pearse AEG 1960 Histochemistry of oxidative enzyme systems in the human thyroid with special reference to Askanazy cells. J Pathol Bacteriol 80: 353–358

Underwood JCE 1987 Introduction to biopsy interpretation and surgical pathology. Springer, Berlin. pp 127–128.

van Slooten H, Scaberg A, Smeenk D, et al 1985 Morphological characteristics of benign and malignant adrenal cortical tumors. Cancer 55: 766–773

Vetto JT, Brennan MF, Woodruf J et al 1993 Parathyroid carcinoma: diagnosis and clinical history. Surgery 114: 882–892

Vickery AL 1981 The diagnosis of malignancy in dyshormonogenetic goitre. Clin Endocrinol Metabolism 10: 317–335

Wang CA, Gaz RD 1985 Natural history of parathyroid carcinoma. Diagnosis, treatment and results. Am J Surg 149: 522–527

Weiss LM 1984 Comparative study of 43 metastasising and non-metastasising adrenocortical tumours. Am J Surg Pathol 8: 163–169

White TJ, Edney JA, Thompson JS et al 1994 Is there a prognostic difference between functional and nonfunctional islet cell tumours? Am J Surg 168: 627–629

Wilson POG, Chalk BT 1996 The neuroendocrine system. In: Bancroft JD, Stevens A (eds) Theory and practice of histological techniques. 4th edn. Churchill Livingstone, Edinburgh. p 274

Wilensky AO, Kaufman PA 1938 Hürthle cell tumor of the thyroid gland. Surg Gynaecol Obstet 66: 1–9

Wolpert HR, Vickery AL, Wang CA 1989 Functioning oxyphil cell adenomas of the parathyroid gland. A study of 15 cases. Am J Surg Pathol 13: 500–504

Yamashita T, Hosoda Y, Kameyama K et al 1992 Peculiar nuclear clearing composed of microfilaments in papillary carcinoma of the thyroid. Cancer 70: 2923–2928

6

Advances in gynaecological pathology

D. G. Lowe   C. H. Buckley   H. Fox

FAMILIAL OVARIAN CANCER

Ovarian cancer is the commonest cause of death from malignancy of the female genital system in the UK and the fifth commonest potentially fatal cancer in women (OPCS mortality statistics 1987). Epithelial ovarian cancer kills more women each year than all other gynaecological cancers combined (Baker & Piver 1994). The incidence is greatest in Sweden and North America (Heintz et al 1985). The disease is commonest in industrialised countries, Japan excepted. Japanese women living in the USA have an incidence rate similar to that of indigenous American women (Heintz et al 1985). Most cases occur in the sixth decade of life with a peak age incidence at 53 years (Piver 1987). In the UK each year 1 in 2500 women over the age of 45 years will develop ovarian cancer (OPCS mortality statistics 1987). The five year survival is only about 17% (Buller et al 1993).

In the UK there are 40–60 cases a year of familial ovarian cancer. These patients and their relatives are currently the subject of a large study funded by the United Kingdom Co-ordinating Committee for Cancer Research (UKCCCR) which involves geneticists, gynaecologists, radiologists, histopathologists and others who are collaborating to identify past and prospective patients and collect tissues, serum and full clinical details from them. The definition of a familial case that is used for inclusion of women into the study is that they must have two or more first or second degree female relatives with ovarian cancer verified by death certificate or histopathology.

It has been recognised for 60 years that ovarian carcinoma can run in families. Lynch (1936) reported three families with familial ovarian cancer from a series of 110 patients. There are several principal ways in which ovarian neoplasms involve families (Table 6.1): the pattern includes malignant epithelial tumours in eight of these syndromes.

The risk in a particular family may be of ovarian carcinoma alone, without associated neoplasia of other organ or tissues. Ovarian cancer may occur with breast cancer alone (Lynch et al 1978, Lynch et al 1981, Prior & Waterhouse 1981) or with Lynch syndrome II, which comprises breast cancer, non-polyposis colorectal cancer, endometrial and ovarian cancer and, occasionally, transitional cell carcinoma (Lynch et al 1989, Lynch et al 1991, Hakala et al

Table 6.1 Familial ovarian neoplasms: clinical setting of ovarian disease

Syndrome or disease and ovarian neoplasm	Associated tumours	References
Ovarian cancer alone	Breast carcinoma	Lynch et al 1978, 1981, Prior & Waterhouse 1981
Peutz-Jeghers' syndrome granulosa cell tumour SCTAT adenocarcinoma fibroma, thecoma Sertoli cell tumour	Hamartomatous intestinal polyposis; minimal deviation adenocarcinoma of the cervix; tumours of the Fallopian tube	Christian 1971, Cantu et al 1980, Young et al 1982, Scully 1982, Young et al 1983, Gilks et al 1989 Spigelman et al 1989
Lynch II syndrome ovarian carcinoma	Non-polyposis colorectal carcinoma; carcinoma of the small intestine and endometrium; transitional cell carcinoma	Lynch et al 1989, Lynch et al 1991, Hakala et al 1991, Ostlere et al 1993
Li-Fraumeni syndrome ovarian carcinoma	Breast carcinoma; soft tissue sarcomas; brain tumours; osteosarcoma.	Sobol et al 1993
Ataxia telangiectasia dysgerminoma gonadoblastoma yolk sac tumour	Smooth muscle tumours of the uterus.	Goldsmith & Hart 1975, Narita & Takagi 1984, Pecorelli et al 1988, Gatti et al 1989
Gorlin's disease (naevoid BCC syndrome) fibroma sclerosing stromal tumour	Basal cell naevi and carcinoma.	Gorlin & Sedano 1971, Lynch 1976, Ismail & Walker 1990, Raggio et al 1983
Cowden's disease adenocarcinoma serous cystadenoma immature teratoma	Carcinoma of the breast, cervix , uteri and endometrium; colorectal polyposis; uterine leiomyomas; facial trichilemmomas; thyroid tumours; lipomas; angiomas; fibrocystic disease of the breast	Carlson et al 1984, Starink 1984, Walton et al 1986, Grattan & Hamburger 1987, Neumann 1991
Torre Muir syndrome adenocarcinoma	Carcinoma of the endometrium, colon, urinary tract and vulva; cutaneous sebaceous neoplasms	Bitran & Pellettiere 1974, Rulon & Helwig 1974, Graham et al 1985
Smith-Lemli-Opitz syndrome yolk sac tumour dysgerminoma		Patsner et al 1989
Adenocarcinoma of ovary	Familial thyroid adenoma	Jensen et al 1974, O'Brien & Wilansky 1981

1991, Ostlere et al 1993). In Li-Fraumeni syndrome, ovarian cancer is one of the many tumours to which such families are prone (Sobol et al 1993). Patients with Peutz-Jeghers' syndrome occasionally develop cystadenocarcinoma of the ovary (Christian 1971). Families with Cowden's disease (Carlson et al 1984, Starink 1984, Walton et al 1986, Grattan & Hamburger 1987, Neumann 1991) and Torre Muir syndrome (Bitran & Pellettiere 1974, Rulon & Helwig 1974, Graham et al 1985) may have members with ovarian adenocarcinoma as well as a wide variety of other benign and malignant neoplasms. Patients with familial thyroid adenomas may sometimes develop ovarian carcinoma (Jensen et al 1974, O'Brien & Wilansky 1981).

Genetic studies

Genetic studies indicate that one locus that is abnormal in familial ovarian cancer is on chromosome 17 in the 17q12-q21 region (Narod et al 1991: Feunteun et al 1993, Flejter et al 1995). There is also evidence that p53 is mutated in the germ line in half of patients with Li-Fraumeni syndrome (Smith & Ponder 1993). Hereditary non-polyposis colorectal cancer may be associated with ovarian cancer and has been linked to loci on chromosomes 2p and 3p.

The tumour suppressor genes BRCA1 and BRCA2 have been cloned (Black 1994). These may be involved in both inherited and sporadic breast and ovarian cancer (Futreal et al 1994). Somatic mutation does not appear to occur in non-familial cases of breast and ovarian tumours but a mutation of BRCA1 is found in nearly half of families who have a high incidence of breast cancer, and in over three-quarters of those with a high incidence of breast and ovary cancer (Miki et al 1994). Numerous different BRCA1 mutations have been described (Shattuck-Eidens et al 1995).

Epidemiology

A woman has a 1.4% chance of developing ovarian cancer during her life. Of all women with ovarian cancer, 5–10% will have a familial association (de Meeus et al 1993), though if detailed family pedigrees are taken the proportion is probably higher than this. It is likely that the rate of gene carriage is also higher, because in some cases the abnormal gene may not result in the development of ovarian cancer. Women in affected families develop ovarian cancer earlier than patients in whom it is a chance event, at 44–55 years rather than 50–59 years (Lewis & Clare Davison 1969, Li et al 1970, Fraumeni et al 1975, Thor et al 1976, Lynch et al 1978, Lurain & Piver 1979, Lynch et al 1981, Franceschi et al 1982, OPCS 1987). In many studies the incidence of bilaterality of ovarian cancer was found to be higher when the affected woman was from a cancer-prone family (Lurain & Piver 1979, Franceschi et al 1982) though bilaterality is not a feature of the tumours in the UKCCCR study. Almost all ovarian tumour types have been described in familial cases, but serous and endometrioid tumours comprised the majority (Liber 1950, Lewis & Clare Davison 1969, Fraumeni et al 1975, Thor et al 1976, Nevo 1978, Lurain & Piver 1979, Piver et al 1984).

Calculation of risk

From the family pedigree it may be possible to assess the risk of inheriting an ovarian cancer gene, though in a particular patient the true risk of cancer will depend not only on having the gene but also on whether it is expressed. Expression may depend on environmental and other unknown factors. In women from families with sporadic cases of primary breast carcinoma there is about double the risk of primary ovarian cancer (Prior & Waterhouse 1981). A family may have a cancer prone genotype that affects different tissues in men and women, and family members without cancer may have progeny who develop cancer (Lynch et al 1981).

The increased risk of death from ovarian cancer in women who have one first degree relative with ovarian cancer is higher when the relative affected is less than 50 years old at the time of diagnosis (Ponder et al 1992). In many cases of familial ovarian cancer there appears to be an autosomal dominant pattern of inheritance, but in some cases rare recessive genes may be responsible (McCrann et al 1974, Fraumeni et al 1975). The cumulative risk of a woman developing ovarian cancer when she has one affected first degree relative is about 2–3 times that of the general population and 3% over her lifetime.

Primary peritoneal carcinoma

Foci of peritoneal neoplasia of ovarian type are seen in up to 40% of patients with borderline epithelial ovarian tumours and there is some evidence that these arise *in situ* and do not represent metastasis (McCaughey 1985). The histological features of localised, well differentiated papillary and glandular neoplasia below the peritoneal surface are characteristic. There is often a disparity between the grade of the peritoneal neoplasia and that of the ovarian tumour, which suggests that there may be a field effect of neoplasia on peritoneal cells over the ovary and elsewhere (Wharton 1959). Psammoma bodies are found in peritoneal endosalpingiosis, peritoneal 'implants' associated with borderline tumours, invasive ovarian carcinoma, and primary peritoneal carcinoma and they cannot alone be used as a differential diagnostic feature (Kannerstein et al 1977).

Women in ovarian cancer families may also develop primary peritoneal carcinoma or serous surface carcinoma of the ovary. The term carcinoma for the peritoneal neoplasm is appropriate — the tumour cells have the structural and immunohistochemical features of malignant epithelial cells and not of mesothelial cells. The diagnosis rests on the demonstration of cancer in the peritoneum, usually of Müllerian epithelial type, without another primary site and without significant involvement of the ovaries. Primary peritoneal carcinoma was first recognised in patients who had had bilateral oophorectomy for histologically proven non-neoplastic disease some years before presenting with peritoneal malignancy of Müllerian type. Ovarian cancer can arise in ectopic ovarian tissue at many sites, including the broad ligament (Scully 1979) and this must also be excluded before a diagnosis of primary peritoneal carcinoma is accepted. Primary peritoneal carcinoma has not been reported in men.

It is likely that peritoneal carcinoma has a similar aetiology to ovarian carcinoma. This presumption is based on the acceptance that the female genital system develops in part from cells lining the coelomic cavity which also form the peritoneum, and also that, by electron microscopy, immunohistochemistry and other techniques, the tumour cells have similar features to their primary ovarian counterparts. Serous carcinoma of the peritoneum is the commonest type and they are often diffuse papillary carcinomas (Foyle et al 1981). Mucinous and clear cell tumours have also been described.

Clinically, patients present with abdominal pain and enlargement. Peritoneal carcinoma is rarely predominantly in or confined to the pelvis, another feature which distinguishes it from ovarian carcinoma (Truong et al 1990). It is usually a high grade carcinoma but invades into the subperitoneal tissues only superficially. The tumour cells stain positive for EMA, cytokeratin, and S100 protein as do ovarian carcinoma cells (Gitsch et al 1992). The prognosis is poor and most patients die from uncontrolled local disease (Truong et al 1990).

Prophylactic oophorectomy

To reduce the risk in women from ovarian cancer prone families, prophylactic oophorectomy when the woman has completed her family has been advocated. There is no evidence that this operation changes the risk of primary peritoneal carcinoma (Chen et al 1985, Lynch et al 1991, Lynch et al 1992). In one series, women from 16 high risk families were treated by prophylactic oophorectomy and followed up for 1–20 years (Tobacman et al 1982). Three developed peritoneal carcinomatosis which histologically was identical with ovarian cancer. Unfortunately, the oophorectomy specimens had not been serially sectioned and so a small ovarian primary was not excluded.

This exemplifies the need for very full sampling of all excised intra-abdominal tissues from these patients. These must be carefully examined histologically for neoplasia and metaplasia, according to the protocol of the UKCCCR Familial Ovarian Study group. This specifies that all neoplasms should be sampled at the rate of one block per centimetre of the tumour's maximum dimension and prophylactic oophorectomy specimens should be serially blocked. Lesions might be only 1–2 mm across and may be non-neoplastic, benign, borderline, or malignant. It is equally important, where possible, to freeze samples of all tissues for genetic and other studies. Blocks should also be taken from the peritoneal surfaces of the Fallopian tubes, uterus and para-uterine tissues in an attempt to identify foci of peritoneal metaplasia or neoplasia.

From the prevalence of asymptomatic ovarian cancer found incidentally in oophorectomy specimens from patients who have pelvic laparotomy and bilateral oophorectomy as part of management of diseases unrelated to the ovary, such as leiomyomas or prolapse, it can be shown that about 5% of all ovarian cancer could be prevented by prophylactic oophorectomy (Speert 1949, Gibbs 1971, Jacobs & Oram 1987). This figure is likely to be higher when women in cancer prone families are considered as a separate group. On the other hand, more than 500 prophylactic oophorectomy operations would be needed to prevent one case of ovarian cancer (Jacobs & Oram 1987).

Prophylactic oophorectomy is unacceptable to many women. Once the gene can be identified in a family, asymptomatic women will be able to make a more informed choice about having a direct gene test. (Jacobs & Oram 1989).

UKCCCR study

Preliminary results are available on 351 patients from whom histological material was taken for prophylaxis, treatment of cancer, or treatment of other conditions such as leiomyoma and adenomyosis. Most of the 200 ovarian tumours were serous or endometrioid cystadenocarcinomas (49%and 13% respectively) and most (63%) were poorly differentiated. Mucinous cystade-nocarcinoma was found in 3%. There were 10 cases (5%) of solid ovarian tumour which closely resembled transitional cell carcinoma of the bladder, and 4 (2%) of carcinosarcoma or pure sarcoma of the ovary.

In those women who had been treated by hysterectomy (119 of the cases so far examined), endometrial polyps, endometrial hyperplasia and endome-trial adenocarcinoma occurred with a prevalence of 11%, 8% and 4%, respectively. Adenomyosis was seen more commonly than would be expected by chance, with a prevalence of 29%.

The surface epithelium of the ovaries, where this could be assessed, varied from being flattened in about 5% to tall columnar with papillary areas in almost 40%. Clefts were present in 54%, and it was in these that epithelial proliferation and metaplastic changes were most evident. Similar changes have been found by other workers (Gusberg & Deligdisch 1984). Stratification of nuclei and pleomorphism have been found in surface inclu-sion cysts, and clear cells with hobnail nuclei have been considered to be dys-plastic (Graham et al 1962, Fraumeni et al 1975). Lynch et al (1981) have also suggested that surface invaginations, small inclusion cysts, and surface papillae constitute atypical changes in ovaries removed prophylactically from women at risk of familial ovarian cancer. Until the results of genetic analysis are available in the UKCCCR study, it seems unwise to over-interpret the significance of these minor and very common changes.

Key points for clinical practice

In the management of a patient with familial ovarian cancer, consideration should be given to the following points:

1. Sampling of prophylactic oophorectomy specimens.

    We have seen very small carcinomas, discovered in apparently normal ovaries removed prophylactically, that might have been missed if only one or two blocks had been taken. The protocol used in the UKCCCR study is to take a block from the centre of each ovary soon after excision for genetic analysis, fix the remaining tissue, and then block it in entirely by serial transverse sections. When a woman has prophylactic oophorectomy and is not in the UKCCCR study, all of the ovarian tissue should be processed.

2. Ovaries with neoplasia should be sampled at the rate of one block per centimetre of the tumour's maximum dimension. When the tumour consists of a unilocular thin-walled cyst, blocks should be taken specifically from any area of thickening, roughening, or papilla formation.

3. Psammoma bodies may be found in endosalpingiosis and are not alone indicative of malignancy.

4. Primary peritoneal carcinoma should be diagnosed only when the ovaries have been removed and shown histologically to be non-neoplastic, or when the ovaries are present and are normal or involved only focally on the surface.

5. At present it is not known specifically which ovarian neoplasms are associated with abnormalities in BRCA1 and BRCA2, but these data will be available shortly.

MICROINVASIVE CARCINOMA OF THE CERVIX

A recent staging announcement by the Federation Internationale d'Obstet-rique et Gynaecologie (FIGO) re-defining Stage I carcinoma of the cervix has stimulated renewed interest in the topic (Shepherd 1995). It is recommended that the new stages should be applied immediately having been ratified by FIGO, UICC and AJCC (Tables 6.2 and 6.3). What does this mean to the histopathologist and, more important, what does it mean to the patient?

    Microinvasive carcinoma of the cervix uteri is, by definition, a histological diagnosis and such a neoplasm is believed to carry little or no risk of metastatic disease. It can therefore usually be treated relatively conservatively. If it is to be distinguished from carcinoma which requires radical therapy, it should be clearly defined, the definition should be agreed, and the diagnosis

Table 6.2 FIGO staging cervical carcinoma (1988)

0	CIN
I	Carcinoma strictly confined to the cervix*
IA	Preclinical – detected only by microscopy IA1 Minimal microscopically evident stromal invasion IA2 Lesions that can be measured: depth should be no greater than 5 mm. Horizontal spread must not exceed 7 mm. Larger lesions are Stage IB**
IB	Lesions greater in size than stage IA2 whether seen clinically or not. Preformed space involvement does not alter the staging but should be recorded to enable future evaluation of its significance to be determined
*	This is the wording used by FIGO, but extension to the corpus is ignored and so strictly is not applicable in the definition
**	Depth of invasion is measured from the base of the epithelium, either surface or crypt, from which invasion occurs

After Shepherd (1989)

should be reproducible by histopathologists. Finally, the distinction should be clinically important and gynaecologists should have confidence in the diagnosis (Lowe 1992).

There are several practical difficulties associated with the designation of microinvasion. First, there is no universally agreed definition of the disease. Second, there are problems in interpretation, recognition and measurement, and third, there are questions as to the most appropriate management of the condition.

Definition

Although the term microinvasive carcinoma is not used in either the 1988 or the 1995 staging announcements from FIGO (Shepherd 1989, 1995), FIGO stage IA cervical carcinoma is usually regarded as synonymous with microinvasive carcinoma.

Stage I carcinoma is limited to the cervix. Rather incongruously, extension to the corpus uteri is disregarded for staging purposes. In both the 1988 and the 1995 FIGO statements stage I is divided into two categories, stage IA and stage IB. Stage IA encompasses invasive lesions that can be diagnosed only on microscopy, whilst stage IB tumours are larger than those coming within the definition of stage IA whether clinically apparent or not. There have been changes in the definitions of both stage IA and stage IB.

Two categories of stage IA carcinoma are described. In 1988, stage IA1 was defined rather loosely as a tumour having minimal microscopically-evident stromal invasion, and came to be known as early stromal invasion, whilst stage IA2 tumours were described as lesions that could be measured,

Table 6.3 FIGO staging cervical carcinoma (1995)

I	Carcinoma strictly confined to the cervix*		
	IA	Lesions detected only microscopically	
		Maximum size 5 mm deep and 7 mm across**	
		Venous or lymphatic permeation does not alter the staging	
		IA1	Invasion of stroma to a maximum of 3 mm** Horizontal axis 7 mm or less
		IA2	Invasion of stroma greater than 3 mm but no greater than 5 mm** Horizontal axis 7 mm or less
	IB	Clinically apparent lesions confined to the cervix or preclinical lesions larger than stage IA allows***	
		IB1	Clinical lesions no greater than 4 cm in size
		IB2	Clinical lesions greater than 4 cm in size
II – IV	Remain the same		

*	Extension to the corpus is ignored [as extension to the corpus is ignored the word *strictly* is not applicable in the definition]
**	Depth of invasion is measured from the base of the epithelium, either surface or crypt, from which invasion occurs
***	All gross lesions, even those with only superficial invasion, are stage IB

After Shepherd (1995)

sometimes termed microcarcinomas. The absence of strict, objective criteria for the recognition of stage IA1 lesions in the 1988 statement led to variations in the diagnosis of this condition and individual interpretation by histopathologists. It was usually agreed, however, that non-confluent foci of invasion in stage IA1 should lie within 1 mm of the epithelium, whether surface or crypt, from which they arose (Kolstad 1989). An indication as to the maximum acceptable width of the lesion was not provided. The new guidelines (Shepherd 1995) rectify this and state that the lesion should not exceed 7 mm in diameter. They have, however, also modified the depth of lesions that should be included in stage IA1 to a maximum depth of 3 mm. Thus some lesions previously in stage IA2 are now to be regarded as stage IA1. The guidelines, however, are not clear on this point, leaving it rather vague as to whether a lesion exactly 3 mm deep should be stage IA1 or IA2. Until there is advice to the contrary, it is suggested that those lesions which are up to and including 3 mm deep should be regarded as stage IA1.

In the 1988 staging announcement, a stage IA2 measurable lesion was not to exceed 5 mm in depth, measured from the base of the epithelium, either surface or glandular, from which it originated, and the horizontal spread was to be no greater than 7 mm. All carcinomas larger than this but still limited to the cervix were to be classified as stage IB whether clinically apparent or not.

In the 1995 announcement, only those lesions greater than 3 mm but less than 5 mm in depth and no more than 7 mm in width are included in stage IA2. Any lesion larger than this, but which is still limited to the cervix, automatically becomes stage IB. This means that those tumours previously classified as stage IB will continue to be described as stage IB as will all clinically visible lesions but even very superficially invasive lesions that exceed 7 mm in diameter will now be classified as stage IB. Some lesions previously described as stage IA, and even stage IA1, will now, therefore, be classified as stage IB and almost certainly treated by radical surgery. This may have serious implications where the patient is young and wishes to preserve her fertility. Stage IB is now subdivided into stage IB1 and stage IB2, respectively, for lesions measuring less than 4 cm in size and more than 4 cm in size.

Whereas in FIGO 1988 we were advised to record, but ignore for staging purposes, all lymphatic and blood vascular permeation in the immediate vicinity of stage IB carcinomas, we are now advised in FIGO 1995 to record this in respect of both stage IA and IB carcinomas so that the significance of this finding can be determined. Not all gynaecological oncologists, however, feel comfortable with ignoring lympho-vascular permeation in their management protocols (Johnson et al 1992).

FIGO is not the only organisation to provide guidelines for the recognition and diagnosis of microinvasive carcinoma of the cervix and there are alternative definitions. The Society of Gynecologic Oncologists (SGO) has a more restrictive view of stage IA carcinoma of the cervix. It defines it as being no more than 3 mm in depth from the base of the epithelium from which invasion occurs and with no histological evidence of vascular permeation. On the other hand, it ignores the width of the lesion (Seski et al 1977). This may be an important omission as there is evidence that the chances of vascular/lymphatic permeation are directly related to the width of the lesion (Copeland et al 1992, Girardi et al 1994). Burghardt (1984) drew attention to the fact that the FIGO and SGO criteria defining microinvasion will not entirely exclude the possibility of metastases and recommended that definitions of microinvasive carcinoma should consider tumour volume, vascular permeation and, although it has yet to be established in a large prospective study, the expression of growth factors. Perhaps the FIGO and SGO guidelines should not be used alone in determining the management of microinvasive carcinoma of the cervix (Burghardt et al 1991).

Unfortunately, the recent FIGO announcement has not taken the opportunity to address the difficulties inherent in any method that measures a three dimensional lesion in only two dimensions. It has ignored the possible implications of tumour differentiation and histological category and ignored advances in our understanding of the molecular biology of the lesions. It could be argued that any system which bases treatment only on the depth of invasion, such as that described by SGO, is potentially dangerous but equally any system which fails to address the biological activity of the neoplasm also has its failings.

The risk of metastatic and recurrent disease

It is difficult to compare published results and to obtain an objective view of the risk of metastasis from microinvasive carcinoma. First, treatment is variable and ranges from cone biopsy to radical hysterectomy with nodal dissection and radiotherapy. Second, the definition of microinvasive carcinoma is not standard and it is clear that the terms early carcinoma, superficial carcinoma, microinvasive carcinoma etc have been used interchangeably but cannot be taken as being synonymous. These terms cover a range of lesions which are generally agreed to be microinvasive (stage IA) whilst others would be regarded as stage IB tumours. Third, in some series, women with incomplete excision of the lesion are included. A comparison of various reports must therefore be interpreted with caution.

Ideally, the definition of microinvasive carcinoma should exclude all cases in which there is a risk of metastatic or recurrent disease. This is, in our present state of knowledge, almost impossible and we should examine the risk to women of treating microinvasive lesions relatively conservatively. The SGO definition of microinvasion is meant to be a guideline to therapy whereas the FIGO guidelines are meant only to allow a comparison between the behaviour of tumours staged according to their guidelines. In fact, FIGO stage frequently forms the basis of management decisions. This being so, its reliability should be examined.

The withdrawal of the 1988 definition of stage IA1 (early stromal invasion) is to be regretted, because though objective criteria for its diagnosis were lacking, and the lesion was perhaps 'limited' rather than 'early', none the less the majority of pathologists and clinicians were happy with the concept and were able to base treatment protocols on it. It was almost universally agreed that, provided the stage IA1 cancer and any associated intraepithelial neoplasm had been completely excised, the patient could be treated conservatively by cone biopsy or loop excision, or, if there were clinical indications, by simple hysterectomy. The reason for such confidence in the diagnosis lies in the fact that metastatic disease is extremely rare (Burghardt et al 1991) though not entirely unknown (Collins et al 1989). The new stage IA1 includes some lesions that will metastasise (Tsukamoto et al 1989, Girardi et al 1994) and the new stage IA2 category will continue to contain a small number of lesions which have metastasised as it always did (Monaghan 1988, Tsukamoto et al 1989, Copeland et al 1992, Sevin et al 1992), and as we know from our own experience (unpublished data).

The overall risk of metastatic disease for invasive lesions no deeper than 0.5 mm is between 1–2% (Averette et al 1976, Ito et al 1986, Monaghan 1988, Tsukamoto et al 1989, Ueki et al 1994). All such lesions come within the present classification of stage IA. Johnson et al (1992) also claim that conservative treatment of microinvasive lesions less than 3 mm deep, in the absence of vascular/lymphatic permeation, is safe. They point out, however, that there is a 2% risk of death in selecting this course of action.

In one study, 14 cases which would now be defined as stage IA1, in that they invaded to a depth of between 0.5–2.8 mm (the diameter of the lesions was not given), were treated by cone biopsy successfully (Morris et al 1993). In these cases there was no evidence of lymphatic or vascular permeation and the excision margins were free from disease. These findings confirmed two larger series (van Nagell et al 1983, Tsukamoto et al 1989). Whilst over a period of time ranging from 1 to 170 months none of Morris's cases developed recurrent invasive neoplasia, two of the cases of described by Copeland et al (1992) progressed to invasive carcinoma, which represents 2.4%.

Sevin et al (1992) examined the risk of nodal metastases in 110 patients who fulfilled the 1988 FIGO criteria for stage IA2 (42 cases), the SGO criteria for microinvasive carcinoma (54 cases) or both the FIGO and SGO criteria (27 cases). There were no nodal metastases or recurrences of tumour in any of these patients, all of whom had been treated by radical hysterectomy and pelvic-aortic node dissection. A review of the literature suggests, however, that the recurrence rate for women with stage IA2 tumours is 4.2% (Sevin et al 1992). As a consequence, these authors recommended that the SGO criteria for microinvasive carcinoma be adopted for management purposes rather than those outlined by FIGO (Shepherd 1989).

Copeland et al (1992) retrospectively studied 59 cases of microinvasive carcinoma that fulfiled the FIGO (1995) guidelines for stage IA2 and found lymph node metastases in only one patient who had a tumour measuring 4.5 mm in depth and 5 mm in width. This represented an incidence of 1%. Other authors have reported that the risk of nodal metastases is 8% for tumours between 3–5 mm in depth (Simon et al 1986).

Burghardt et al (1991) evaluated 486 patients with stage IA (FIGO 1988) disease of which 344 were stage IA1 and 101 stage IA2. All the cases were followed for 5 years or longer. During that time, one patient who had previously had stage IA1 disease, re-presented with stage IIB carcinoma. As a consequence of their experience they disputed the FIGO recommendations and stated that whilst treatment of stage IA1 disease (early stromal invasion) can be conservative, treatment of stage IA2 disease needs to be individualised.

Recognition of microinvasive carcinoma and problems with histopathological interpretation

The 1995 FIGO guidelines are not going to be of help to the histopathologist in diagnosing microinvasive carcinoma or in interpreting the histological appearances, yet all management is based ultimately on the opinion of the histopathologist. There are no caveats about measuring ulcerated carcinomas and no advice on what to do when the epithelium from which the carcinoma has arisen cannot be identified, as is often the case. No help has been offered in making the decision as to whether a lesion is actually invasive or the appearances are the result of cross cutting. The description of a gross lesion also needs clarification. Does it mean a palpable lesion, a lesion visible to the colposcopist or a lesion visible to the histopathologist examining the dissected specimen?

It is welcome that the recording of vascular/lymphatic permeation is to be extended to stage IA carcinomas and retained for stage IB lesions. Although various reports have given different results in respect to the significance of this finding, we shall not be able to understand its full significance until the data are complete.

A practical difficulty remains, however, in that the histopathologist is given no guidance on where measurements should be made. Does the width include all foci of invasion including those at the margin of the lesion which are only 'early stromal invasion' or only suspicious of invasion, or does it include only the confluent measurable area? A defined method of measuring width in melanoma has been established and this could have been applied to cervical tumours.

There is no advice on cutting the cone biopsy so that the histopathologists can be sure that they have seen the maximum width of the lesion. This can be very difficult to identify if the cone has been cut radially, yet there is no recommendation that the cone should be received intact and cut in parallel slices (Anderson 1986).

Should multifocal disease be treated differently? Some authors (Hopkins & Morley 1994) suggest that radical therapy may be indicated in such cases. If that is so, how should one define multifocal disease? Should we count as multifocal all cases where there is more than one tongue of invasive tissue or is it necessary for the invasive foci to be separated by normal tissue?

In our experience, a growing problem is the increasing number of adenocarcinomas of the cervix that are encountered. If the criteria for the recognition for microinvasive squamous cell carcinoma leave something to be desired then the criteria for microinvasive adenocarcinoma are non-existent. Moreover, the problems of interpretation are harder than they are for squamous carcinoma and the distinction between adenocarcinoma in situ (CGIN) and well-differentiated adenocarcinoma may be impossible to make. If we are still in a quandary over the recognition of microinvasive adenocarcinoma and its distinction from CGIN, how much greater is the problem in distinguishing extensive CGIN from stage IB carcinoma.

Management of microinvasive carcinoma

There seems to be some agreement that lesions encompassed by the term early stromal invasion can be treated by local therapy (Burghardt et al 1991, Girardi et al 1994).

Some stage IA1 lesions (Shepherd 1995) may be treated by local means provided that the patient has been counselled about the risk of metastatic disease and the treatment will need to be individualised. SGO stage IA may not exclude cases with metastatic disease but deaths have been reported in women fulfilling these criteria even when treated by simple or radical hysterectomy (Taki et al 1979, Yajima & Noda 1979). Two cases described by Sevin et al (1992) in which there were metastases were regarded as microinvasive but would now be described as stage IB as their width exceeded 7 mm. Women with stage IA2 disease will need to be managed individually (Girardi et al 1994) and many authors think that these cases should always be treated radically (Copeland et al 1992).

Key points for clinical practice

1. Until the prognostic implications of the new staging guidelines are fully evaluated, it may be appropriate for the histopathologist to continue to identify those cases of stage IA1 carcinoma (FIGO 1995) which would have been previously described as 'early stromal invasion' (FIGO 1988).

2. The new stages should be introduced into reporting practice. It may be useful, however, to maintain a parallel register of the old and new categories in order to compare the pathological findings and to compare the outcomes. Only in this way will we see the practical effects of the changes.

3. Closed cone biopsies should be cut in parallel blocks according to the guidelines described by Anderson (1986) and only when a cone is received already opened should radial sampling be undertaken.

4. Those invasive lesions which are ulcerated and cannot, therefore, be accurately measured should continue to be excluded from the category of microinvasive carcinoma. Their management will remain a problem and almost certainly be decided on an individual basis.

5. The diameter of a microinvasive carcinoma should include the tongues of 'early stromal invasion' at its margins.

6. The greatest width of a lesion may lie across several blocks and may not be represented in the section containing the largest piece of tumour.

7. The presence or absence of vascular/lymphatic permeation should be recorded in all cases of microinvasive carcinoma as it may accompany 'early stromal invasion' as well as small confluent lesions.

8. The differentiation and type of microinvasive carcinoma should be accurately determined by carrying out PAS/Alcian Blue stains.

9. The time has come to examine microinvasive tumours for the presence of growth factors and oncogene over-expression if high risk lesions are to be distinguished from low risk ones.

NEW CONCEPTS OF ENDOMETRIOSIS

Endometriosis appears to be a reasonably straightforward disease and, certainly in histopathological terms, this is to a considerable extent true. Nevertheless, views on and concepts about this condition have undergone significant changes during the last decade. The basic histopathology of endometriosis and the diagnostic problems which the disease may present have been discussed in detail (Clement 1990, Czernobilsky 1995) and this brief review will address only selected aspects of this disease.

It is becoming progressively clear that under the general title of endometriosis there are three separate entities:

- pelvic peritoneal endometriosis

- endometriotic cysts of the ovary

- endometriotic nodules of the rectovaginal septum

Pelvic peritoneal endometriosis

Pathogenesis and incidence

Pelvic endometriosis probably can develop as a result of metaplasia in peritoneal tissues (Fujii 1991, Nakamura et al 1993, Nakayama et al 1994, Lauchlan 1994) but, nevertheless, there is now widespread acceptance that pelvic peritoneal endometriosis is usually due to retrograde menstruation with regurgitation of viable endometrial tissue onto the pelvic peritoneum (Haney 1991). Retrograde menstruation is a virtually universal phenomenon (Halme et al 1984) and viable endometrial cells are present in the peritoneal fluid of more than 70% of women (Kruitwagen et al 1991). The question is therefore why endometriosis does not develop in all women and the answer is that it probably does at some time during their reproductive lives (Evers 1994). It is currently believed that the early superficial non-invasive lesions of pelvic endometriosis are unstable and that whilst a minority progress to an invasive lesion, most will spontaneously regress. Repeated laparoscopies have indeed confirmed that early endometriotic lesions appear and disappear with a constantly changing pattern (Wiegerinck et al 1993).

The reported incidence of detectable pelvic endometriosis is as high as 20% in asymptomatic, normal women (Moen & Muus 1991, Vercellini & Crosignani 1993) but this simply describes the incidence of endometriotic lesions in a given population at any one time. A few months later the same incidence would be found in the same population but the lesions would mostly be in other women. Furthermore, reported incidences of pelvic endometriosis are based upon the frequency with which lesions are visible at laparoscopic examination, but biopsies of macroscopically normal pelvic peritoneum have shown detectable microscopic endometriosis in 13–25% of women (Murphy et al 1986, Nisolle et al 1990). Therefore, minimal pelvic endometriosis is not, in the true sense of the word, a disease but rather an event that occurs intermittently in most, and probably all, women (Koninckx 1994).

Development of endometriotic lesions

There is abundant evidence that the cells shed from menstrual endometrium can be fully viable (Wardle & Hull 1993). For such cells to attach to the pelvic peritoneum and establish an endometriotic focus, they must adhere to the peritoneal tissue, break down the local extracellular matrix, and migrate into the tissue. Regurgitated endometrial cells obtained from the peritoneal fluid express integrins and E-cadhedrin, though there may be a temporary loss of these cell adhesion molecules during the actual process of regurgitation (Van der Linden et al 1994). These molecules are also expressed in endometriotic tissue (Bridges et al 1994) and clearly play an important role in the attachment of shed endometrial tissue to the peritoneum. Early endometriotic lesions invade the peritoneal extracellular matrix and products of local proteolysis and tissue recycling, such as the amino-terminal propeptide of type III collagen, accumulate in the peritoneal fluid of women with early active lesions (Spuijbroek et al 1992).

Subsequent development of the endometrial implant depends upon its ability to establish a blood supply. Angiogenic factors are present at a higher concentration in the peritoneal fluid of women with endometriosis than in the fluid of women without (Oosterlynck et al 1993). Epidermal growth factor (EGF) has emerged as the strongest candidate for the principal angiogenic and growth factor in early endometriosis. EGF is produced in endometriotic tissue (Haining et al 1991); EGF receptors are present in such tissue (Prentice et al 1992); and EGF significantly stimulates protein synthesis in endometriotic stromal cells (Mellor & Thomas 1994). It is unlikely, however, that EGF is the only factor involved in the initial growth of the endometriotic implant. The roles of other factors, such as transforming growth factors α and β, interleukin-6, interleukin-8, colony-stimulating factor and fibroblast growth factors have not yet been fully defined (Smith 1991, Oosterlynck et al 1994, Rier et al 1995, Ryan et al 1995).

Regression and progression of endometriotic lesions

The natural history of pelvic endometriotic lesions is for them to regress. The peritoneal response against the implants is directed towards their destruction and removal by peritoneal macrophages undoubtedly plays an important part in this. Persistence and progression of endometriotic foci may therefore be taken as a failure of pelvic cleansing mechanisms. Genetic factors play a role in this failure — a familial tendency to develop endometriosis has been firmly established (Simpson et al 1980, Lamb et al 1986, Moen & Magnus 1993, Moen 1995) and there is high concordance of the disease in monozygotic twins (Moen 1994). This has prompted the suggestion that there may be a gene specifically coding for a predisposition to endometriosis which is heterozygous in women with mild endometriosis and homozygous in women with severe disease (Gleicher 1995).

The failure to prevent progression of endometriotic foci, whether genetically based or not, is almost certainly due either to an inadequate immunological response to the ectopic tissue or to an excessive degree of regurgitation of endometrial tissue, to an extent that it overwhelms the peritoneal defence mechanisms. In terms of an inadequate immunological reaction, emphasis has been placed on a diminished macrophage response (Dmowski et al 1991, Evers 1993) and on decreased natural killer (NK) cell mediated cytotoxicity as key factors in the progression of endometriotic lesions (Oosterlynck et al 1991, Hill 1992, Oosterlynck et al 1992, Garzetti et al 1993). It is of note that NK cell activity is normal in women with non-progressive lesions and diminished only in women with progressive disease (Brosens 1994). Circumstances in which excessive endometrial regurgitation occurs include a deficient uterotubal control mechanism (Bartosik et al 1986), a narrow cervical os (Barbieri et al 1992) and congenital abnormalities of the uterus in which there is an outflow obstruction (Olive & Henderson 1987, Fedele et al 1992).

Pelvic peritoneal endometriosis in relation to a patient's diminished capacity for reproduction

It has long been held, virtually as a dogma, that endometriosis, even of a minor degree, is associated with an increased incidence of infertility (Kistner 1979) and this belief has prompted a plethora of explanatory theories which include disorders of ovulation, abnormalities of peritoneal prostaglandin synthesis, stimulation of an autoimmune disorder and altered peritoneal macrophage activity (Halme & Surrey 1990). Thomas (1991) critically reviewed the evidence for an association between endometriosis and diminished fertility, however, and came to the iconoclastic, though scientifically impeccable, conclusion that in the absence of mechanical damage, endometriosis does not cause infertility and that treatment of endometriosis, unless it involves the lysis of adhesions, is of no benefit for future fertility.

Claims that endometriosis is associated with a high incidence of spontaneous abortion (Naples et al 1981, Olive et al 1982) have not been confirmed (Pittaway et al 1988, Regan et al 1989). Similarly, the belief that rates of successful pregnancy after in vitro fertilization are lower in women with endometriosis than in women without (Wardle et al 1985) have not withstood the test of time and greater experience (Oehninger & Rosenwaks 1990).

Ovarian endometriotic cysts

It has long been clear that there is a fundamental difference between pelvic peritoneal endometriosis and ovarian endometriotic cysts. The incidence of pelvic endometriosis declines with age whilst that of ovarian endometriotic cysts increases (Redwine 1987). It is distinctly uncommon for progressive pelvic disease to co-exist with ovarian cystic lesions (Koninckx & Martin 1992). Most important, many endometriotic cysts of the ovary do not fulfil the diagnostic criteria for endometriosis — they have a lining of epithelial cells of endometrioid type but lack an endometrial stromal component.

These observations have prompted the suggestion that many ovarian endometriotic cysts are, in reality, endometrioid cystadenomas (Czernobilsky 1982) and this hypothesis has recently received striking support from the demonstration that many, though not all, such cysts are monoclonal in nature (Nilbert et al 1995). If it is accepted that many endometriotic cysts are neoplastic, then an obvious lacuna in the scheme of ovarian tumours would be filled: there has never been any obvious reason why benign ovarian serous neoplasms should be so common whilst benign endometrioid tumours were apparently so rare.

Atypia is seen with modest frequency in the epithelial lining of ovarian endometriotic cysts (Czernobilsky & Morris 1979), this being characterized by nuclear pleomorphism and hyperchromasia, eosinophilic cytoplasm, tufting and stratification. Such changes are often thought to be reactive in nature but Ballouk et al (1994) found that the abnormal glandular epithelium had a diploid DNA content in cases of mild atypia, and found DNA aneuploidy in three of six cases of severe atypia. This is in accord with the neoplastic nature of ovarian endometriotic cysts and strongly suggests that cysts showing such atypia are the equivalent of mucinous and serous tumours of borderline malignancy.

Nodular rectovaginal endometriosis

Recently, it has been suggested that the nodular form of endometriosis which occurs in the rectovaginal septum is a separate and discrete entity (Brosens 1994, Donnez et al 1995). This view is based on the observation that smooth muscle appears to be an integral component of these lesions whilst endometrial stromal tissue is either scanty or absent. An incorrect analogy has therefore been drawn with myometrial adenomyosis and an unconvincing origin from Müllerian rests has been suggested. The true nature and origin of these nodules remains to be determined.

Endometriosis as a premalignant lesion

Malignant neoplasms can arise in extragonadal endometriosis. Endometrioid adenocarcinoma, clear cell carcinoma and endometrial stromal sarcoma can arise from endometriotic foci in sites such as the rectovaginal septum, vagina, large intestine, urinary bladder, omentum and pleura (Brooks & Wheeler, 1977, Czernobilsky 1995). Such tumours are, however, distinctly rare and it is a further indication of the basic difference between the pelvic and ovarian forms of the disease that malignant neoplasms occur with a very much greater frequency in ovarian than in extra-ovarian endometriosis (Scully et al 1966, Mostoufizadeh & Scully 1980, Heaps et al 1990). It has, however, proved difficult to quantify the contribution of endometriosis to ovarian neo-plasia, largely because of an over-reliance on the criteria laid down by Sampson (1925) for the recognition that adenocarcinoma has arisen in endometriosis. These require the observation of a direct transition from benign endometriotic epithelium to malignant tissue. This criterion is clearly unduly stringent as a rapidly growing adenocarcinoma may easily obliterate evidence of a preceding endometriotic focus.

Russell & Bannatyne (1989) considered that between 5–10% of endometrioid adenocarcinomas of the ovary arise from endometriotic foci, with endometriosis being present elsewhere in the same ovary in a further 5–10% of such neoplasms. Vercellini et al (1993) found that, amongst 556 patients undergoing surgery for ovarian cancer, there was a low incidence of associated endometriosis in those patients who had serous or mucinous neo-plasms but an incidence of 21–26% in those with endometrioid or clear cell adenocarcinoma.

Toki et al (1996) used a combined scoring system, consisting of both clin-ical and histological findings, to assess the association between endometriosis and ovarian adenocarcinoma in 235 patients. Overall, 21.3% of all carcino-mas were associated with endometriosis: again, the co-existence of the two lesions was low in cases of serous and mucinous tumours but was 30% in endometrioid adenocarcinomas and 50% in clear cell carcinomas. The carci-nomas associated with endometriosis occurred at an earlier age and were at an earlier clinical stage at presentation than those in which there was no asso-ciated endometriosis.

From this it is apparent that there is a significant association between endometriosis and ovarian adenocarcinoma. It could be argued that this sim-ply demonstrates an undue tendency towards instability of the peritoneum in some women but a more likely reason for this association is that more ovar-ian adenocarcinomas than previously realised arise in foci of endometriosis.

REFERENCES

Anderson M C 1986 Premalignant and malignant disease of the cervix. In: Fox H (ed) Haines and Taylor: Obstetrical and gynaecological pathology. 3rd edn. Churchill Livingstone, Edinburgh. p 282
Averette H E, Nelson J H Jr, Ng A B et al 1976 Diagnosis and management of microinvasive (stage IA) carcinoma of the uterine cervix. Cancer 38: 414–425
Baker T R, Piver M S 1994 Etiology, biology, and epidemiology of ovarian cancer. Seminars in Surg Oncol 10: 242–248
Ballouk F, Ross J S, Wolf B C 1994 Ovarian endometriotic cysts: an analysis of cytologic atypia and DNA ploidy patterns. Am J Clin Pathol 102: 415–419

Barbieri R L, Callery M, Perez S E 1992 Directionality of menstrual flow: cervical os diameters: a determinant of retrograde menstruation. Fertil Steril 57: 727–730

Bartosik D, Jacobs S L, Kelly L J 1986 Endometrial tissue in peritoneal fluid. Fertil Steril 46: 796–800

Bitran J, Pellettiere E W 1974 Multiple sebaceous gland tumors and internal carcinoma: Torre's syndrome. Cancer 33: 835–836

Black D 1994 Familial breast cancer. BRCA1 down, BRCA2 to go. Curr Biol 4:1023–1024

Bridges J E, Prentice A, Roche Wet al 1994 Expression of integrin adhesion molecules in endometrium and endometriosis. Br J Obstet Gynaecol 101; 696–700

Brooks J J, Wheeler J E 1977 Malignancy arising in extragonadal endometriosis: a case report and summary of the world literature. Cancer 40: 3065–3073

Brosens I A 1994 Is mild endometriosis a progressive disease? Hum Reprod 9: 2209–2211

Buller R E, Anderson B, Connor J P et al 1993 Familial ovarian cancer. Gynecol Oncol 51: 160–166

Burghardt E 1984 Microinvasive carcinoma in gynecological pathology. Clin Obstet Gynaecol 11: 239–257

Burghardt E, Girardi F, Lahousen M et al 1991 Microinvasive carcinoma of the uterine cervix (International Federation of Gynecology and Obstetrics Stage IA). Cancer 67: 1037–1045

Cantu J M, Rivera H, Ocampo- Campos R et al 1980 Peutz-Jeghers syndrome with feminizing Sertoli cell tumor. Cancer 46: 223–228

Carlson G J, Nivatvongs S, Snover D C 1984 Colorectal polyps in Cowden's disease (multiple hamartoma syndrome). Am J Surg Pathol 8: 763 770

Chen K T K, Schooley J L, Flam M S 1985 Peritoneal carcinomatosis after prophylactic oophorectomy in familial ovarian cancer syndrome. Obstet Gynecol 66: 93S–94S

Christian C D 1971 Ovarian tumors: an extension of the Peutz–Jeghers syndrome. Am J Obstet Gynecol 15: 529–534

Clement P B 1990 Pathology of endometriosis. In: Rosen PR, Fechner RE (eds) Pathology annual, part 1, vol 25. Appleton & Lange, Norwalk, pp 245–295.

Collins H S, Burke T W, Woodward J E et al 1989 Widespread lymph node metastases in a patient with microinvasive cervical carcinoma. Gynecol Oncol 34: 219–221

Copeland L J, Silva E G, Gershenson D M et al 1992 Superficially invasive squamous cell carcinoma of the cervix. Gynecol Oncol 45: 307–312

Czernobilsky B 1982 Endometrioid neoplasia of the ovary: a reappraisal. Int J Gynecol Pathol 203–210

Czernobilsky B 1995 Endometriosis. In: Fox H (ed) Haines and Taylor: Obstetrical and gynaecological pathology 4th Edition. Churchill Livingstone, Edinburgh, pp 1043–1062.

Czernobilsky B, Morris W J 1979 A histologic study of ovarian endometriosis with emphasis on hyperplastic and atypical changes. Obstet Gynecol 53: 318–323.

de Meeus J B, Bennouna C, Marechaud M et al 1993 Cancer familial de l'ovaire. A propos d'une famille regroupant 6 cas index. J Gynecol Obstet Biol Reprod 22: 749–756

Dmowski W P, Braun D, Gebel H 1991 The immune system in endometriosis. In: Thomas EJ, Rock JA (eds) Modern approaches to endometriosis. Kluwer, Dordrecht. pp 97–111

Donnez J, Nisolle M, Casanas–Roux F et al 1995 Rectovaginal septum, endometriosis or adenomyosis: laparoscopic management in a series of 231 patients. Hum Reprod 10: 630–635

Evers J L H 1993 The immune system in endometriosis: introduction. In: Brosens IA, Donnez J (eds) The current status of endometriosis. Parthenon, Carnforth, pp 223–233

Evers J L H 1994 Endometriosis does not exist: all women have endometriosis. Hum Reprod 9: 2206–2211

Fedele L, Bianchi S, Di Nola G et al 1992 Endometriosis and non-obstructive Müllerian anomalies. Obstet Gynecol 79: 515–517

Feunteun J, Narod SA, Lynch HT et al 1993 A breast–ovarian cancer susceptibility gene map to chromosome 17q 21. Am J Hum Genet 52: 736–742

Flejter W L, Bennett-Baker P, Barcroft C L et al 1995 Region-specific cosmids and STRPs identified by chromosome microdissection and FISH. Genomics. 25:413–20

Foyle A, Al Jabi M, McCaughey W T E 1981 Papillary peritoneal tumors in women. Am J Surg Pathol 5:241–249

Franceschi S, Vecchia C, Mangioni C 1982 Familial ovarian cancer: eight more families. Gynecol Oncol 13: 31–36

Fraumeni J F, Grundy G W, Creagan E Tet al 1975 Six families prone to ovarian cancer.

Cancer 36: 364–369

Fujii S 1991 Secondary Müllerian system and endometriosis. Am J Obstet Gynecol 165: 219–225

Futreal P A, Liu Q, Shattuck-Eidens D et al 1994 BRCA1 mutations in primary breast and ovarian carcinomas. Science 266: 120–2

Garzetti G G, Ciavattini A, Provincial I M et al 1993 Natural killer cell activity in endometriosis: correlation between serum estradiol levels and cytotoxicity. Obstet Gynecol 81: 685–688

Gatti R A, Nieberg R, Boder E 1989 Uterine tumors in ataxia-telangiectasia. Gynecol Oncol 32: 257–260

Gibbs E K 1971 Suggested prophylaxis for ovarian cancer. Am J Obstet Gynecol 15: 756–765

Gilks C B, Young R H, Aguirre P et al 1989 Adenoma malignum (minimal deviation adenocarcinoma) of the uterine cervix. A clinicopathological and immunohistochemical analysis of 26 cases. Am J Surg Pathol 13: 717–729.

Girardi F, Burghardt E, Pickel H 1994 Small FIGO stage Ib cervical cancer. Gynecol Oncol 55: 427–432

Gitsch G, Tabery U, Feigl W et al 1992 The differential diagnosis of primary peritoneal papillary tumors. Arch Gynecol Obstet 251:139–44

Gleicher N 1995 Immune dysfunction — a potential target for treatment in endometriosis. Br J Obstet Gynaecol 102 (Suppl 12): 4–7.

Goldsmith C I, Hart W R 1975 Ataxia telangiectasia with ovarian gonadoblastoma and contralateral dysgerminoma. Cancer 36: 1838–1842

Gorlin R J, Sedano H O 1971 The multiple nevoid basal cell carcinoma syndrome revisited. Birth Defects 7: 140–148

Graham J B, Graham R M, Schueller E F 1962 Preclinical detection of ovarian cancer. Cancer 17: 1414–1419

Graham R, McKee P, McGibbon D et al 1985 Torre–Muir syndrome. An association with isolated sebaceous carcinoma.. Cancer 55: 2868–2873

Grattan C E H, Hamburger J 1987 Cowden's disease in two sisters, one showing partial expression. Clin Exp Dermatol 12: 360–363

Gusberg S, Deligdisch L 1984 Ovarian dysplasia: a study of identical twins. Cancer 54: 1–4

Haining R E, Cameron I T, van Papendorp C et al 1991 Epidermal growth factor in human endometrium: proliferative effects in culture and immunocytochemical localization in normal and endometriotic tissues. Hum Reprod 6: 1200–1205

Hakala T, Mecklin J P, Forss M et al 1991 Endometrial carcinoma in cancer family syndrome. Cancer 68: 1656–1659

Halme J, Surrey E S 1990 Endometriosis and infertility: the mechanisms involved. In: Chadha DR, Buttram VC (eds) Current concepts in endometriosis. Liss, New York. pp 157–178

Halme J, Hammond M G, Hulka J F et al 1984 Retrograde menstruation in healthy women and in patients with endometriosis. Obstet Gynecol 64: 151–154

Haney A F 1991 The pathogenesis and aetiology of endometriosis. In: Thomas EJ, Rock JA (eds) Modern approaches to endometriosis. Kluwer, Dordrecht. pp 3–19

Heaps J M, Nieberg R K, Berek J S 1990 Malignant neoplasms arising in endometriosis. Obstet Gynecol 75: 1023–1028

Heintz A P M, Hacker N F, Lagasse L D. Epidemiology and aetiology of ovarian cancer: a review. Obstet Gynecol 1985;66:127–135

Hill J A 1992 Immunology and endometriosis. Fertil Steril 58: 262– 264

Hopkins M P, Morley G W 1994 Microinvasive squamous cell carcinoma of the cervix. J Reprod Med 39; 671–673

Ismail S, Walker S M 1990 Bilateral virilizing sclerosing stromal tumours of the ovary in a pregnant woman with Gorlin's syndrome: implications for pathogenesis of ovarian stromal neoplasms. Histopathology 17: 159–163

Ito T, Yago H, Kuribayashi M, Ohsawa H 1986 Colposcopy in dysplasia, carcinoma in situ and microinvasive cancer of the cervix–systematic diagnosis. Nippon Sanka Fujinka Gakkai Zasshi 38: 168–176

Jacobs I, Oram D 1987 Prophylactic oophorectomy. Br J Hosp Med 38:440–449

Jacobs I, Oram D 1989 Prevention of ovarian cancer: a survey of the practice of prophylactic oophorectomy by fellows and members of the Royal College of Obstetricians and Gynaecologists. Br J Obstet Gynaecol 96: 510–515

Jensen R D, Norris H J, Fraumeni J F 1974 Familial arrhenoblastoma and thyroid adenoma.

Cancer 33: 218–223

Johnson N, Lilford R J, Jones S E et al 1992 Using decision analysis to calculate the optimum treatment for microinvasive cervical cancer. Br J Cancer 65: 717–722

Kannerstein M, Chung J, McCaughey W T E et al 1977 Papillary tumors of the peritoneum in women: mesothelioma or papillary carcinoma. Am J Obstet Gynecol 127: 306–314

Kistner R 1979 Management of endometriosis in the infertile patient In: Wallach EE, Kempers RD (eds) Modern trends in infertility and conception control. Williams & Wilkins, Baltimore. pp 35–40

Kolstad P 1989 Follow–up study of 232 patients with stage Ia1 and 411 patients with stage Ia2 squamous cell carcinoma of the cervix (microinvasive carcinoma). Gynecol Oncol 33: 265–272

Koninckx P R 1994 Is mild endometriosis a disease? Is mild endometriosis a condition occurring intermittently in all women? Hum Reprod 9: 2202–2211

Koninckx P R, Martin D 1992 Deep endometriosis: a consequence of infiltration or retraction or possible adenomyosis externa? Fertil Steril 58: 924–928

Kruitwagen R F P M, Poels L G, Willemsen W N P et al 1991 Endometrial epithelial cells in peritoneal fluid during the early follicular phase. Fertil Steril 55: 297–303

Lamb K, Hoffman R G, Nichols T R 1986 Family trait analysis: a case control study of 43 women with endometriosis and their best friends. Am J Obstet Gynecol 154: 596–601

Lauchlan S C 1994 The secondary Müllerian system revisited. Int J Gynecol Pathol 13: 73–79

Lewis A C W, Clare Davison B C 1969 Familial ovarian cancer. Lancet 1969;2:235–237

Li F P, Rapoport A H, Fraumeni J F et al 1970 Familial ovarian cancer. JAMA 214: 1559–1561

Liber A F 1950 Ovarian cancer in mother and five daughters. Arch Pathol 49: 280–290

Lowe DG 1992 Microinvasive carcinoma of the lower female genital tract. In: Lowe DG, Fox H (eds). Advances in gynaecological pathology. Churchill Livingstone, Edinburgh. pp 145–162

Lurain J R, Piver M S 1979 Familial ovarian cancer. Gynecol Oncol 8: 185–192

Lynch F W A 1936 A clinical review of 110 cases of ovarian carcinoma. Am J Obstet Gynecol 32: 753–61

Lynch H T, Harris R E, Guirgis H A et al 1978 Familial association of breast/ovarian cancer. Cancer 41: 1543–1549

Lynch H T, Albano W, Black L et al 1981 Familial excess of cancer of the ovary and other anatomic sites. JAMA 245: 261–264

Lynch H T, Bowtra C, Lynch J F 1986 Familial peritoneal ovarian carcinomatosis: a new clinical entity? Med Hypoth 21: 171–177

Lynch H T, Bowtra C, Wells I C et al 1987 Hereditary ovarian cancer: clinical and biomarker studies. In Piver M S (ed) Ovarian malignancies: diagnostic and therapeutic advances. Churchill Livingstone, Edinburgh. pp 81–108

Lynch H T, Smyrk T C, Lynch P M et al 1989 Adenocarcinoma of the small bowel in Lynch syndrome II. Cancer 64: 2178–2183

Lynch H T, Richard J D, Amin M et al 1991 Variable gastrointestinal and urologic cancers in Lynch syndrome II. Dis Colon Rectum 34: 891–5

Lynch H T, Cavalieri R J, Lynch J F et al 1992 Gynecologic cancer clues to Lynch syndrome II diagnosis: a family report. Gynecol Oncol 44:198–203

McCaughey W T E 1985 Papillary peritoneal neoplasms in females. Pathol Ann 20: 389–404

McCrann D J, Marchant D J, Bardawil W A 1974 Ovarian carcinoma in three teenage siblings. Obstet Gynecol 43: 132–137

Mellor S J, Thomas E J 1994 The actions of estradiol and epidermal growth factor in endometrial and endometriotic stroma in vitro. Fertil Steril 62: 507–513

Miki Y, Swensen J, Shattuck–Eidens D et al 1994 A strong candidate for the breast and ovarian cancer susceptibility gene BRCA1. Science 266: 66–71

Moen M H 1994 Endometriosis in monozygotic twins. Acta Obstet Gynecol Scand 73: 59–62

Moen M H 1995 Is mild endometriosis a disease? Why do women develop endometriosis and why is it diagnosed? Hum Reprod 10: 8– 12

Moen M H, Muus K M 1991 Endometriosis in pregnant and non–pregnant women at tubal sterilization. Hum Reprod 6: 699–702

Moen M H, Magnus P 1993 The familial risk of endometriosis. Acta Obstet Gynecol Scand 72: 560–564

Monaghan J M 1988 Management decision using clinical and operative staging in cervical cancer. Clin Obstet Gynaecol 2: 737–746

Morris M, Mitchell M F, Silva E G et al 1993 Cervical conization as a definitive therapy for early invasive squamous carcinoma of the cervix. Gynecol Oncol 51: 193–196

Mostoufizadeh M, Scully RE 1980 Malignant tumors arising in endometriosis. Clin Obstet Gynecol 23: 951–953

Murphy A A, Green W R, Bobbie D et al 1986 Unsuspected endometriosis documented by scanning electron microscopy in visually normal peritoneum. Fertil Steril 46: 522– 524

Nakamura M, Katabuchi H, Tohya T et al 1993 Scanning electron microscopic and immunohistochemical studies of pelvic endometriosis. Hum Reprod 8: 2218–2226

Nakayama K, Masuzawa H, Li S F et al 1994 Immunohistochemical analysis of the peritoneum adjacent to endometriotic lesions using antibodies for Ber–EP4 antigen, estrogen receptors, and progesterone receptors: implication of peritoneal metaplasia in the pathogenesis of endometriosis. Int J Gynecol Pathol 13:348– 358

Naples J D, Batt R E, Sadigh J 1981 Spontaneous abortion rate in patients with endometriosis. Obstet Gynecol 57: 509–512

Narita T, Takagi K 1984 Ataxia–telangiectasia with dysgerminoma of right ovary, papillary carcinoma of thyroid and adenocarcinoma of pancreas. Cancer 54: 1113–1116

Narod S A, Feunteun J, Lynch H T et al 1991 Familial breast–ovarian cancer locus on chromosome 17q 12–q23. Lancet 388: 82–83

Neumann S 1991 Cowden-Syndrom mit einem Ovariantumor (Multiple Hamartome Syndrom). Chirurg 62: 629–630

Nevo S 1978 Familial ovarian cancer: a problem in genetic counselling. Clin Genet 14: 219–222

Nilbert M, Pejovic T, Mandahl N et al 1995 Monoclonal origin of endometriotic cysts. Int J Gynecol Cancer 5: 61–63

Nisolle M, Paindaveine B, Bourdon A et al 1990 Histologic study of peritoneal endometriosis in infertile women. Fertil Steril 53: 984–988

O'Brien P K, Wilansky D L 1981 Familial thyroid nodulation and arrhenoblastoma. Am J Clin Pathol 75: 578–581

Oehninger S, Rosenwaks Z 1990 In vitro fertilization and embryo transfer: an established and successful therapy for endometriosis. In: Chadha DR, Buttram VC (eds) Current concepts in endometriosis. Liss, New York. pp 319–335.

Olive D L, Henderson D Y 1987 Endometriosis and Müllerian anomalies. Obstet Gynecol 69: 412–415

Olive D L, Franklin R R, Gratkins R V 1982 The association between endometriosis and spontaneous abortion. J Reprod Med 27: 333–338

Oosterlynck D J, Cornillie F J, Waer M et al 1991 Women with endometriosis show a defect in natural killer activity resulting in a decreased cytotoxicity to autologous endometrium. Fertil Steril 56: 45–51

Oosterlynck D J, Meuleman C, Waer M et al 1992 The natural killer activity of peritoneal fluid lymphocytes is decreased in women with endometriosis. Fertil Steril 58: 292– 295

Oosterlynck D J, Meuleman C, Sobis H et al 1993 Angiogenic activity of peritoneal fluid from women with endometriosis. Fertil Steril 59: 778–782

Oosterlynck D J, Meuleman C, Waer M et al 1994 Transforming growth factor–beta activity is increased in peritoneal fluid from women with endometriosis. Obstet Gynecol 83: 287–292

OPCS mortality statistics (1987) (England and Wales) HMSO London

Ostlere L S, Houlston R S, Laing J H et al 1993 Risk of cancer in relatives of patients with cutaneous melanoma. Int J Dermatology 32: 719–721

Patsner B, Mann W J, Chumas J 1989 Malignant mixed germ cell tumor of the ovary in a young woman with Smith-Lemli-Opitz syndrome. Gynecol Oncol 33: 386–388

Pecorelli S, Sartori E, Favalli G et al 1988 Ataxia-telangiectasia and endodermal sinus tumor of the ovary: report of a case. Gynecol Oncol 29: 240–244

Pittaway D E, Vernon C, Fayez J A 1988 Spontaneous abortion in women with endometriosis. Fertil Steril 50: 711–715

Piver M S. 1987 Epidemiology of ovarian cancer. In: Piver M S (ed) Ovarian malignancies: diagnostic and therapeutic advances. Churchill Livingstone, Edinburgh, pp 1–10

Piver M S, Mettlin C J, Tsukada Y et al 1984 Familial ovarian cancer registry. Obstet Gynecol 64: 195–199

Ponder B A J, Peto J, Easton D F 1992 Familial ovarian cancer. In: Sharp F, Mason WP, Creasman W (eds) Ovarian cancer 2: biology, diagnosis, and management. Chapman &

Hall, London pp 3–7

Prentice A, Thomas E J, Weddell A et al 1992 Epidermal growth factor receptor expression in normal endometrium and endometriosis: an immunohistochemical study: Br J Obstet Gynaecol 99: 395–398

Prior P, Waterhouse J A H 1981 Multiple primary cancers of the breast and ovary. Br J Cancer 44:628–636

Raggio M, Kaplan A L, Harberg J F 1983 Recurrent ovarian fibromas with basal cell nevus syndrome (Gorlin syndrome). Obstet Gynecol 61: 95s–96s

Redwine D B 1987 The distribution of endometriosis in the pelvis by age groups and fertility. Fertil Steril 47: 173–175

Regan R, Braude P R, Tembath P L 1989 Influence of past reproductive performance on risk of spontaneous abortion. Postgrad Med J 299: 541–545

Rier S E, Zarmakoupis P N, Hu X et al 1995 Dysregulation of interleukin–6 responses in ectopic endometrial stromal cells: correlation with decreased soluble receptor levels in peritoneal fluid of women with endometriosis. J Clin Endocrinol Metab 80: 1431–1437

Rulon D B, Helwig E B 1974 Cutaneous sebaceous neoplasms. Cancer 33: 82–102.

Russell P, Bannatyne P 1989 Surgical pathology of the ovaries. Churchill Livingstone, Edinburgh

Ryan I P, Tseng J F, Schriock E D et al 1995 Interleukin–8 concentrations are elevated in peritoneal fluid of women with endometriosis. Fertil Steril 63: 929–932

Sampson J A 1925 Endometrial carcinoma of the ovary, arising in endometrial tissue in that organ. Arch Surg 10: 1–72

Scully R E 1982 Sex cord stromal tumors. In: Blaustein A (ed) Pathology of the female genital tract, 2nd edn. Springer Verlag, New York, pp 598 – 599

Scully R E 1979 Tumours of the ovary and maldeveloped gonads. Armed Forces Institute of Pathology, Washington DC

Scully R E, Richardson G S, Barlow J F 1966 The development of malignancy in endometriosis. Clin Obstet Gynecol 9: 384–411

Seski J C, Murray R A, Morley G 1977 Microinvasive squamous carcinoma of the cervix: definition, histologic analysis, late results of treatment. Obstet Gynecol 50: 410–414

Sevin B U, Nadji M, Averette H E et al 1992 Microinvasive carcinoma of the cervix. Cancer 70: 2121–2128

Shattuck-Eidens D, McClure M, Simard J et al 1995 A collaborative survey of 80 mutations in the BRCA1 breast and ovarian cancer susceptibility gene. Implications for presymptomatic testing and screening. JAMA 273: 535–41

Shepherd J H 1989 Revised FIGO staging for gynaecological cancer. Br J Obstet Gynaecol 96: 889–892

Shepherd J H 1995 Staging announcement. FIGO staging of gynecologic cancers; cervical and vulva. Int J Gynecol Cancer 5: 319 [Erratum 1995 Int J Gynecol Cancer 5: 465]

Simon N L, Gore H, Shingleton H M et al 1986 Study of superficially invasive carcinoma of the cervix. Obstetrics and Gynecology 68: 19–24

Simpson J L, Elias S, Malinak L R, Buttram V C 1980 Heritable aspects of endometriosis. I. Genetic studies. Am J Obstet Gynecol 137: 327–331

Smith SA, Ponder B A 1993 Predisposing genes in breast and ovarian cancer: an overview. Tumori 79; 291–296

Smith SK 1991 The endometrium and endometriosis. In: Thomas EJ, Rock JA (eds) Modern approaches to endometriosis. Kluwer, Dordrecht pp 57–77

Sobol H, Mazoyer S, Smith S A et al 1993 Familial ovarian carcinoma: pedigree studies and preliminary results from linkage analysis. Bull Cancer (Paris) 80:121–34

Speert H 1949 Prophylaxis of ovarian cancer. Ann Surg 29: 468–475

Spigelman A D, Murday V, Phillips R K 1989 Cancer and the Peutz–Jeghers syndrome. Gut 30: 1588–1590

Spuijbroeck M D E H, Dunselman G A J, Menheere P P C A et al 1992 Early endometriosis invades the extracellular matrix. Fertil Steril 58: 929–933

Starink T M 1984 Cowden's disease: analysis of fourteen new cases. J Am Acad Dermatol 11: 1127–1141

Taki I, Sugimori H, Matsuyama T et al 1979 Treatment of microinvasive carcinoma. Obstet Gynecol Surv 34: 839–843

Thomas EJ 1991 Endometriosis and infertility. In: Thomas EJ, Rock JA (eds) Modern approaches to endometriosis. Kluwer, Dordrecht, pp 113–128

Thor L, Persson B H, Kjessler B 1976 Familial ovarian cancer. Uppsala J Med Sci 81: 189–191

Tobacman J K, Tucker M A, Kase R et al 1982 Intra abdominal carcinomatosis after prophylactic oophorectomy in ovarian cancer–prone families. Lancet 9: 795–797

Toki T, Fujii S, Silverberg S G 1996 A clinicopathologic study on the association of endometriosis and carcinoma of the ovary using a scoring system. Int J Gynecol Cancer 6: 68—73

Truong L D, Maccato M L, Awalt H et al 1990 Serous surface carcinoma of the peritoneum: a clinicopathologic study of 22 cases. Hum Pathol. 21:99–110

Tsao S W, Mok C H, Knapp R C et al 1993 Molecular genetic evidence of a unifocal origin for human serous ovarian carcinomas. Gynecol Oncol 48: 5–10

Tsukamoto N, Kaku T, Matsukuma K et al 1989 The problem of Stage Ia (FIGO, 1985) carcinoma of the uterine cervix. Gynecol Oncol 34: 1–6

Ueki M Okamoto Y, Misaki O et al 1994 Conservative therapy for microinvasive carcinoma of the uterine cervix. Gynecol Oncol 53: 109–113

van Nagell J R, Greenwell N, Powell D F et al 1983 Microinvasive carcinoma of the cervix. Am J Obstet Gynecol 145: 981–991

van der Linden P J Q, van der Linden E P M, de Goeij A F P M et al 1994 Expression of integrins and E–cadherin in cells from menstrual effluent, endometrium, peritoneal fluid, peritoneum and endometriosis. Fertil Steril 61: 85–90

Vercellini P, Crosignani P G 1993 Epidemiology of endometriosis. In: Brosens IA, Donnez J (eds) The current status of endometriosis: research and management. Parthenon, Carnforth, pp 111–130

Vercellini P, Parazzini F, Bolis C et al 1993 Endometriosis and ovarian cancer. Am J Obstet Gynecol 169: 181–182

Walton B J, Morain W D, Baughman R D et al 1986 Cowden's disease: a further indication for prophylactic mastectomy. Surgery 99: 82–86

Wardle P G, Hull M G R 1993 Is endometriosis a disease? Clin Obstet Gynaecol 7: 673–685

Wardle P G, Mitchell J D, McLaughlin E A et al 1985 Endometriosis and ovulatory disorder: reduced fertilization in vitro compared with tubal and unexplained fertility. Lancet 2: 236–239

Wharton L R. Two cases of supernumerary ovary and one of accessory ovary with an analysis of previously reported cases. Am J Obstet Gynecol 1959;78:1101–1118

Wiegerinck M Λ H M, van Dop P A, Brosens I A 1993 The staging of peritoneal endometriosis by the type of active lesion in addition to the revised American Fertility Society classification. Fertil Steril 60: 461–464

Yajima A, Noda K 1979 The results of treatment of microinvasive carcinoma (stage Ia) of the uterine cervix by means of simple and extended hysterectomy. Am J Obstet Gynecol 135: 685–688

Young R H, Welch W R, Dickersin G R et al 1982 Ovarian sex cord tumor with annular tubules: review of 74 cases including 27 with Peutz–Jeghers syndrome and 4 with adenoma malignum of the cervix. Cancer 50: 1384–1402

Young R H, Dickersin G R, Scully R E 1983 A distinctive ovarian sex cord–stromal tumor causing sexual precosity in the Peutz–Jeghers syndrome. Am J Surg Pathol 7: 233–243

7

Tumours of odontogenic epithelium

D. G. MacDonald   R. M. Browne

Tumours of odontogenic epithelium are infrequent, but can pose problems because of the number of different entities and the variability of their features.

Odontogenic epithelium is concerned with tooth formation which involves a complex series of interactions of epithelium and adjacent mesenchyme. The odontogenic epithelium is derived from the primitive ectoderm of the stomatodeum. The epithelium forms the enamel organ, from which enamel develops, but it is also involved in determining the shape of the tooth roots. On completion of tooth development, residues of odontogenic epithelium are found at any point where it has been previously active, but particularly in the periodontal ligament. There are no immunocytochemical techniques which specifically identify odontogenic epithelium. The enamel proteins, amelogenin and enamelin have been demonstrated in some tumours, but these reflect functional differentiation (Saku et al 1992). Specific gene expression may prove helpful in the future (Snead et al 1992).

CLASSIFICATION OF ODONTOGENIC TUMOURS

The sequence of inductive influences between odontogenic epithelium and ectomesenchyme is reflected in tumours and forms the basis of their classification. After the epithelium of the enamel organ has formed, dentine formation is initiated in the mesenchyme of the related dental papilla and then enamel formation starts. Some tumours involving odontogenic epithelium are undoubtedly neoplasms, but some are hamartomas. The classification and relative frequency of tumour types is shown in Table 7.1. The majority of tumours can be accommodated within this classification, but occasional tumours do not fit in readily. From a pragmatic standpoint, the great majority of tumours involving odontogenic epithelium are benign neoplasms or hamartomas. Malignant neoplasms almost always show clear cytological evidence of malignancy. The presence of calcified dental tissues is usually associated with less aggressive behaviour. There is overlap in the microscopic features of a number of lesions involving odontogenic epithelium and it is important that the detailed clinical presentation and radiographic features are taken account of in diagnosis.

Table 7.1. Relative frequency of tumours with odontogenic epithelium shown as a % of all odontogenic tumours (after Regezi et al 1978)

ameloblastoma	12
squamous odontogenic tumour	<1
calcifying epithelial odontogenic tumour	<1
clear cell odontogenic tumour	<<1
ameloblastic fibroma	2
ameloblastic fibrodentinoma, ameloblastic fibro-odontome	2
odontoameloblastoma	<<1
adenomatoid odontogenic tumour	3
calcifying odontogenic cyst	2
complex odontome	41
compound odontome	33
malignant odontogenic neoplasms	
all types	<<1

ODONTOGENIC EPITHELIAL RESTS

The debris of Malassez are the odontogenic epithelial rests found in periodontal ligament. They are small nests of histologically bland, stratified squamous epithelium. Following tooth extraction, these nests may be left within bone and require to be distinguished from neoplastic epithelium. Rarely, the epithelial rests have a clear cell appearance. Similar epithelial rests may also be seen in the gingiva. If these rests are more extensive and form small epithelial masses, sometimes with keratinisation, the diagnosis of gingival odontogenic epithelial hamartoma may be appropriate. This lesion requires to be differentiated from peripheral ameloblastoma and from odontogenic fibroma which is a fibrous proliferation within which strands of odontogenic epithelium are present.

Epithelial rests in dental follicles and opercula

With completion of enamel formation, the enamel organ decreases in size. In unerupted teeth, most commonly third molar and upper canine, an enlarged dental follicle is sometimes found. The reduced enamel epithelium is cuboidal or low columnar (Fig. 7.1a) and there are often quite extensive strands of inactive looking epithelium in a loose connective tissue (Fig. 7.1b). This epithelium is distinguished from ameloblastoma by the lack of peripheral pallisading and stellate reticulum-like appearance. A not infrequent error is for the enlarged dental follicle to be misdiagnosed as an ameloblastic fibroma (Kim & Ellis 1993). In the opercula related to partially erupted lower third molars, or the tissues overlying other unerupted teeth (Philipsen et al 1992b) a variety of appearances may be seen which simulate odontogenic tumours. The small size of these structures and their situation should allow the histopathologist to avoid misdiagnosis.

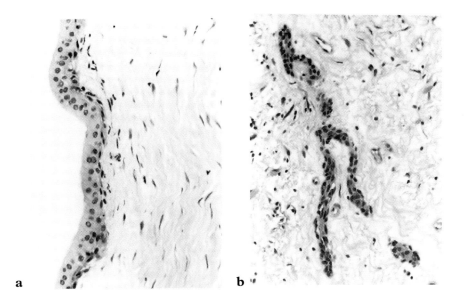

a   b

Fig. 7.1 (a) Reduced enamel epithelium in a follicle related to an unerupted tooth. H & E ×
200. **(b)** Strands of inactive odontogenic epithelium in the connective tissue of a dental follicle
related to an unerupted tooth. H & E × 200

AMELOBLASTOMA

Clinical and radiographic features

Ameloblastoma is the most frequent odontogenic neoplasm. A recent review
of published cases (Reichart et al 1995) confirms that the tumour occurs at
any age, but the peak incidence is in the fourth decade. Most tumours present as slow growing, painless swellings in the mandible. Ameloblastomas are
locally destructive tumours which have a deserved reputation for recurrence
and persistence if not adequately treated by surgical resection. Radiographically the lesions are usually multilocular, but some 6% appear unilocular. Some 2% of ameloblastomas are peripheral in location. Maxillary
ameloblastomas account for some 15%, occur at an older age and have a
poorer prognosis because of earlier spread to extra-bony soft tissues and adjacent structures (Nastri et al 1995).

Histopathology

Ameloblastomas are classified as epithelial neoplasms without inductive
effects on other dental tissues. The range of histological variation both within
and between tumours is much greater than is often suggested by standard
textbooks. Classically, two main histological patterns are recognised. The fol-

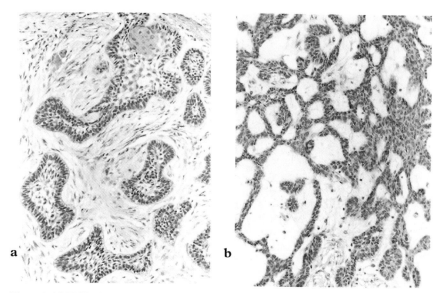

Fig. 7.2 (a) Follicular ameloblastoma. Note the peripheral palisaded layer of cells, often with the nuclei located towards the looser, stellate reticulum, areas. H & E × 120. **(b)** Plexiform ameloblastoma. Even the more extensive areas of epithelium may fail to show the typical features of peripheral palisading and stellate reticulum seen in follicular ameloblastoma. H & E × 120

licular pattern (Fig. 7.2a) comprises epithelial islands with peripheral palisaded cells and central looser areas resembling the stellate reticulum of the tooth germ. The plexiform pattern consists of strands and cords of epithelium of variable appearance. Where the epithelial aggregates are large, peripheral palisading and stellate reticulum areas may be found, but sometimes the dominant feature is strands of epithelium not showing obvious odontogenic features (Fig. 7.2b). Many ameloblastomas show a mixture of follicular and plexiform areas. Ueno et al (1989) have reported a higher incidence of recurrence following surgery in follicular ameloblastomas. Cytologically, ameloblastomas appear bland. Mitoses are infrequent and if many are seen, the possibility of malignant ameloblastoma should be considered.

Other histological variants of ameloblastoma have been described. Acanthomatous ameloblastomas show follicles with peripheral palisading which lack the separation of cells seen in stellate reticulum and exhibit squamous metaplasia, sometimes with well-formed keratin. Tumours with particularly marked keratinisation have been designated as keratoameloblastomas (Norval et al 1994). Altini et al (1991) described a further rare variant designated as a papilliferous keratoameloblastoma. Granular cells with prominent eosinophilic cytoplasm, which comprises numerous enlarged lysosomes, are a well documented feature of some ameloblastomas and occasionally are so dominant as to mask the typical features. A basaloid variant has also been identified (Kramer et al 1992).

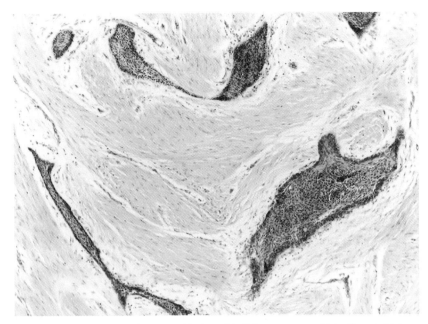

Fig. 7.3 Desmoplastic ameloblastoma with the epithelial component widely dispersed in a collagenous stroma. Some peripheral palisading is evident. The centres of the epithelial strands and nests show squamous metaplasia, an appearance that can be classified as an acanthomatous ameloblastoma. H & E × 75

There has been recent interest in the desmoplastic ameloblastoma, first described as a distinctive entity by Eversole et al (1984). In this tumour, the islands of follicular ameloblastoma are widely dispersed in a collagenous stroma of varying cellularity (Fig. 7.3). There may be associated reactive bone formation which can give rise to radiographic appearances resembling a fibro-osseous lesion (Philipsen et al 1992a, Kaffe et al 1993). The desmoplastic histology may be associated with other histological patterns or may be the only pattern. Desmoplastic ameloblastoma differs from conventional ameloblastoma in being more frequent in the anterior parts of the jaws and lacking the clear predilection for the mandible. It is not yet apparent whether the prognosis differs significantly from conventional ameloblastoma.

Clear cells have been described as a component of ameloblastomas (Waldron et al 1985, Muller & Slootweg 1986). These are similar to the clear cell odontogenic tumour, but occur in association with more typical areas of ameloblastoma which should allow the differential diagnosis to be made from other clear cell neoplasms. Waldron et al (1985) felt that the clear cells were associated with an aggressive tumour type, but there have been too few cases reported to substantiate this.

Unicystic ameloblastomas are an infrequent variant, but merit separate discussion because they present at a younger age and have a better prognosis. The site distribution is the same as for conventional ameloblastomas. The pre-operative diagnosis is usually of some other type of odontogenic cyst and the correct diagnosis is made only after histological examination. Ackermann et al (1988) distinguished three histological variants. The cyst may show ameloblastoma restricted to the epithelial lining, there may be intraluminal growth or there may be spread into the connective tissue capsule. In the last instance, it was recommended that the lesions be treated as for conventional ameloblastoma. In all three types, parts of the cyst lining may be stratified squamous epithelium, not identifiable as ameloblastoma. Gardner & Corio (1983, 1984) drew particular attention to plexiform unicystic ameloblastomas and the need to identify the intraluminal growth of nodules of plexiform tumour.

Peripheral ameloblastomas are confined to the soft tissues or produce only some saucerisation of underlying bone. El-Mofty et al (1991) and Nauta et al (1992) confirm earlier reports that peripheral ameloblastomas show the same histological features as intra-osseous ameloblastomas, but are less aggressive. Most peripheral ameloblastomas show continuity with the surface epithelium (Batsakis et al 1993).

Differential diagnosis

Apart from the wide range of features characteristic of ameloblastomas, these tumours may occasionally co-exist with other tumour types. This, and other aspects of variability in ameloblastomas have been emphasised by Raubenheimer et al (1995).

SQUAMOUS ODONTOGENIC TUMOUR

This rare tumour was described as a distinct entity by Pullon et al (1975).

Clinical features

Squamous odontogenic tumour presents as an osteolytic lesion adjacent to teeth. An extra-osseous case has been reported (Baden et al 1993). Clinical swelling is infrequent and attention may be drawn to the lesion because of loosening of the teeth or pain thought to be of dental origin. Most reported cases have been in young adults with equal numbers in upper and lower jaw. Sometimes multiple lesions occur and a familial tendency has also been noted (Leider et al 1989). The lesions, although not as aggressive as ameloblastomas, can be quite destructive and recurrence after surgery is recorded (Pullon et al 1975).

Histopathology

The tumour consists of islands and strands of histologically bland stratified squamous epithelium. This lacks a peripheral palisaded basal layer and shows no evidence of stellate reticulum appearance (Fig. 7.4). Within some

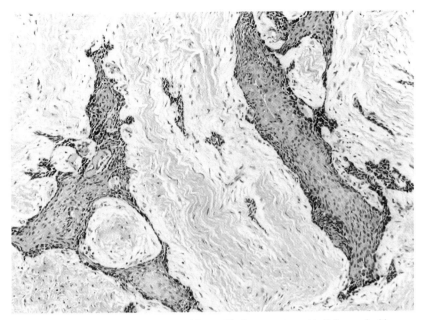

Fig. 7.4 Squamous odontogenic tumour with stratified squamous epithelial nests lacking any features of ameloblastoma. H & E × 110

epithelial nests vacuolation, apparent duct-like spaces and occasional small foci of keratin formation may be present. Dystrophic calcification is sometimes seen and crystalloid structures have been reported (Goldblatt et al 1982). The stroma is variably cellular, collagenous connective tissue lacking the features of ameloblastic fibroma.

Squamous odontogenic tumours are thought to arise principally from the debris of Malassez in the periodontal ligament. The study of cytokeratins reported by Tatemoto et al (1989) gives support to this concept.

Differential diagnosis

The main differential diagnoses are from ameloblastoma and primary intra-osseous carcinoma. The bland nature of the epithelium serves to distinguish it from a carcinoma and the lack of ameloblastoma features has already been noted. Some authors have described areas of epithelial proliferation resembling squamous odontogenic tumour in various cysts of dental origin, but it is now accepted that these should not be regarded as squamous odontogenic tumours.

CALCIFYING EPITHELIAL ODONTOGENIC TUMOUR

The eponymous name of Pindborg tumour has been applied to this benign neoplasm since the first description of the lesion as a separate entity by

Pindborg in 1955 and later in more detail (Pindborg 1958). The first substantial review was by Franklin & Pindborg (1976) and Pindborg et al (1991) have updated knowledge.

Clinical features

The clinical features are similar to ameloblastoma, occurring over a wide age range. One or more unerupted teeth have been associated with the tumour in about half of the reported cases and the tumours are almost always intra-osseous. Radiographically, the lesions are similar to ameloblastomas, but with variable amounts of calcification within the lesion.

Histopathology

Calcifying epithelial odontogenic tumours show great histological variabilty. The tumour cells are usually eosinophilic with well-defined cytoplasm and often show obvious intercellular bridges. They may form large sheets, appear as cribriform areas or as small separate nests. A striking feature is marked variation in cell size and nuclear pleomorphism (Fig. 7.5), sometimes with hyperchromatism and prominent nucleoli. Multinucleated tumour cells may be present. These features can give a distinct impression of malignancy, but an important point is that they are not associated with equivalent mitotic activity, mitotic figures being infrequent.

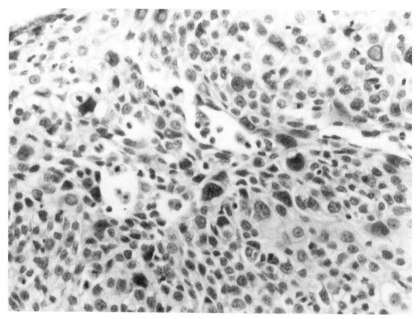

Fig. 7.5 Calcifying epithelial odontogenic tumour highlighting the degree of anisonucleosis and nuclear pleomorphism which can give rise to a false interpretation of malignancy. H & E × 360

Within the sheets of epithelial cells, eosinophilic homogeneous areas are found which stain positively for amyloid. Calcification occurs in these areas. In addition, calcified tissue resembling cementum (El-Labban 1990) and bone (Slootweg 1991) has also been reported. Cases lacking calcification are on record (Takata et al 1993) and calcification is usually not an obvious feature in the rare extra-osseous cases. A small number of clear cell variants of calcifying epithelial odontogenic tumour have been reported which may be associated with more typical appearances. The recurrence rate following surgery is higher in clear cell variants and perineural invasion is recorded (Hicks et al 1994). This is at variance with the concept of a benign neoplasm and there is a growing awareness that clear cells in any odontogenic neoplasm need to be viewed with suspicion.

Differential diagnosis

Calcifying epithelial odontogenic tumours present a real danger of wrong diagnosis for the unwary. The cytological features suggest malignancy and misdiagnosis as mucoepidermoid carcinoma or other salivary gland neoplasm is possible. The clear cell variant may also be mistaken for a range of primary and metastatic clear cell neoplasms.

CLEAR CELL ODONTOGENIC TUMOUR

This tumour type appears in the WHO classification (Kramer et al 1992) as a benign neoplasm, but it is now being recognised as a more sinister lesion. Hansen et al (1985) first described three cases which had originally been thought to be metastatic clear cell neoplasms. Although they thought that these tumours were benign, subsequent reports indicated that such neoplasms can be locally invasive and even metastasise. Current opinion is that the clear cell odontogenic tumour should be redesignated as a carcinoma (Bang et al 1989). Whether or not a benign variant exists remains to be determined.

Clinical features

Clear cell odontogenic tumours present as swellings which may be associated with loosening of teeth. Only a small number of cases has been documented (Sadeghi & Levin 1995). They appear more often in the mandible than the maxilla and more often in elderly patients. Radiographically, there is an ill defined radiolucency which may be multilocular. Metastases to adjacent lymph nodes have been reported in a third of cases and local recurrence in a similar proportion. Pulmonary metastasis has been reported, but this has been in cases with multiple recurrence and more than one episode of surgery. Whether or not these were true haematogenous metastases is still in doubt.

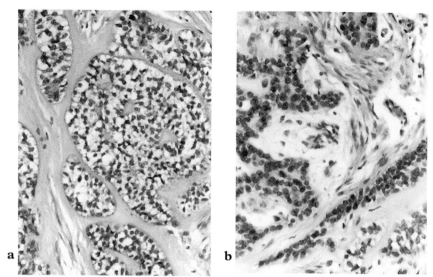

Fig. 7.6 (a) Clear cell odontogenic tumour. H & E × 130. **(b)** Area of basaloid cells in clear cell odontogenic tumour. H & E × 205

Histopathology

Most authors report tumours dominated by nests and cords of cells with vacuolated nuclei and clear or faintly eosinophilic cytoplasm (Fig. 7.6a). Only occasionally is peripheral palisading seen. There is no amyloid, calcification or mucus production. Glycogen may be demonstrated by PAS staining. A second population of epithelial cells may form part of the tumour. This comprises smaller cells with scant eosinophilic cytoplasm and a basaloid appearance (Fig. 7.6b) . Mitotic activity is usually reported as present, but not marked. The tumour infiltrates and destroys bone, and nerve-related spread is recorded (Piatelli et al 1994). Bang et al (1989) reported a case that had an associated cystic component.

Differential diagnosis

The differential diagnosis is from other clear cell tumours either metastatic or primary, particularly salivary gland tumours. Clear cell variants of ameloblastoma and calcifying epithelial odontogenic tumour are distinguished by the finding of areas characteristic of these lesions.

AMELOBLASTIC FIBROMA, AMELOBLASTIC FIBRO-DENTINOMA AND AMELOBLASTIC FIBRO-ODONTOMA

These form a rare group of tumours involving epithelial and mesenchymal growth, sometimes regarded as mixed odontogenic tumours (Hansen &

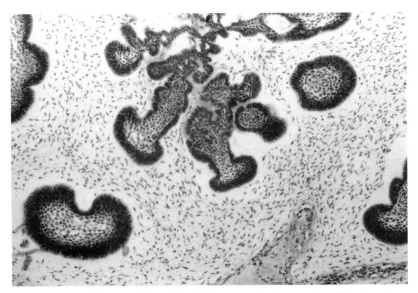

Fig. 7.7 Ameloblastic fibroma with typical cellular connective tissue and proliferation of odontogenic epithelium resembling ameloblastoma. H & E × 110

Ficarra 1988) Ameloblastic fibroma is a benign neoplasm, but the other two lesions may be hamartomas.

Clinical features

These tumours are usually diagnosed in the first two decades of life. They present as a painless swelling of the jaws, most often in the molar region of the mandible. Tumours occasionally arise in adjacent soft tissues. Radiographically, the lesions are typically well-circumscribed with varying radio-opacity and are often associated with unerupted teeth. Occasionally, growth may be rapid (Sawyer et al 1982).

Histopathology

All lesions contain sheets and strands of epithelium which are similar to those of ameloblastoma and are usually scattered uniformly throughout a loose, cellular fibrous stroma. Mitotic figures are uncommon. The fibrous tissue contains little obvious collagen although, around the epithelial islands, there are cell-free halos which may become hyalinised. Sometimes hyalinisation is widespread. Separation from the surrounding bone is abrupt and sometimes a distinct capsule is present.

In ameloblastic fibroma (Trodahl 1972, Zallen et al 1982), the epithelium forms strands only a few cells thick with some localised thickenings which resemble the follicular areas of ameloblastoma (Fig. 7.7). Occasionally, a

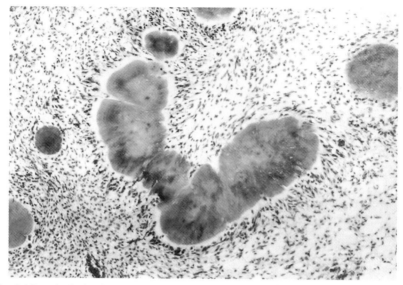

Fig. 7.8 Dysplastic dentine formation within the cellular ectomesenchymal component of an ameloblastic fibro-dentinoma. H & E × 110

variable number of fibroblasts show granular cytoplasm, the so-called granular cell ameloblastic fibroma. Sometimes there are myxomatous areas. The matrix, except the hyaline areas, stains intensely for collagen VI which might provide a marker for the tumour (Becker et al 1992).

In the ameloblastic fibro-dentinoma (van Wyk & van der Vyer 1983, Ulmansky et al 1994), the epithelial strands are usually only two or three cells thick, and foci of dentine formation are present (Fig. 7.8). The dentine is usually poorly formed with few tubules, the presence of orderly orthodentine being exceptional. There is often a clear surface layer of poorly staining non-mineralised matrix, but the interface with the adjacent odontoblast-like cells is irregular with some cells being trapped within the matrix. In more mature tumours, the epithelium is less conspicuous, the fibrous tissue less cellular and the mineralised matrix progressively abundant.

In ameloblastic fibro-odontoma (Miller et al 1976, Slootweg 1980), the overall composition of the lesion is similar to ameloblastic fibro-dentinoma, but the tissue inductive processes have progressed to the formation of enamel adjacent to the dentine matrix. The epithelium related to the enamel has the features of an enamel organ and there is resemblance to a developing tooth. Areas of structureless mineralisation may also be present.

Differential diagnosis

The ameloblastic fibroma does not usually present a difficult diagnosis. Multiple tissue sections may need to be examined to be certain that an apparent ameloblastic fibro-dentinoma is not a fibro-odontoma. Distinction from an odontome can be made by the presence of the ameloblastoma-like epithelium in association with the distinctive fibrous tissue.

ODONTOAMELOBLASTOMA

In this very rare tumour, which is most often reported in childhood, there is an odontoma-like mass in association with typical follicular or plexiform ameloblastoma (LaBriola et al 1980, Thompson et al 1990, Gunbay et al 1993) These tumours behave as ameloblastomas and require to be distinguished from other types of mixed odontogenic tumours.

ADENOMATOID ODONTOGENIC TUMOUR

Although recognised since 1948 (Stafne 1948), the adenomatoid odontogenic tumour was first fully documented by Philipsen & Birn (1969) and has since been comprehensively reviewed by Toida et al (1991) and by Philipsen et al (1991). There is debate about whether the tumour is a hamartoma (Kramer et al 1992) or a benign neoplasm, which probably arises most often from reduced enamel epithelium after completion of tooth crown formation.

Clinical features

Adenomatoid odontogenic tumour is a slow growing, expansile tumour which is usually symptomless and rarely more than 3 cm in diameter. Approximately three quarters of cases are associated with an unerupted tooth, most frequently the maxillary canine. Diagnosis often follows investigation of eruption failure of this tooth. The tumour is more frequent in the anterior parts of the jaws and is more common in maxilla than mandible. Extra-osseous location is rare. Two-thirds of tumours are diagnosed in the second decade of life and presentation beyond the third decade is unusual. Females are affected approximately twice as often as males.

Radiographically, the presentation is of a well defined radiolucency which, in about two-thirds of cases, shows speckled radio-opaque foci. When associated with an unerupted tooth, the lesion commonly appears as a dentigerous cyst. The roots of adjacent teeth may be displaced, but root resorption is unusual.

Histopathology

Microscopically, the tumour is a well-circumscribed mass which is variably cystic. Two cell populations are present in varying amounts. Sheets and strands of small-darkly-stained cells are mixed with larger paler cells in follicular groups (Fig. 7.9a) with the central cells orientated radially. Within these, tubular or duct-like structures are a typical feature (Fig. 7.9b). The cells lin-

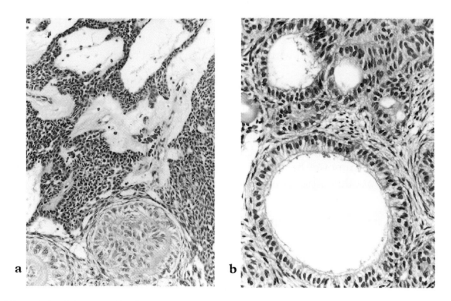

Fig. 7.9 (a) Adenomatoid odontogenic tumour clearly showing the two different patterns of epithelial differentiation. H & E × 140. **(b)** Typical duct-like areas in an adenomatoid odontogenic tumour. H & E × 220

ing these structures have oval, vesicular nuclei usually positioned away from the lumen, resembling pre-ameloblasts. The lumen is either empty or contains eosinophilic amorphous coagulum around the periphery which has been variously reported as keratin, vimentin and amelogenin positive. The small dark cells sometimes have a cribriform pattern, among which the stroma is tenuous and the blood vessels show degenerative changes (El-Labban & Lee 1988). Areas of mineralisation are often present, usually as small rounded acellular masses, but less frequently as dysplastic dentine or cementum-like matrix. Laminated bodies, sometimes with amyloid, may also be seen occasionally (El-Labban 1992). Melanin pigmentation has been reported (Takeda 1989).

When cystic, a variable part of the lining may be stratified squamous epithelium and study of multiple blocks may be required for correct diagnosis. Some adenomatoid odontogenic tumours show features of calcifying epithelial odontogenic tumour, suggesting a combined lesion (Damm et al 1983, Chanda et al 1987). The benign clinical behaviour is not altered in these circumstances.

Differential diagnosis

In most instances the diagnosis of adenomatoid odontogenic tumour is straightforward. The infrequent finding of features of other odontogenic tumour types in mixed or hybrid tumours needs to be remembered.

CALCIFYING ODONTOGENIC CYST

First described as an entity by Thoma & Goldman (1946), this tumour was designated as calcifying odontogenic cyst by Gorlin et al (1962). Comprehensive reviews have been published by Praetorius et al (1981), Buchner (1991) and Hong et al (1991). Besides the cystic form, a solid variant of similar histological structure exists which has been variably reported as calcifying ghost cell odontogenic tumour (Fejerskov & Krogh 1972) dentinogenic ghost cell tumour (Praetorius et al 1981) and epithelial odontogenic ghost cell tumour (Ellis & Shmookler 1986). It is not clear whether the solid form is a separate entity or one extreme of a range.

Clinical features

Approximately 90% of calcifying odontogenic cysts are intra-osseous with no predilection for either jaw. They cause painless swellings in any part of the tooth-bearing area, but most often in the maxillary incisor and canine regions. They occur over a wide age range, the peak incidence being in the second decade. Beyond the age of 50, the tumour is more likely in the mandible.

Radiographically, there is a well circumscribed radiolucency which is usually unilocular, but occasionally multilocular. Scattered radio-opacities are present in about 60% of cases and one third are associated with an odontome or unerupted tooth. Root resorption of adjacent teeth is not uncommon.

Approximately 10% of calcifying odontogenic cysts are extra-osseous. A painless mucosal swelling, approximately 1 cm in size, is the usual presentation. Saucerisation of the underlying bone may be evident radiographically (Buchner et al 1991).

Histopathology

There is a range of histological appearances from a cyst with a characteristic regular epithelial lining, through cysts with more proliferative epithelium, to a solid tumour mass. It is not established from which residues of odontogenic epithelium the tumour arises, but it is likely that it takes origin from more than one.

Microscopically, the presence of ghost cells is the key diagnostic feature, although they also occur infrequently in other tumours. Ghost cells (Fig. 7.10a) are large epithelial cells with granular eosinophilic cytoplasm and a non-staining area centrally representing the ghost image of the degenerated nucleus. Some cells react positively for amelogenins (Mori et al 1991) and enamelins (Saku et al 1992), but negatively for keratins (Kakudo et al 1989). Similar ghost cells are characteristic of pilomatrixoma (calcifying epithelioma of Malherbe). The ghost cells become increasingly numerous towards the luminal surface of the epithelium and may fuse together forming quite extensive sheets, or undergo dystrophic mineralisation.

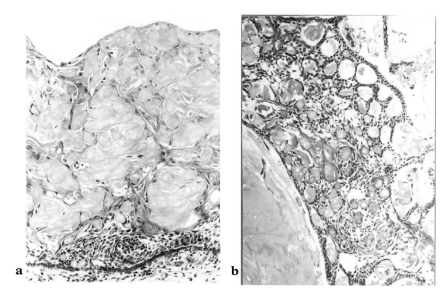

Fig. 7.10 (a) Cyst lining in a calcifying odontogenic cyst showing a thick layer of ghost cells overlying an area resembling ameloblastoma. H & E × 125. **(b)** Complex mixture of epithelial proliferation, ghost cells and dysplastic dentine in a dentinogenic ghost cell tumour (solid variant of calcifying odontogenic cyst). H & E × 125

The cyst linings are variable with some parts being unremarkable stratified squamous epithelium while other areas can resemble an ameloblastoma. Satellite cysts may be present (Takeda et al 1990). Melanin pigmentation is occasionally found. Areas of dystrophic mineralisation or poorly mineralised dentinoid, often closely apposed to the epithelial basement membrane, are more common in lesions with proliferative epithelium which have islands and sheets of epithelium within the fibrous tissue. The admixture of keratinous sheets, mineralised matrix and fibrous stroma, sometimes containing multi-nucleate giant cells, can produce a complex appearance (Fig. 7.10b). Van Gieson's method and rhodamine B, which latter gives the ghost cells a yellow fluorescence, are helpful in distinguishing the components. Amyloid is usually absent (Buchner & David 1976). A clear cell variant has also been reported (Ng & Siar 1985). Approximately 10% of lesions with the histological features of calcifying odontogenic cyst are solid or have only small cystic areas (Praetorius et al 1981, Buchner 1991).

Differential diagnosis

Most calcifying odontogenic cysts present little difficulty in diagnosis. Ghost cells occur rarely in other forms of odontogenic tumour, including ameloblastomas, ameloblastic fibro-odontomes and odontomes, but are more frequent in craniopharyngiomas. For a diagnosis of calcifying odontogenic cyst, the other characteristic epithelial and connective tissue changes are required. When areas with the appearance of other forms of odontogenic tumour are also present, the relative proportions determine whether the diagnosis is that of calcifying odontogenic cyst or some form of mixed odontogenic tumour. Rarely, carcinomas have been reported in association with calcifying odontogenic cyst . Otherwise recurrence is unusual, but it is more likely in the solid forms (Colmenero et al 1990).

ODONTOMES

Odontomes, the most frequent form of odontogenic tumour, are hamartomas which contain the three mineralised dental tissues: enamel, dentine and cementum. A spectrum exists ranging from compound odontomes, containing multiple small teeth, to complex odontomes in which the dental tissues form a disorganised mass.

Clinical features

Odontomes are usually diagnosed in the first two decades of life (Kaugars et al 1989), when they may interfere with the normal eruption of a tooth or cause displacement of the roots of adjacent teeth. They are usually less than 2 cm in diameter, although occasionally they can be of much greater size. If undetected in early life, a later infective episode often brings them to attention. Complex odontomes are more commonly found in the molar region of the mandible, and compound odontomes in the anterior part of the maxilla (Budnick 1976).

Radiographically, odontomes are well circumscribed mineralised masses. They are usually diagnosed when maturing, but if observed at an early developmental stage will be more radiolucent because of the lack of mineralised tissue. Approximately half are associated with an unerupted tooth (Kaugars et al 1989).

Histopathology

Complex odontomes are made up of a mixture of enamel, dentine and cementum, in normal embryonic relationship to each other, but bearing no morphological resemblance to a tooth. Enamel matrix may be retained in demineralised sections if it is not fully mineralised (Fig. 7.11). Remnants of odontogenic epithelium and ectomesenchyme may be present, and these are more abundant in developing lesions. Occasionally, cystic degeneration may occur in the epithelium. Ghost cells are said to occur in about 10% of odontomes (Sedano & Pindborg 1975).

Compound odontomes consist of numerous denticles scattered throughout a stroma of mature fibrous tissue. Again, residues of odontogenic epithelium and ectomesenchyme are often present, particularly in developing lesions.

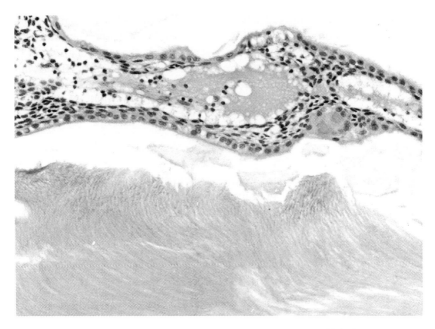

Fig. 7.11 Odontogenic epithelium and enamel matrix in an odontome. H & E × 215

Differential diagnosis

The diagnosis of mature complex and compound odontomes presents little difficulty. However, the immature developing lesions may be histologically difficult to differentiate from ameloblastic fibro-odontome. Enucleation is curative.

ODONTOGENIC KERATOCYST

The odontogenic keratocyst, first described by Phillipsen (1956), is classified with odontogenic cysts, accounting for 8–10% of such cysts. It has a reputation for recurrence after surgery and is included in this discussion of odontogenic tumours because, in many respects, it behaves like a neoplasm. Indeed a few authors have suggested that it is a neoplasm (Toller 1972, Ahlfors et al 1984). There are a number of comprehensive reviews (Brannon 1976, 1977, Forsell 1980, Browne 1996).

Clinical features

Odontogenic keratocysts are developmental cysts, most common in the second and third decades of life, but diagnosed in all age groups. They usually occur in the mandible, particularly the molar and ramus regions, and are often associated with an unerupted tooth. The cyst tends to grow within bone, causing little or no expansion, and may reach a large size before diagnosis. Chronic infection with discharge into the mouth may occur. The cysts are usually solitary, but may be multiple, in which case they are usually in patients with the naevoid basal cell carcinoma syndrome (Gorlin's syndrome).

Radiologically, odontogenic keratocysts are varied in appearance with no consistent relationship to teeth. They may be multilocular cysts, and as such are included in the radiographic differential diagnosis of many odontogenic tumours.

Histopathology

The walls of odontogenic keratocysts are frequently thin and friable resulting in fragmentary specimens being submitted to the histopathologist. The epithelial lining is characteristically thin and uniform with cuboidal or columnar basal cells, sometimes exhibiting reverse polarity with their nuclei away from the basement membrane. There is a surface layer of parakeratin (Fig. 7.12) which is often very thin with a typical corrugated appearance. The fibrous tissue capsule is usually free from inflammatory cell infiltrate but if areas of the cyst do become inflamed, the characteristic keratinisation can be lost and hyaline bodies may be present. Epithelial rests or satellite cysts may be found in the capsule, these being more numerous in cysts from patients with the naevoid basal cell carcinoma syndrome. Mitotic figures are quite

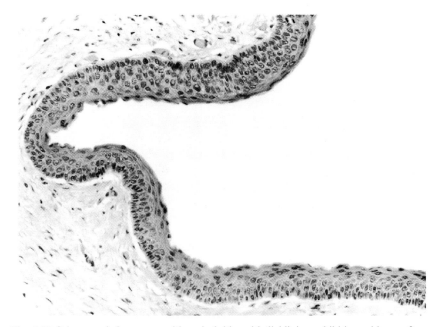

Fig. 7.12 Odontogenic keratocyst with typical thin epithelial lining exhibiting evidence of palisading of basal cells and thin parakeratotic surface layer. H & E × 170

common and marker studies with Ki67 (Li et al 1995) and p53 (Li et al 1996) substantiate the growth potential of the lesion.

Small areas of orthokeratinisation may be present and occasionally the entire cyst lining shows this pattern of keratinisation. These orthokeratinised variants lack the other features of odontogenic keratocysts and are not so destructive, rarely recurring following enucleation (Wright 1981, Crowley et al 1992,). For these reasons, most authorities feel that the orthokeratinised variant is not a subtype of odontogenic keratocyst (Vuhahula et al 1993).

Recurrence is frequent following enucleation, varying from 10–60% in different reports. There is no evidence that cysts which recur are more aggressive than those that do not, although cysts from syndromatic patients do tend to show greater proliferative activity. The friable nature of the cyst wall increases the risk of epithelial remnants being left in the bone cavity. Removal of cysts in one piece greatly reduces the risk of recurrence. Excision of mucosa overlying the cyst, particularly in the mandibular molar region, also reduces the risk of recurrence as this tissue often contains epithelial residues and microcysts. Pretreatment of the lining epithelium by Carnoy's fluid (Voorsmit et al 1981) or a cryogenic agent such as liquid nitrogen (Pogrel 1993) can reduce the risk of recurrence.

Occasional instances of malignant transformation in the epithelial lining of odontogenic keratocysts have been reported, although there is as yet no evidence that this risk is greater in keratocysts than in other forms of jaw cysts.

Differential diagnosis

Aspiration biopsy is useful for the diagnosis of odontogenic keratocysts. The presence of low soluble protein (>4 mg/100 ml) and epithelial squames is almost pathognomonic of the condition (Browne 1976). Histological diagnosis usually presents no difficulty unless the cyst is infected and large areas of the epithelial lining have dedifferentiated to non-keratinised stratified squamous epithelium. Identification of the orthokeratinised variant is important in view of its less aggressive behaviour. Other types of odontogenic cyst may occasionally undergo keratin metaplasia, but this usually affects only a small part of the wall and the epithelium lacks the other features characteristic of the odontogenic keratocyst. Rarely, intra-osseous epidermoid cysts occur. Sometimes unicystic ameloblastomas exhibit areas of keratinizing squamous metaplasia, but these will always show other features characteristic of this tumour. A similar comment may be made about the rare intra-osseous mucoepidermoid carcinomas.

MALIGNANT ODONTOGENIC NEOPLASMS

Malignant odontogenic tumours are rare. It is therefore not surprising that the classification of these lesions is still not entirely satisfactory and remains based upon interpretation of sporadic case reports. Occasional examples of malignant variants of most of the benign odontogenic tumours have been reported.

Infiltration of malignant tumours into the jaw bones is usually a consequence of direct invasion by a squamous cell carcinoma arising from the adjacent mucosa or it represents a metastatic deposit of carcinoma from a primary tumour elsewhere, most commonly in the bronchus, breast, thyroid, prostate, kidney or colon. Differentiation of these tumours from malignant odontogenic tumours is usually not a problem, except in the case of clear cell tumours.

Malignant ameloblastoma

The occurrence of malignant ameloblastomas has been recognised for some time. Many early reports were based on secondary pulmonary deposits, which developed following surgery for the primary tumour. These lesions, however, were often cytologically benign and many of them probably represented spread of tumour cells by aspiration at the time of surgery. However, ameloblastomas exhibiting cytological features of malignancy and producing metastases to sites other than the lung, have now been reported (Buff et al 1980, Jephcote 1981, Dorner et al 1988, Laughlin 1989). It has been suggested that primary tumours showing cytological features of malignancy should be designated ameloblastic carcinoma and that those that are cytologically benign, but are found subsequently to metastasise should be designated malignant amelobastoma (Elzay 1982, Slootweg & Muller 1984, Corio et al 1987). This distinction is probably unnecessary.

Clinically and radiologically there are no reliable distinguishing features between an ameloblastoma and a malignant ameloblastoma. Occasionally paraesthesia or numbness is present (Bruce & Jackson 1991). Metastases may not develop until many years after treatment of the primary tumour (Ramadar et al 1990). Some cases of malignant ameloblastoma have been associated with hypercalcaemia (Harada et al 1989, Laughlin 1989).

The epithelial cells show a variable degree of pleomorphism and they may be of plexiform or follicular pattern sometimes with central necrosis. Sometimes the primary tumour appears cytologically benign. A clear cell component may be present (Waldron et al 1985). The metastatic tumour is often less well differentiated than the primary tumour.

The prognosis of malignant ameloblastoma appears to be poor (Waldron 1988) although, because of the small number of cases on record, accurate survival data are not available.

Primary intra-osseous carcinoma

Rarely, malignant neoplasms with the histological features of a squamous cell carcinoma arise *de novo* within the jaws (Shear 1969, Elzay 1982, To et al 1991). These lesions most probably arise from residues of the dental lamina, although origin from other residues of epithelium cannot be discounted (Takeda 1991). They are more common in males from the fifth decade onwards, and in the posterior part of the mandible, though they may arise in any part of the jaw and at any age. Paraesthesia of the mental nerve may be present. Radiographically, the lesions are radiolucent and often poorly defined. A pathological fracture may be present (To et al 1991). Lymph node metastases are present in approximately one third of cases. (Suei et al 1994).

Histologically, primary intra–osseous carcinomas may have an alveolar or plexiform pattern and exhibit varying degrees of cellular pleomorphism and keratinisation. The peripheral cells may exhibit a tendency to palisading of their nuclei. Rarely, reactive osseous metaplasia is present (Bennett et al 1993).

The prognosis of this form of carcinoma is not good (Waldron & Mustoe 1989) with an estimated 5 year survival of 30–40% (To et al 1991).

Malignant change in odontogenic cysts

The relatively frequent occurrence of odontogenic cysts in the jaws and the fact that they may be symptomless for prolonged periods of time make it likely that malignant transformation in the epithelial lining occurs from time to time. This event is more frequent than the development of a primary intra-osseous carcinoma. Such neoplasms, always squamous cell carcinomas, are usually diagnosed from the fifth decade onwards, more commonly in males and in the posterior part of the mandible (Eversole et al 1975). They most frequently develop in residual cysts. Some authors have suggested that cysts showing keratinising squamous metaplasia have a greater risk of undergoing malignant change (Browne & Gough 1972, Areen et al 1981, Van der Waal et al 1985). Such cysts are not odontogenic keratocysts, although these latter have occasionally been reported to undergo malignant change, either in solitary lesions (Ward & Cohen 1963, Macleod & Soames 1988, Minic 1992) or in Gorlin's syndrome (Moos & Rennie 1987). Change in the ploidy of the cells has been demonstrated in sequential biopsies in an odontogenic keratocyst (High et al 1987).

Clinically, the patient complains of pain and swelling and there may be associated paraesthesia of an involved nerve. Radiologically, the radiolucency may be at least partially well circumscribed, evidence presumably of the pre-existing cyst, but it is usually poorly defined in parts and there may be a pathological fracture. Lymph node metastases are present in some 20% of cases (Eversole et al 1975).

Histologically, the unequivocal demonstration of malignant transformation in the epithelial lining of an odontogenic cyst is dependent upon the examination of numerous blocks and the demonstration of a transition of the one to the other. The malignant component may be predominant so that only a small part of the cyst of origin remains. The carcinomas are usually well differentiated squamous cell tumours with numerous keratin pearls. The associated cyst lining usually shows dysplasia, at least in those areas adjacent to the neoplasm, and may be keratinised.

Although these carcinomas are generally regarded as low grade tumours, their prognosis may be poor. A two year survival of 53% has been quoted (Eversole et al 1975).

Malignant variants of other odontogenic epithelial tumours

The rare occurrence of malignant forms of other kinds of odontogenic tumour is confirmed from the publication of occasional case reports in the literature. Because of their rarity it is not possible to make any meaningful analysis of their behaviour or diagnosis. Malignant variants of a number of odontogenic epithelial tumours have been reported, including dentinogenic ghost cell tumours (Ellis & Shmookler 1986, Grodjesk et al 1987, McCoy et al 1992) and calcifying epithelial odontogenic tumour (Basu et al 1984).

Ameloblastic fibrosarcoma

In ameloblastic fibrosarcoma the ectomesenchymal component shows the histological features of malignancy, although the epithelium appears benign. Painful swelling is the usual complaint. These lesions are more common in males than females and in the mandible than the maxilla, with a mean age of 26 (Wood et al 1988). Radiologically there are no distinguishing features.

Histologically, although the ectomesenchymal tissues exhibit the typical features of malignant cells, there are often areas of more benign appearance suggesting that at least some of the lesions develop in a previously benign form of neoplasm (Leider et al 1972, Altini et al 1985).

Local recurrence is common following surgery which appears to be the treatment of choice. Distant metastasis occurs occasionally both to the regional lymph nodes (Howell & Burkes 1977) and to the lungs (Chomette et al 1983).

Ameloblastic fibrodentinosarcoma and ameloblastic fibro-odontosarcoma

Both these entities are extremely rare and there are little documented data on them (Howells & Burkes 1977, Takeda et al 1990).

Odontogenic carcinosarcomas

Rarely, an odontogenic tumour is reported in which both the epithelial and ectomesenchymal components are cytologically malignant (Yoshida et al 1989, Tanaka et al 1991, Shinoda et al 1992). The behaviour of these lesions is uncertain.

KEY POINTS FOR CLINICAL PRACTICE

1. Odontogenic epithelium is found in a range of situations from developmental rests to malignant neoplasms.

2. A wide range of histological appearances can be assumed by odontogenic epithelium.

3. The classsification of odontogenic tumours contains both hamartomas and neoplasms.

4. Wide variations in histological appearances can be found within individual tumour types.

5. Clear cells in odontogenic tumours usually indicate an aggressive or malignant variant.

REFERENCES

Ackermann G L, Altini M, Shear M 1988 The unicystic ameloblastoma: a clinicopathological study of 57 cases. J Oral Pathol 17: 541–546

Ahlfors E, Larsson A, Sjogren S 1984 The odontogenic keratocyst: a benign cystic tumor? J Oral Maxillofac Surg 42: 10–19

Altini M, Slabbert H D, Johnston T 1991 Papilliferous keratoameloblastoma. J Oral Pathol Med 20: 46–48

Altini M, Thompson S H, Lowrie J F et al 1985 Ameloblastic sarcoma of the mandible. J Oral Maxillofac Surg 43: 789–794

Areen R G, McClatchey K D, Baker H L 1981 Squamous cell carcinoma developing in an odontogenic cyst. Report of a case. Arch Otolaryngol 107: 568–569

Baden E, Doyle J, Meas M et al 1993 Squamous odontogenic tumour. Oral Surg Oral Med Oral Pathol 75: 733–738

Bang G, Koppang H S, Hansen L S et al 1989 Clear cell odontogenic carcinoma: report of three cases with pulmonary and lymph node metastases. J Oral Pathol Med 18: 113–118

Basu M K, Matthews J B, Sear A J et al 1984 Calcifying odontogenic tumour: a case showing features of malignancy. J Oral Pathol 13: 310–319

Batsakis J G, Hicks M J, Flaitz C M 1993 Peripheral epithelial odontogenic tumors. Ann Otol Rhinol Laryngol 102: 322–324.

Becker J, Reichert P A, Schuppan D et al 1992 Ectomesenchyme of ameloblastic fibroma reveals a characteristic distribution of extracellular matrix proteins. J Oral Pathol Med 21: 156–159

Bennett J H, Jones I, Speight P M 1993 Odontogenic squamous cell carcinoma with osseous metaplasia. J Oral Pathol Med 22: 286–288

Brannon R B 1976 The odontogenic keratocyst. A clinicopathologic study of 312 cases. Part 1. Clinical features. Oral Surg Oral Med Oral Pathol 42: 54–72

Brannon R B 1977 The odontogenic keratocyst. A clinicopathological study of 312 cases. Part II. Histological features. Oral Surg Oral Med Oral Pathol 43: 233–255

Browne R M 1976 Some observations on the fluids of odontogenic cysts. J Oral Pathol 5: 74–87

Browne R M 1996 Per(cyst)ent growth: the odontogenic keratocyst 40 years on. Ann Roy Coll Surg Engl 76: 426–433

Browne R M, Gough N G 1972 Malignant change in the epithelial lining of odontogenic cysts. Cancer 29: 1199–1207

Bruce R A, Jackson I T 1991 Ameloblastic carcinoma: a report of an aggressive case and review of the literature. J Craniomaxillofac Surg 19: 276–271

Buchner A 1991 The central (intraosseous) calcifying odontogenic cyst; analysis of 215 cases. J Oral Maxillofac Surg 49: 330–339

Buchner A, David R 1976 Amyloid-like material in odontogenic tumors. J Oral Surg 34: 320–332

Buchner A, Merrell P W, Hansen L S et al 1991 Peripheral (extraosseous) calcifying odontogenic cyst. Oral Surg Oral Med Oral Pathol 72: 65–70

Budnick S D 1976 Compound and complex odontomes. Oral Surg Oral Med Oral Pathol 42: 501–506

Buff S J, Chen J T, Ravin C C et al 1980 Pulmonary metastasis from ameloblastoma of the mandible: report of a case and review of the literature. J Oral Surg 38: 374–376

Chanda Y, Mochiyuki K, Sugimura M 1987 Odontogenic tumour with combined characteristics of adenomatoid odontogenic and calcifying epithelial odontogenic tumours. Pathol Res Pract 182: 647–657

Chomette G, Auriol M, Guilbert F et al 1983 Ameloblastic fibrosarcoma of the jaws – report of three cases. Pathol Res Pract 178: 40–47

Colmenero C, Patron M, Colmenero B 1990 Odontogenic ghost cell tumors. The neoplastic form of calcifying odontogenic cyst. J Craniomaxillofac Surg 18: 215–218

Corio R L, Goldblatt L I, Edwards P A et al 1987 Ameloblastic carcinoma: a clinicopathologic study and assessment of eight cases. Oral Surg Oral Med Oral Pathol 64: 570–576

Crowley T E, Kaugars G E, Gunsolley J C 1992 Odontogenic keratocysts: a clinical and histologic comparison of the parakeratin and orthokeratin variants. J Oral Maxillofac Surg 50: 22–26

Damm D D, White D K, Drummond J F et al 1983 Combined epithelial odontogenic tumor: adenomatoid odontogenic tumor and calcifying odontogenic tumor. Oral Surg Oral Med Oral Pathol 55: 487–496

Dorner L, Sear A J, Smith G T 1988 A case of ameloblastic carcinoma with pulmonary metastasis. Br J Oral Maxillofac Surg 26: 503–510

El-Labban N G 1990 Cementum-like material in a case of Pindborg tumor. J Oral Pathol Med 19: 166–169

El-Labban N G 1992 The nature of the eosinophilic and laminated masses in the adenomatoid odontogenic tumour: a histochemical and ultrastructural study. J Oral Pathol Med 21: 75–81

El-Labban N G, Lee K W 1988 Vascular degeneration in adenomatoid odontogenic tumour: an ultrastructural study. J Oral Pathol 17: 298–305

El-Mofty S K, Gerard N O, Farish S E et al 1991 Peripheral ameloblastoma: a clinical and histologic study of 11 cases. J Oral Maxillofac Surg 49: 970–974

Ellis G L, Shmookler B M 1986 Aggressive (malignant?) epithelial odontogenic ghost cell tumor. Oral Surg Oral Med Oral Pathol 61: 471–478

Elzay R P 1982 Primary intraosseous carcinoma of the jaws. Review and update of odontogenic carcinomas. Oral Surg Oral Med Oral Pathol 54: 299–303

Eversole L R, Sabes W R, Rovin S 1975 Aggressive growth and neoplastic potential of odontogenic cysts. Cancer 35: 270–282

Eversole L R, Leider A S, Hansen L S 1984 Ameloblastomas with pronounced desmoplasia. J Oral Maxillofac Surg 42: 735–740

Fejerskov O, Krogh J 1972 The calcifying ghost cell odontogenic tumor – or the calcifying odontogenic cyst. J Oral Pathol 1: 273–287

Forssell K 1980 The primordial cyst. A clinical and radiographic study. Proc Finn Dent Soc 76: 129–174

Franklin C D, Pindborg J J 1976 The calcifying epithelial odontogenic tumor. Oral Surg Oral Med Oral Pathol 42: 753–765

Gardner D G, Corio R L 1983 The relationship of plexiform unicystic ameloblastoma to conventional ameloblastoma. Oral Surg Oral Med Oral Pathol 56: 54–60

Gardner D G, Corio R L 1984 Plexiform unicystic ameloblastoma. A variant of ameloblastoma with a low-recurrence rate after enucleation. Cancer 53: 1730–1735

Goldblatt L I, Brannon R B, Ellis G L 1982 Squamous odontogenic tumor. Oral Surg Oral Med Oral Pathol 54: 187–196

Gorlin R J, Pindborg J J, Clausen F P et al 1962 The calcifying odontogenic cyst – a possible analogue of the cutaneous calcifying epithelioma of Malherbe. Oral Surg Oral Med Oral Pathol 15: 1235–1243

Grodjesk J E, Dolinsky J B, Schneider L D et al 1987 Odontogenic ghost cell carcinoma. Oral Surg Oral Med Oral Pathol 63: 576–581

Gunbay T, Gunbay S, Oztop F 1993 Odontoameloblastoma: report of a case. J Clin Pediatr Dent 18: 17–20

Hansen L S, Ficarra G 1988 Mixed odontogenic tumors: an analysis of 23 new cases. Head Neck Surg 10: 330–343

Hansen L S, Eversole L R, Green T L et al 1985 Clear cell odontogenic tumor – a new histologic variant with aggressive potential. Head Neck Surg 8: 115–123

Harada K, Suda S, Kayano T et al 1989 Ameloblastoma with metastasis to the lung and associated hypercalcemia. J Oral Maxillofac Surg 47: 1083–1087

Hicks M J, Flaitz C M, Wong M E K et al 1994 Clear cell variant of calcifying epithelial odontogenic tumor: case report and review of the literature. Head Neck 16: 272–277

High A S, Quirke P, Hume W J 1987 DNA-ploidy studies in a keratocyst undergoing subsequent transformation. J Oral Pathol 16: 135–138

Hong S P, Ellis G L, Hartman K S 1991 Calcifying odontogenic cyst. Oral Surg Oral Med Oral Pathol 72: 56–64

Howell R M, Burkes E J 1977 Malignant transformation of ameloblastic fibro-odontoma to ameloblastic fibrosarcoma. Oral Surg Oral Med Oral Pathol 43: 391–401

Jephcote C H J 1981 Ameloblastoma with pulmonary metastases: a case report. Br J Oral Surg 19: 38–42

Kaffe I, Buchner A, Taicher S 1993 Radiologic features of desmoplastic variant of ameloblastoma. Oral Surg Oral Med Oral Pathol 76: 525–529

Kakudo K, Mushimoto K, Shirasu R et al 1989 Calcifying odontogenic cysts: co-expression of intermediate filament proteins and immunohistochemical distribution of keratins, involucrin and filaggrin. Pathol Res Prac 185: 891–899

Kaugars G E, Miller M E, Abbey L M 1989 Odontomas. Oral Surg Oral Med Oral Pathol 67: 771–778

Kim J, Ellis G L 1993 Dental follicular tissue: misinterpretation as odontogenic tumors. J Oral Maxillofac Surg 51: 762–767

Kramer I R H, Pindborg J J, Shear M 1992 Histological typing of odontogenic tumours. Springer Verlag, Berlin

LaBriola J D, Steiner M, Bernstein M L et al 1980 Odontoameloblastoma. J Oral Surg 38: 139–143

Laughlin E H 1989 Metastasising ameloblastoma. Cancer 64: 776–780

Leider A S, Nelson J F, Trodahl J N 1972 Ameloblastic fibrosarcoma of the jaws. Oral Surg Oral Med Oral Pathol 33: 559–569

Leider A S, Jonker L A, Cook H E 1989 Multicentric familial squamous odontogenic tumor. Oral Surg Oral Med Oral Pathol 68: 175–181

Li T J, Browne R M, Matthews J B 1995 Epithelial proliferation in odontogenic keratocyst: a comparative immunocytochemical study of Ki67 in simple, recurrent and basal cell naevus syndrome (BCNS) associated lesions. J Oral Pathol Med 24: 221–226

Li T J, Browne R M, Prime S S et al 1996 p53 expression in odontogenic keratocyst epithelium. J Oral Pathol Med 25: 249–255

McCoy B P, O'Carroll H K, Hall J M 1992 Carcinoma arising in a dentinogenic ghost cell tumor. Oral Surg Oral Med Oral Pathol 74: 371–378

Macleod R I, Soames J V 1988 Squamous cell carcinoma arising in an odontogenic keratocyst. Br J Oral Maxillofac Surg 26: 52–57

Miller A S, Lopez C F, Pullon P A et al 1976 Ameloblastic fibro-odontoma. Oral Surg Oral Med Oral Pathol 41: 354–365

Minic A J 1992 Primary intraosseous squamous cell carcinoma arising in a mandibular keratocyst. Int J Oral Maxillofac Surg 21: 163–165

Moos K F, Rennie J S 1987 Squamous cell carcinoma arising in a mandibular keratocyst in a patient with Gorlin's syndrome. Br J Oral Maxillofac Surg 25: 280–284

Mori M, Yamada K, Kasai T et al 1991 Immunohistochemical expression of amelogenins in odontogenic tumors and cysts. Virchows Arch A Pathol Anat Histopathol 418: 319–325

Muller H, Slootweg P J 1986 Clear cell differentiation in an ameloblastoma. J Maxillofac Surg 14: 158–160

Muller S, Waldron C A 1991 Primary intraosseous squamous carcinoma. Int J Oral Maxillofac Surg 20: 362–365

Nastri A L, Weisenfeld D, Radden B G et al 1995 Maxillary ameloblastoma; a retrospective study of 13 cases. Br J Oral Maxillofac Surg 33: 28–32

Nauta J M, Panders A K, Schoots C J F et al 1992 Peripheral ameloblastoma. A case report and review of the literature. Int J Oral Maxillofac Surg 21: 40–44

Ng K H, Siar C H 1985 Clear cell change in a calcifying odontogenic cyst. Oral Surg Oral Med Oral Pathol 60: 417–419

Norval E J G, Thompson I O C, van Wyk C W 1994 An unusual variant of keratoameloblastoma. J Oral Pathol Med 23: 465–467

Philipsen H P 1956 Om keratocyster (kolesteatom) i kaeberne. Tandlaegebladet 60: 963–981

Philipsen H P, Birn H 1969 The adenomatoid odontogenic tumour. Acta Pathol Microbiol Scand 75: 375–398

Philipsen H P, Reichert P A, Zhang K H et al 1991 Adenomatoid odontogenic tumor: biologic profile based on 499 cases. J Oral Pathol Med 20: 149–158

Philipsen H P, Ormiston I W, Reichert P A 1992a The desmo- and osteoplastic ameloblastoma. Int J Oral Maxillofac Surg 21: 352–357

Philipsen H P, Thosaporn W, Reichert P A et al 1992b Odontogenic lesions in opercula of permanent molars delayed in eruption. J Oral Pathol Med 21: 38–41

Piattelli A, Sesenna E, Trisi P 1994 Clear cell odontogenic carcinoma. Report of a case with lymph node and pulmonary metastases. Oral Oncol, Eur J Cancer 30B: 278–280

Pindborg J J 1955 Calcifying epithelial odontogenic tumor. Acta Pathol Microbiol Scand Supp 3: 71

Pindborg J J 1958 A calcifying epithelial odontogenic tumor. Cancer 2: 838–843

Pindborg J J, Vedtofte P, Reibel J et al 1991 The calcifying epithelial odontogenic tumor. A review of recent literature and report of a case. APMIS Suppl 23: 152–157

Pogrel M A 1993 The use of liquid nitrogen cryotherapy in the management of locally aggressive bone lesions. J Oral Maxillofac Surg 51: 269–273

Praetorius F, Hjortling-Hansen E, Gorlin R J et al 1981 Calcifying odontogenic cyst. Acta Odontol Scand 39: 227–240

Pullon P A, Shafer W G, Elzay R P et al 1975 Squamous odontogenic tumor. Oral Surg Oral Med Oral Pathol 40: 616–630

Ramadar K, Jose C C, Subhaskins J et al 1990 Pulmonary metastases from ameloblastoma of the mandible treated with cisplatin, adriamycin and cyclophosphamide. Cancer 65: 1475–1479

Raubenheimer E J, van Heerden W F P, Noffke C E E 1995 Infrequent clinicopathological findings in 108 ameloblastomas. J Oral Pathol Med 24: 227–232

Regezi J A, Kerr D A, Courtney R M 1978 Odontogenic tumors: analysis of 706 cases. J Oral Surg 36: 771–778

Reichert P A, Philipsen H P, Sonner S 1995 Ameloblastoma: biological profile of 3677 cases. Oral Oncol, Eur J Cancer 31B: 86–99

Sadeghi E M, Levin S 1995 Clear cell odontogenic carcinoma of the mandible: report of a case. J Oral Maxillofac Surg 53: 613–616

Saku T, Okabe H, Shimokawa H 1992 Immunohistochemical demonstration of enamel proteins in odontogenic tumors. J Oral Pathol Med 21: 113–119

Sawyer D R, Nwoku A L, Mosadomi A 1982 Recurrent ameloblastic fibroma. Report of two cases. Oral Surg Oral Med Oral Pathol 53: 19–23

Sedano H O, Pindborg J J 1975 Ghost cell epithelium in odontomas. J Oral Pathol 4: 27–30

Shear M 1969 Primary intra-alveolar epidermoid carcinoma of the jaw. J Pathol 97: 645–651

Shinoda T, Iwata H, Nakamura A et al 1992 Cytologic appearance of carcinosarcoma. A case report. Acta Cytol 36: 132–136

Slootweg P J 1980 Epithelio-mesenchymal morphology in ameloblastic fibro-odontoma: a light and electron microscope study. J Oral Pathol 9: 29–40

Slootweg P J 1991 Bone and cementum as stromal features in Pindborg tumor. J Oral Pathol Med 20: 93–95

Slootweg P G, Muller H 1984 Malignant ameloblastoma or ameloblastic carcinoma. Oral Surg Oral Med Oral Pathol 57: 168–176

Snead M L, Luo W, Hsu D D J et al 1992 Human ameloblastoma tumors express the amelogenin gene. Oral Surg Oral Med Oral Pathol 74: 64–72

Stafne E C 1948 Epithelial tumors associated with developmental cysts of the maxilla. Oral Surg Oral Med Oral Pathol 1: 887–894

Suei Y, Tanimoto K, Taguchi A et al 1994 Primary intraosseous carcinoma: review of the literature and diagnostic criteria. J Oral Maxillofac Surg 52: 580–583

Takata T, Ogawa I, Miyauchi M et al 1993 Non-calcifying Pindborg tumor with Langerhans cells. J Oral Pathol Med 22: 378–383

Takeda Y 1989 Pigmented adenomatoid odontogenic tumour. Virchows Archiv A Pathol Anat Histopathol 415: 571–575

Takeda Y 1991 Intraosseous squamous cell carcinoma of the maxilla: probably arisen from non-odontogenic epithelium. Br J Oral Maxillofac Surg 29: 392–394

Takeda Y, Kuroda M, Suzuki A 1990 Ameloblastic odontosarcoma (ameloblastic fibro-odontosarcoma) in the mandible. Acta Pathol Jpn 40: 832–837

Takeda Y, Suzuki A, Yamamoto H 1990 Histopathologic study of epithelial components in the connective tissue wall of unilocular type of calcifying odontogenic cyst. J Oral Pathol Med 19: 108–113

Tanaka T, Olkubo T, Fujitsuka H 1991 et al Malignant mixed tumor (malignant ameloblastoma and fibrosarcoma) of the maxilla. Arch Pathol Lab Med 115: 84–87

Tatemoto Y, Okada Y, Mori M 1989 Squamous odontogenic tumor: immunohistochemical identification of keratins. Oral Surg Oral Med Oral Pathol 67: 63–67

Thoma K H, Goldman H M 1946 Odontogenic tumors: a classification based on observations of the epithelial, mesenchymal and mixed varieties. Am J Pathol 12: 433–471

Thompson I O C, Phillips V M, Ferreira R et al 1990 Odontoamelobastoma: a case report. Br J Oral Maxillofac Surg 28: 347–349

To E H W, Brown J S, Avery B S et al 1991 Primary intraosseous carcinoma of the jaws. Three new cases and a review of the literature. Br J Oral Maxillofac Surg 29: 19–25

Toida M, Hyodu I, Okudo T et al 1991 Adenomatoid odontogenic tumor: report of two cases and survey of 126 cases in Japan. J Oral Maxillofac Surg 48: 404–409

Toller P A 1972 Newer concepts of odontogenic cysts. Int J Oral Surg 1: 3–16

Trodahl J N 1972 Ameloblastic fibroma. A survey of cases from the Armed Forces Institute of Pathology. Oral Surg Oral Med Oral Pathol 33: 547–558

Ueno S, Mushimoto K, Shirasu R 1989 Prognostic evaluation of ameloblastoma based on histologic and radiographic typing. J Oral Maxillofac Surg 47: 11–15

Ulmansky M, Bodner L, Praetorius F et al 1994 Ameloblastic fibrodentinoma: report of two new cases. J Oral Maxillofac Surg 52: 980–984

van der Waal I, Rauhanaa R, van der Kwast W A M et al 1985 Squamous cell carcinoma arising in the lining of odontogenic cysts. Int J Oral Surg 14: 146–152

van Wyk C W, van der Vyver P C 1983 Ameloblastic fibroma with dentinoid formation/immature dentinoma. J Oral Pathol 12: 37–46

Voorsmit R A C A, Stoelinga P J W, van Haelst U J G M 1981 The management of keratocysts. J Maxillofac Surg 9: 228–236

Vuhahula V E, Nikai H, Ijuhin N et al 1993 Jaw cysts with orthokeratinization: analysis of 12 cases. J Oral Pathol Med 22: 35–40

Waldron C A 1988 Odontogenic tumors and selected jaw cysts. In: Gnepp D R (ed) Pathology of the head and neck. Churchill Livingstone, Edinburgh pp 403–458

Waldron C A, Mustoe T A 1989 Primary intraosseous carcinoma of the mandible with probable origin in an odontogenic cyst. Oral Surg Oral Med Oral Pathol 67: 716–724

Waldron C A, Small I A, Silverman H 1985 Clear cell ameloblastoma – an odontogenic carcinoma. J Oral Maxillofac Surg 43: 707–717

Ward T G, Cohen B 1963 Squamous carcinoma in a mandibular cyst. Br J Oral Surg 1: 8–12

Wood R M, Markle T L, Barker B F et al 1988 Ameloblastic fibrosarcoma. Oral Surg Oral Med Oral Pathol 66: 74–77

Wright J M 1981 The odontogenic keratocyst: orthokeratinised variant. Oral Surg Oral Med Oral Pathol 51: 609–618

Yoshida T, Shingaki S, Nakajima T et al 1989 Odontogenic carcinoma with sarcomatous proliferation. A case report. J Craniomaxillofac Surg 17: 139–142

Zallen R D, Preshar M H, McClary S A 1982 Ameloblastic fibroma. J Oral Maxillofac Surg 40: 513–517

8

Salivary gland tumours

R. H. W. Simpson

Tumours of the salivary glands occur with enough frequency that even the less common types will be seen now and again by all surgical pathologists. For example, a typical English district general hospital such as Exeter, with a catchment population of 325 000, yields about 40 new cases each year. Most of these present few problems in identification, but in a significant minority difficulties can arise. It is beyond the scope of this chapter to discuss every tumour in detail, particularly those that are well-established, and it is intended to concentrate on some of the newer and perhaps less familiar entities.

CLASSIFICATION

Salivary gland tumours exhibit a wide variety of microscopic appearances, even within one particular lesion, and this has caused considerable problems in categorization and diagnosis. This is illustrated by the plethora of classification systems developed over the years: from 1954 to 1986 six different schemes were proposed (Foote & Frazell 1954, Evans & Cruickshank 1970, Thackray & Sobin 1972, Thackray & Lucas 1974, Batsakis 1979, Seifert et al 1986), of which that described in the first edition of the World Health Organization (WHO) 'Blue Book' (Thackray & Sobin 1972) was perhaps the most widely adopted. Whilst these classifications at the time clearly represented major advances in our understanding of salivary gland neoplasia, it duly became apparent that there were considerable areas of difficulty in practice, compounded by the discovery of several new and distinct clinicopathological entities. An updated classification was clearly needed, and two new ones correct many, but not all, of the earlier defects.

The AFIP morphologic classification of Ellis & Auclair (1991) and the revised WHO classification (Seifert & Sobin 1991) (Table 8.1) both recognize several types of adenoma and replace the imprecise term 'monomorphic adenoma'. There are separate categories for several new carcinomas formerly grouped together as adenocarcinoma, and both rightly upgrade acinic cell and mucoepidermoid 'tumours' to the genuine (and often fatal) carcinomas they undoubtedly are. The major difference between the two classifications is that the AFIP divides carcinomas into low, intermediate and high grades of malignancy. Whilst this has some advantages, it is liable to lead to confusion when several examples of the same entity appear in more than one grade.

167

Table 8.1 Revised WHO histological classification of salivary gland tumours and tumour-like lesions

---

1 Adenomas

1.1	Pleomorphic adenoma		
1.2	Myoepithelioma (myoepithelial adenoma)		
1.3	Basal cell adenoma		
1.4	Warthin tumour (adenolymphoma)		
1.5	Oncocytoma (oncocytic adenoma)		
1.6	Canalicular adenoma		
1.7	Sebaceous adenoma		
1.8	Ductal papilloma –	1.8.1	Inverted ductal papilloma
		1.8.2	Intraductal papilloma
		1.8.3	Sialadenoma papilliferum
1.9	Cystadenoma –	1.9.1	Papillary cystadenoma
		1.9.2	Mucinous cystadenoma

2 Carcinomas

2.1	Acinic cell carcinoma
2.2	Mucoepidermoid carcinoma
2.3	Adenoid cystic carcinoma
2.4	Polymorphous low grade adenocarcinoma (terminal duct adenocarcinoma)
2.5	Epithelial-myoepithelial carcinoma
2.6	Basal cell adenocarcinoma
2.7	Sebaceous carcinoma
2.8	Papillary cystadenocarcinoma
2.9	Mucinous adenocarcinoma
2.10	Oncocytic carcinoma
2.11	Salivary duct carcinoma
2.12	Adenocarcinoma (not otherwise specified)
2.13	Malignant myoepithelioma (myoepithelial carcinoma)
2.14	Carcinoma in pleomorphic adenoma
2.15	Squamous cell carcinoma
2.16	Small cell carcinoma
2.17	Undifferentiated carcinoma
2.18	Other carcinomas

3 Non-epithelial tumours

4 Malignant lymphomas

5 Secondary tumours

6 Unclassified tumours

7 Tumour-like lesions

7.1	Sialadenosis
7.2	Oncocytosis
7.3	Necrotizing sialometaplasia (salivary gland infarction)
7.4	Benign lymphoepithelial lesion
7.5	Salivary gland cysts
7.6	Chronic sclerosing sialadenitis of submandibular gland (Küttner tumour)
7.7	Cystic lymphoid hyperplasia in AIDS

Both these classifications represent great improvements on their predecessors, and I would certainly advocate the adoption of one or other by all diagnostic surgical histopathologists. Which one depends on personal choice, but my own preference is for the WHO one as it is more concise but still allows most tumours to be correctly classified.

ADENOMAS

Myoepithelioma

Whether or not myoepithelioma is a true biological entity is open to debate, but most commentators believe that it represents one end of a spectrum that also includes pleomorphic adenoma and non-membranous forms of basal cell adenoma. Nevertheless, myoepithelioma displays particular microscopic features that pose specific practical problems in identification and differential diagnosis, and on this basis it can be accepted as a separate diagnostic category (Simpson et al 1995). As such, it can be defined as a neoplasm composed completely, or almost completely, of myoepithelial cells.

Most cases present as a well circumscribed mass, usually 1–5 cm in diameter, in either major or minor salivary glands. Microscopically, there are several typical appearances, reflecting the different forms that non-neoplastic myoepithelial cells may take. Solid, myxoid and reticular growth patterns may be seen, and the component cells may be spindle-shaped, plasmacytoid (hyaline) or, less frequently, clear or epithelioid. Many of these tumours show more than one growth pattern or cell type. Benign myoepitheliomas do not usually show invasiveness, necrosis, cytological pleomorphism, or more than an isolated mitotic figure, though such features are seen in malignant myoepitheliomas (Di Palma & Guzzo 1993). The stroma is usually scanty, fibrous or myxoid, and it may occasionally contain chondroid material (Dardick et al 1989) or mature fat cells (Ng & Ma 1995). Extracellular collagenous crystalloids are seen in 10–20% of plasmacytoid cell type myoepitheliomas, (as well as sometimes in myoepithelial-rich pleomorphic adenomas). These crystalloids measure about 50–100 μm in diameter and consist of radially-arranged needle-shaped fibres composed of collagen types I and III, which stain red with the van Gieson method (Skálová et al 1992).

Scanty small ducts may be present (usually less than 5% of the tumour tissue) in otherwise typical myoepitheliomas, and their presence reflects the probable common precursor cell of both epithelial and myoepithelial cells in the terminal duct (Barnes et al 1985). Immunohistochemically, almost all tumours express S100 protein, as well as low molecular weight cytokeratins. Alpha smooth muscle actin positivity is seen in most spindle cell myoepitheliomas, but only occasionally in the plasmacytoid cell type (Simpson et al 1995). Electron microscopic studies have also confirmed both epithelial and smooth muscle differentiation (Sciubba & Brannon 1982).

Although neither growth pattern nor cell type appear to be of prognostic significance, several studies have shown that tumours of the minor glands are usually composed of plasmacytoid cells, whilst those of the parotid predominantly comprise spindle cells. The clear cell variant of myoepithelioma can occur in both major and minor glands (Simpson & Kitara-Okot 1995), but is rare: of a series of 40 myoepitheliomas, clear cells constituted the predominant pattern in only one (Dardick et al 1989). The behaviour of myoepithelioma is similar to that of pleomorphic adenoma, and complete excision should be curative. Malignant change in a benign lesion has been described (Adam et al 1994, Alós et al 1995), but too little information is available about the percentage of cases involved. However, it is probably not very different from that of pleomorphic adenoma (see below).

Basal cell adenoma

Most tumours previously included under monomorphic adenoma (other types) are now termed basal cell adenoma. The revised WHO classification recognizes four histopathological subtypes – solid, tubular, trabecular and membranous. However, it is probable that, in reality, there are only two – membranous and non-membranous – and that these are different enough from each other to be considered as separate biological entities.

Non-membranous basal cell adenomas have an equal sex incidence, arise mostly in the major glands, do not recur after excision, and have a low rate of malignant transformation (about 4%). It is likely that they represent part of the spectrum of myoepithelioma and pleomorphic adenoma. The tumours are ovoid, well circumscribed masses in which nests and trabeculae of basaloid cells are surrounded by a distinct thin PAS positive basement membrane. The component cells may take two forms – one is small with scanty cytoplasm and a round, deeply basophilic nucleus, and the other is larger with amphophilic or eosinophilic cytoplasm and an ovoid paler staining nucleus. These two types are intermixed, but the smaller cells tend to be arranged around the periphery of the nests and trabeculae, giving the appearance of palisading. Ductal differentiation may or may not be apparent. There is little pleomorphism and mitotic figures are rare. The stroma varies in amount and cellularity, but S100 positive spindle cells may be numerous.

Membranous basal cell adenoma (dermal analogue tumour) occurs predominantly in men, and is often multicentric. Most arise in the major glands, and also on occasion within intraparotid lymph nodes. Microscopically, they are not encapsulated and appear multinodular, often with a jigsaw-like pattern. The most characteristic feature is deposition of large amounts of hyaline basement membrane material, which is brightly eosinophilic and PAS positive. It surrounds the epithelial cell islands and blood vessels, and is present within the former as small droplets (Fig. 8.1). As in the non-membranous tumours, the epithelial cells may be small and dark with peripheral palisading, or large and pale. There is little pleomorphism or mitotic activity. In about 40% of cases, membranous basal cell adenoma is associated with synchronous and often multiple skin appendage tumours of sweat gland or hair

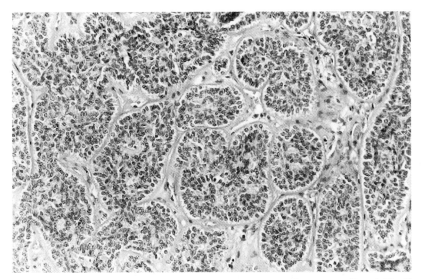

Fig 8.1. Membranous basal cell adenoma showing cylindroma– like groups of basaloid cells surrounded by eosinophilic basement membrane material. H&E × 160.

follicle origin, usually cylindromas or eccrine spiradenomas. According to the review of Batsakis et al (1991) 24% of cases of membranous basal cell adenoma recurred after surgery, probably reflecting multicentricity and, in addition, malignancy in the form of basal cell adenocarcinoma developed in 28%.

Whilst the evidence for two different entities of basal cell adenoma is strong, it is not always easy in practice to separate them. My own policy is first to make the diagnosis of basal cell adenoma, and then allocate the tumour to the membranous or non-membranous type on the basis of the amount of basement membrane material, also considering other factors such as multicentricity or history of skin tumours. However, this is not always possible in every case, particularly where basement membrane material is noticeable but not excessive. It is best to describe such cases as basal cell adenoma, indeterminate type, and advise prolonged follow-up of the patient.

The most important differential diagnosis of basal cell adenoma, particularly the non-membranous type, is adenoid cystic carcinoma. Useful pointers to adenoma include lack of invasiveness and cytological pleomorphism, low mitotic activity, and whorled eddies of epithelial cells, none of which are seen in adenoid cystic carcinoma. The membranous type of basal cell adenoma often closely resembles basal cell adenocarcinoma (see below), in which cytological pleomorphism and mitotic figures may be absent. Adenomas may be poorly circumscribed but lack the true invasiveness of the malignant counterpart.

Canalicular adenoma

Another tumour with a basaloid appearance is canalicular adenoma. Its location is almost exclusively intraoral, particularly affecting the upper lip

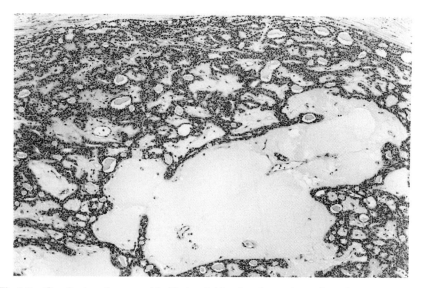

Fig 8.2.   Canalicular adenoma with thin basaloid trabeculae set in a pale oedematous stroma. H&E × 80.

(Kratochvil 1991). As a result, most tumours present when small – rarely more than 2 cm in diameter. It has a characteristic morphology of anastomosing bi-layered strands of darkly staining epithelial cells set in a loose vascular stroma (Fig. 8.2). There is no pleomorphism or significant mitotic activity. Not infrequently, they are multifocal (Daley 1984), and can thus mimic the true invasiveness of a cribriform adenoid cystic carcinoma. The lack of destructiveness and the presence of blood vessels in the cribriform spaces are the best guides to canalicular adenoma. They also display uniform strong positivity for S100 protein, whereas this is negative or only patchily expressed in adenoid cystic carcinoma.

CARCINOMAS

Polymorphous low grade adenocarcinoma (terminal duct carcinoma)

Tumours that earlier classifications described simply as adenocarcinoma of the salivary gland are now recognized to include several distinct clinicopathological entities. Amongst these, polymorphous low grade adenocarcinoma (PLGA) was first identified by Batsakis et al (1983) and by Freedman & Lumerman (1983). The vast majority of cases arise in intraoral minor salivary glands, particularly in the palate where it is the second commonest malignancy after adenoid cystic carcinoma. Much less frequently, cases have been described in the parotid, sometimes as the malignant component of a carcinoma in pleomorphic adenoma (Tortoledo et al 1984), but also *de novo*

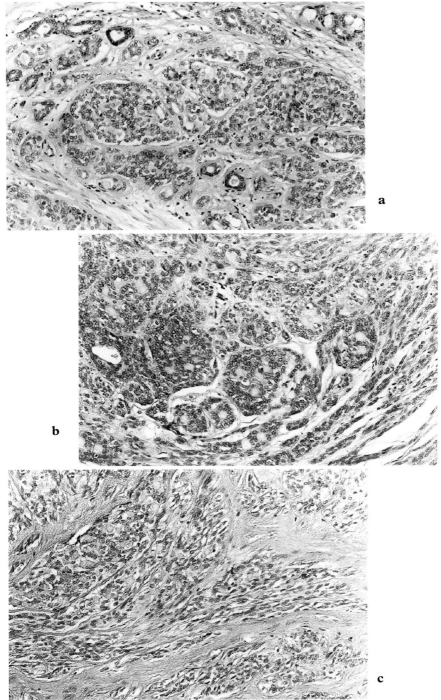

Fig 8.3 a–c. Polymorphous low grade adenocarcinoma – three different areas from the same tumour, illustrating the morphological diversity and cytological uniformity. H&E × 160.

(Kemp et al 1995). Microscopically, PLGA is characterized by cytological uniformity and morphological diversity (Fig. 8.3). It has cells with regular bland nuclei arranged in a variety of patterns, including ducts, cribriform and solid structures and diffuse infiltration with Indian filing, at times reminiscent of lobular carcinoma of the breast, particularly when there is concentric growth around nerves. The stroma also varies from fibromyxoid to densely hyaline, but the chondroid matrix of a pleomorphic adenoma is not seen. Immunohistochemistry shows positivity for epithelial markers such as cytokeratin and epithelial membrane antigen (EMA), as well as for S100 protein and vimentin. The pattern may be patchy, reflecting the morphological diversity and possibly, areas of varying differentiation. As its name suggests, the behaviour of PLGA is malignant but of low aggressiveness; according to a recent literature review, there is a recurrence rate of 21%, regional nodal metastasis in 6.5%, distant metastasis in 1.8%, and death due to cancer in 0.9% (Kemp et al 1995).

The most important differential diagnosis is adenoid cystic carcinoma, in which even the tubulo-trabecular type (grade 1) pursues a much more aggressive and eventually fatal course in over 60% of cases (Szanto et al 1984). Both tumours invade surrounding tissue including bone. At a cytological level, however, the nuclei in adenoid cystic carcinoma are seen to be more hyperchromatic, angulated, pleomorphic and densely packed: in contrast, the nuclei in PLGA are uniform with finely speckled chromatin. They frequently display vacuolation not unlike papillary carcinoma of the thyroid (Simpson et al 1991c), which electron microscopy shows to be due to cytoplasmic indentations (Dardick & van Nostrand 1988). In addition, the proliferation marker MIB 1, which recognizes Ki-67 on paraffin sections, may be of some help: in a series of 14 PLGAs, between 0.2 and 6.4% of nuclei stained for MIB 1, in contrast to 20 adenoid cystic carcinomas where positivity ranged from 11.3 to 56.7% (Simpson & Skálová 1995).

Closely related to PLGA is a tumour described as low grade papillary adenocarcinoma (Mills et al 1984). Exactly how closely related is still an unresolved question, as indeed is the place of papillary cystadenocarcinoma, which is accorded a separate category in the revised WHO classification. Most but not all studies (Colmenero et al 1992) have shown that these papillary carcinomas are slightly but significantly more aggressive. For example, figures from a review of admittedly only a few cases, give a local recurrence rate of 47%, cervical lymph node metastasis in 40%, distant metastasis in 7% and death due to disease in 13% (Batsakis & El-Naggar 1991). Some authors have therefore advocated that it should be completely separated from PLGA (Wenig & Gnepp 1991). However, others including Batsakis & El-Naggar (1991) considered that they all lie within the same spectrum. Probably the best approach is that of Slootweg (1993) who, in a series of 22 cases, tabulated the various histopathological features and concluded that papillary structures formed part of the spectrum of PLGA, as they were often seen in lesions with lobular, cribriform, and tubulo-trabecular areas. However, in two of the tumours in this series papillary structures constituted the only component, and it was concluded that these should be classified separately as papillary cystadenocarcinoma.

Epithelial-myoepithelial carcinoma

Another of the more recently established forms of adenocarcinoma is epithelial-myoepithelial carcinoma. This tumour had been previously described as glycogen-rich clear cell adenoma (Corridan 1956, Feyrter 1963) and was illustrated as such in the first edition of the WHO classification, before its true nature as a malignant tumour (Epithelial-myoepitheliales Schaltstück-carcinom) was first recognized by Donath et al (1972).

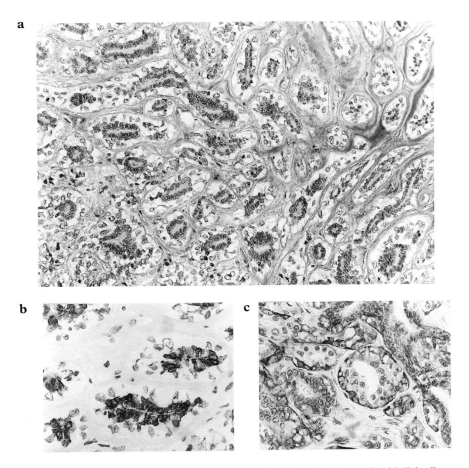

Fig 8.4. (a) Epithelial-myoepithelial carcinoma showing ducts lined by small epithelial cells surrounded by clear myoepithelial cells and an outer rim of basement membrane material. PASD × 160. (b) The inner cells express cytokeratin. AE1 × 240. (c) The outer cells express myoepithelial marker αSMA × 240.

It occurs predominantly in the parotid, though cases have been reported in the submandibular gland, intra-oral minor salivary glands, the maxillary antrum (Batsakis et al 1992) and the bronchus (Nistal et al 1994), as well as arising in a pleomorphic adenoma (Littman & Alguacil-Garcia 1987). The microscopic appearance is characterized by small ductular lumina lined by two layers of cells with striking immunohistochemical differences (Fig. 8.4), which are also reflected ultrastructurally (Brocheriou et al 1991). The inner layer comprises cytokeratin positive epithelial cells, and it is surrounded by an outer mantle of myoepithelial cells which express α smooth muscle actin. S100 protein also stains the outer cells strongly, but is less specific and sometimes reacts with the inner layer (Skálová & Michal 1990, Jones et al 1992). The outer cells are in turn surrounded by a rim of PAS positive basement membrane material of variable thickness. This pattern is reproduced throughout most of the tumour, though each element may vary in prominence among cases as well as within any given lesion. Grossly the tumours often appear to be well circumscribed, but microscopy usually reveals invasion of blood vessels, nerves or surrounding salivary tissue. Cytological pleomorphism is not usual, but mitotic figures can be quite numerous in places.

The most characteristic appearance of epithelial-myoepithelial carcinoma is that of a clear cell tumour, due to plentiful cytoplasmic glycogen within myoepithelial cells. In contrast, the epithelial cells are small and cuboidal, and on occasion may be difficult to identify unless highlighted by cytokeratin staining. The differential diagnosis of tumours with this appearance encompasses a wide range of other salivary neoplasms composed of optically clear cells (Table 8.2).

Table 8.2 Salivary tumours that may display prominent clear cells

Tumours	Characteristics
Benign	
Oncocytic hyperplasia }	PTAH +, mitochondria ++ on EM
Oncocytoma }	
Myoepithelioma	S100 +, CK +, αSMA variable
Pleomorphic adenoma	Myxochondroid stroma, ducts, myoepithelial cells
Sebaceous adenoma	Foam cells, lipid+
Malignant	
Acinic cell carcinoma	PASD + granules, PTAH −
Mucoepidermoid carcinoma	Goblet (mucinous), squamous & intermediate cells
Epithelial-myoepithelial ca.	Double lining of ducts:– inner CK +, outer S100 +, αSMA +
Sebaceous carcinoma	Foam cells, lipid +.
Malignant myoepithelioma	Collagenous spherules +, areas of necrosis usual
	Spindle cells ±, S100 +, αSMA+ (most cells)
Hyalinizing (monomorphic)	
clear cell carcinoma	Single population. CK +, S100 negative
Metastatic renal carcinoma	Vascular. Abdominal ultrasound +

Less frequently, other patterns of epithelial-myoepithelial carcinoma can occur, and the diagnosis may not at first be obvious. This is particularly the case when prominent basement membrane material forms a dense hyaline stroma in which the bi-layered ducts are relatively inconspicuous. This can be mistaken for a pleomorphic adenoma (Simpson et al 1991b), but in doubtful cases adequate sampling should demonstrate invasive behaviour.

Diagnostic difficulties can also arise on occasions when one element of an epithelial-myoepithelial carcinoma appears to dedifferentiate and overgrows much of the rest of the lesion. This can take the form of a high grade adenocarcinoma or a sarcomatoid spindle cell neoplasm of myoepithelial type (Simpson et al 1991b). Another unusual feature of epithelial-myoepithelial carcinoma is that apparent collision tumours, though uncommon, seem to arise more frequently than would be expected purely by chance. For example, Corio (1991) described a parotid neoplasm composed of epithelial-myoepithelial, adenoid cystic and basal cell adenocarcinomatous areas. In addition, and possibly related, is the unusual case reported by Di Palma (1994) of a typical epithelial-myoepithelial carcinoma in a parotid gland which also contained multiple nodules of intercalated duct hyperplasia. This suggests a probable ductal origin of the tumour. Furthermore, it is possible to speculate that this could be the reason for the appearance of some of the combination tumours, as two or more hyperplastic foci may differentiate along diverging pathways and then become neoplastic.

The behaviour of epithelial-myoepithelial carcinoma has up to now generally been considered low grade, and in a literature review of 67 cases by Batsakis et al (1992), recurrences were noted in 31%, cervical lymph node metastasis in 18%, distant metastasis in 7%, and death attributable to the neoplasm in 7%. Subsequently, however, in a disturbing series reported by Fonseca & Soares (1993), 50% recurred and 40% of patients died of cancer. The only morphological feature found to be correlated to a poor prognosis was the presence of nuclear atypia in more than 20% of the tumour cells.

From these studies and my own observations, it is likely that epithelial-myoepithelial carcinoma encompasses a broader range of appearances than has up to now been accepted, and consequently, this tumour does not always have the relatively indolent growth that initial reports suggested.

Basal cell adenocarcinoma

This is a malignant tumour with the architecture and cytology of basal cell adenoma but it shows infiltration. Most cases of basal cell adenocarcinoma are found in the parotid gland in patients over 50 years of age. There is an equal sex incidence. It is not clear what proportion arises *de novo* or in pre-existing lesions, but Batsakis & Luna (1991) suggested in their review that 11 out of 37 (29.7%) developed from a pre-existing basal cell adenoma of membranous type. Microscopically, the general morphological and cytological appearances are almost identical to basal cell adenoma and likewise, four growth patterns are recognized – solid, tubular, trabecular and membranous – though these are not thought to have prognostic significance. The tumour islands contain a mixture of large and small basaloid cells, with the latter sometimes demonstrating peripheral palisading, though this is less marked than in the benign counterpart. The large cells sometimes form eddies, and the tumour islands may also contain small tubules. The amount of basement membrane material varies but can be marked, especially in the membranous variant. Occasional cases show cytological pleomorphism but generally this is absent, and mitotic figures are usually sparse. The most reliable indicator of malignancy is infiltration of the surrounding gland, and less frequently of blood vessels and nerves.

The differential diagnosis of basal cell adenocarcinoma includes solid forms of adenoid cystic carcinoma, which are much more aggressive neoplasms with cytological pleomorphism and plentiful mitotic figures; these are generally associated with other growth patterns such as cribriform structures. The tumours described by Gallimore et al (1994) appear to fall in between and possibly represent a rare high grade form of basal cell adenocarcinoma.

Apart from the study of Gallimore et al (1994), the behaviour of most basal cell adenocarcinomas is low grade. In the series of Ellis & Wiscovitch (1990), 7 out of 29 tumours recurred, three metastasized to lymph nodes and lungs, and one patient died of disseminated disease. It is possible, however, that this may be a slight underestimate of the true malignant potential as follow up periods were short in some cases.

Salivary duct carcinoma

This tumour may not be as rare as previously thought (Di Palma et al 1993, Hellquist et al 1994). Most patients are over 50 years old and there is an approximately 3:1 male predominance. Salivary duct carcinoma arises almost exclusively in the major glands, especially the parotid, though very occasionally cases have been described in the minor glands of the palate (Delgado et al 1993), buccal mucosa (Pesce et al 1986), maxilla (Kumar et al 1993) and larynx (Ferlito et al 1981), as well as in a pre-existing pleomorphic adenoma (Grenko et al 1995). Microscopically, salivary duct carcinoma bears a striking resemblance to ductal carcinoma of the breast (Fig. 8.5). This similarity is seen not only in the invasive element, but also in the *in situ* change in ducts, where all of the features of the mammary equivalent can be reproduced, from Roman bridges to comedo-necrosis. Both *in situ* and invasive carcinoma show considerable nuclear pleomorphism and nucleoli may be prominent. The tumour cells possess plentiful cytoplasm which is usually eosinophilic. Mitotic figures are often numerous, and other markers of cell proliferation, such as nuclear expression of MIB 1 are high (Hellquist et al 1994). The stroma is often densely sclerotic, comprising fibrous and, to a lesser extent, elastic tissue. PAS positive mucin may be present in small quantities, but if copious, an alternative diagnosis such as high grade

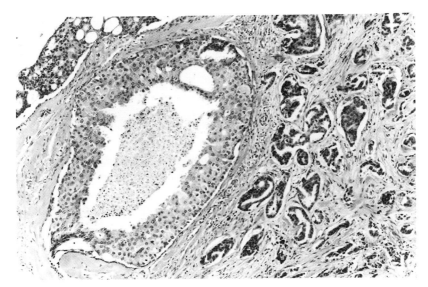

Fig 8.5. Salivary duct carcinoma showing invasive and *in situ* comedo-carcinoma; note the close resemblance to ductal breast cancer. H&E × 80.

mucoepidermoid carcinoma must be considered. This is, however, more of academic interest than of practical value, as both are aggressive malignancies with poor survival rates. A more important differential diagnosis is metastatic carcinoma, particularly from the prostate or breast. Positive staining for Prostate Specific Antigen (PSA) has been reported in a range of primary salivary gland neoplasms (van Krieken 1993), but these findings have not been confirmed. Metastatic breast carcinoma is microscopically identical to salivary duct carcinoma and differentiation must be made on clinical grounds.

The prognosis of salivary duct carcinoma is poor, and most series have shown that more than 70% of patients die of disease, usually within three years. There are no clinical or histopathological prognostic indicators: size was at one time considered to be important, and it was suggested that tumours with a diameter of less than 3 cm had a better prognosis (Hui et al 1986). However, several fatal lesions with a diameter of 2 cm or less have been reported (Brandwein et al 1990, Simpson et al 1991a, Colmenero Ruiz et al 1993, Grenko et al 1995). Determination of tumour DNA ploidy has not been found to have prognostic significance (Barnes et al 1994, Grenko et al 1995), but it is possible that MIB 1 activity might do so (Hellquist et al 1994).

Despite the morphological resemblance of salivary duct carcinoma to breast carcinoma, Hellquist et al (1994) were unable to show convincing evidence of either progesterone or oestrogen receptors, though equivocal nuclear staining was seen in a few cases. Therefore, any role for hormonal therapy or drugs such as tamoxifen is uncertain and treatment remains surgical excision followed by radiotherapy to the tumour bed.

Malignant myoepithelioma (myoepithelial carcinoma)

This tumour can be defined as a malignant epithelial neoplasm in which the predominant differentiation of the tumour cells is myoepithelial. As such, it has been accorded a separate category in both new classifications. Although relatively few cases have been described, malignant myoepithelioma may be less rare than previously supposed. The largest series to date is the ten cases of Di Palma & Guzzo (1993); of these, eight occurred in the parotid and two were intra-oral. The sex incidence was about equal.

There is a similar range of histological appearances to benign myoepithelioma, the malignant counterpart also being composed of spindle cells (sometimes their shape is more round or stellate) or plasmacytoid cells which express S100 protein, vimentin, cytokeratin and sometimes α smooth muscle actin. For the diagnosis of malignancy, the presence of cytological abnormalities, an increased mitotic rate, necrosis and, particularly, invasiveness are the most useful criteria.

Clear cells have occasionally been described as a minor component in malignant myoepithelioma (Tortoledo et al 1984, Takeda 1992, Di Palma & Guzzo 1993) and may rarely be the predominant cell type (Klijanienko et al 1989, Ogawa et al 1991, Cassidy & Connolly 1994, Michal et al 1996). This variant may also arise in both major and minor glands. Microscopy shows lobules made up of relatively uniform clear cells, sometimes with a minor component of spindle cells, in addition to plentiful basement membrane material, foci of collagenous spherulosis and zones of necrosis. Ducts are absent or scanty, and areas with the dimorphic appearance of epithelial-myoepithelial carcinoma are lacking.

Whatever its cell type, malignant myoepithelioma can arise either *de novo* or in a recurrent pleomorphic adenoma. Tumours arising *de novo* tend to be more aggressive locally and have a greater metastatic potential whilst a tumour that develops in a benign lesion often has a long clinical history and shows only local aggressiveness. Di Palma & Guzzo (1993) suggested that there was a continuum from pleomorphic adenoma with a tendency to recur through to frankly malignant myoepithelioma capable of metastasis.

Hyalinizing (monomorphic) clear cell carcinoma

The unqualified terms 'clear cell tumour' and 'clear cell carcinoma' are not diagnostic entities, because a wide range of growths in the salivary glands may be microscopically characterized by non-mucinous clear cells. Such tumours or tumour-like lesions are mostly variants of established entities, but the existence of a carcinoma composed entirely of a single population of clear cells was first recognized by Skorpil (1937, 1940), who called it 'lamprocytic' carcinoma. Although a few isolated reports appeared afterwards, it was Chen (1983) who proposed dividing clear cell carcinomas into dimorphic (i.e. epithelial-myoepithelial carcinoma) and monomorphic types. Even then,

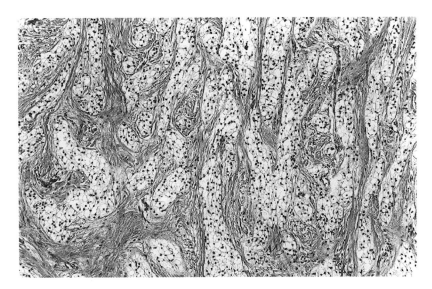

Fig 8.6.   Hyalinizing clear cell carcinoma showing invasive groups of a monomorphic population of clear cells separated by hyaline fibrous bands. H&E × 160.

uncertainty about the nature of the latter has persisted, compounded by inconsistent results with immunohistochemistry, especially for S100 protein. This problem can be resolved by considering monomorphic clear cell carcinoma as comprising not one but two distinct entities – one myoepithelial and the other epithelial.

Clear cell malignant myoepithelioma has been discussed above. In contrast, several studies have shown that there is a low grade carcinoma composed of a single population of clear epithelial cells often set in a dense stroma, hence the accepted term, hyalinizing clear cell carcinoma (Simpson et al 1990, Ogawa et al 1991, Milchgrub et al 1994). It was not included in the revised WHO classification, but it is now accepted as an entity by Seifert (1995). Most cases arise in the minor salivary glands of adults, and though some tumours appear grossly circumscribed, all are in fact invasive. Microscopy shows sheets and ribbons of box-like cells with distinct borders and apparently empty cytoplasm (Fig. 8.6). They vary in size and may be relatively small, particularly at the invasive edge. Nuclei also are small and uniform, but may on occasions show a minor degree of pleomorphism. Mitotic figures are generally rare. The stroma may be inconspicuous or there may be dense hyalinizing fibrous bands. Special stains show variable amounts of glycogen in the cytoplasm of tumour cells, and some extracellular mucin may be present, possibly reflecting overwhelmed non-neoplastic mucinous salivary glands. Immunohistochemistry shows positivity for epithelial markers, especially cytokeratins, but S100 protein and α smooth muscle actin are not expressed. This is in contrast to myoepithelial neoplasms with clear cell change, which express either or both of these markers. Electron microscopy of hyalinizing clear cell carcinoma shows no evidence of myoepithelial differentiation but some display squamous features such as desmosomes. In addition, four out of six cases studied by Milchgrub et al (1994) showed microvilli protruding into intracytoplasmic lumina.

The behaviour of hyalinizing clear cell carcinoma is generally that of a low grade malignant tumour, but cervical lymph node metastases can occur (Mohamed 1976, Milchgrub et al 1994). Local excision is probably adequate treatment in most patients.

The differential diagnosis encompasses other tumours in the salivary glands composed of optically clear cells, most of which are malignant (Table 8.2). There are exceptions, for example oncocytic lesions, especially multifocal nodular oncocytic hyperplasia, which is not even neoplastic. Similarly, a clear cell variant of benign myoepithelioma undoubtedly exists but it is rare. Amongst malignant tumours, many that were previously called clear cell tumour or carcinoma are now recognized to be epithelial-myoepithelial carcinoma, as discussed above. In addition, several primary malignancies of the salivary glands have clear cell variants. It is a relatively rare pattern in acinic cell carcinoma, occurring in 6% of cases (Ellis & Corio 1983). The clarity is possibly only a fixation artefact, and cells with characteristic zymogen granules are always found. In mucoepidermoid carcinoma, many of the clear cells contain mucin, but others do not. If the latter are plentiful, the tumour can closely resemble hyalinizing clear cell carcinoma (Ogawa et al 1992). Arguably, the most important differential diagnosis is metastatic disease. Clear cell variants of melanoma and thyroid carcinoma can be excluded immunohistochemically with S100 protein, HMB 45 and thyroglobulin, but renal cell carcinoma is more of a problem. The prominent vascularity is often a useful clue, but other morphological and immunohistochemical features are inconsistent. In practice, the best approach is to look for a primary tumour in the kidneys by appropriate imaging techniques.

MALIGNANCY IN PLEOMORPHIC ADENOMA
(Malignant mixed tumour)

Pleomorphic adenoma may recur if surgery has been inadequate, but a different process altogether is that of secondary malignant change. This is a well recognized event, occurring in 3–4% of all pleomorphic adenomas. It is partly dependent on time, as the risk increases from 1.5% with a 5 year history of a benign tumour to 9.5% after more than 15 years. The nature of the malignancy may take one of four forms in descending order of frequency: carcinoma, malignant myoepithelioma, carcinosarcoma and metastasizing pleomorphic adenoma.

Several different types of purely epithelial malignancy can develop in a pleomorphic adenoma, though acinic cell carcinoma probably does not and adenoid cystic and mucoepidermoid carcinomas do so only rarely. The commonest patterns are poorly differentiated ductal and undifferentiated carcinomas (Nagao et al 1981). In the malignant areas, epithelial cells display an increased nuclear-cytoplasmic ratio and frequent mitotic figures, which may be abnormal. Not all carcinomas are aggressive, as polymorphous low grade adenocarcinoma may occur. Histological type certainly has prognostic implications, but probably more important is the extent of the invasion beyond the capsule of the original benign tumour. In the series of Tortoledo et al (1984), no patient died if the carcinoma was restricted to the pre-existing pleomorphic adenoma or showed invasion of less than 0.6 cm beyond the capsule. In contrast, all patients whose neoplasm extended to more than 0.8 cm died as a consequence. These included one patient with a polymorphous low grade adenocarcinoma, though eight other patients with tumours of the same type that were less invasive survived.

Considering the predominance of myoepithelial cells in pleomorphic adenomas, it is surprising that so few examples of malignant myoepithelioma arising from them have been reported. The largest series is five cases of Di Palma & Guzzo (1993), whilst Tortoledo et al (1984) reported three cases. These figures may represent an underestimate. Nagao et al (1981) reported 48 cases of carcinoma in pleomorphic adenomas; of these, 56% were described as 'undifferentiated carcinoma', which they suggested were perhaps of myoepithelial origin. The evidence was based on some not altogether specific ultrastructural similarities to myoepithelial cells. These findings remain unconfirmed, and this area warrants further investigation, including immunohistochemical studies.

True malignant mixed tumour (i.e. carcinosarcoma) is extremely rare, and only eight examples were found in the AFIP Registry (Gnepp & Wenig 1991). About half of all reported cases had a history of a previous pleomorphic adenoma. Microscopy shows malignancy of both the epithelial and mesenchymal elements – the former is usually a high grade adenocarcinoma and the latter is most often a chondrosarcoma, or occasionally a fibrosarcoma or osteosarcoma. About 60% of all reported patients with carcinosarcoma died of disseminated disease.

Metastasizing pleomorphic adenoma is very rare. Systemic dissemination of an apparently unremarkable pleomorphic adenoma occurs, the reason for this behaviour being unknown. Retrospective analysis of various histological variables (e.g. mitotic count, infiltrative growth) and flow cytometry has failed to identify criteria that predict the development of metastases. Secondary deposits may be found in lymph nodes and in distant sites such as lungs, kidneys and bones, and the outcome may be fatal (Wenig et al 1992).

Several questions about malignancy in a pleomorphic adenoma remain unanswered. These include, in particular, the proportion of malignant myoepitheliomas, the importance of the histopathological subclassification of the carcinomatous element, and whether invasion beyond 0.8 cm. is really the prognostic milestone that has been proposed. New techniques may in due course provide some of the answers but they have so far been disappointing. For example, a study of 10 carcinomas ex pleomorphic adenoma with known clinical outcome showed no significant association of prognosis with c-*erb*B-2 expression or amplification (Müller et al 1994). Perhaps, more promisingly, Deguchi et al (1993) found that activation of c-*myc* and *ras* p21 proto-oncogenes and p53 mutation may play important rôles in the malignant transformation of pleomorphic adenoma, but they did not relate these findings to clinical outcome.

In practice, the diagnosis of malignancy in a pleomorphic adenoma can be made with certainty only if there is true extracapsular invasion, abnormal mitotic figures, or metastasis. Cellular atypia, increased mitotic activity, necrosis and haemorrhage are worrying but do not in themselves confirm malignancy. Nevertheless, these features should always raise suspicion, and such tumours must be sampled as completely as possible.

ONCOCYTOMA AND ONCOCYTIC LESIONS

Oncocytic change was first named as such (*onkocyten*) by Hamperl (1931) to describe cells with abundant eosinophilic and granular cytoplasm, subsequently seen by electron microscopy to be due to numerous mitochondria. Tumours composed of such cells are seen in many organs, such as the kidney, thyroid and parathyroid. In the salivary glands, oncocytic cells characterize the epithelial element of Warthin's tumour. They are also found now and again in a variety of tumours such as pleomorphic adenoma (Palmer et al 1990), basal cell adenoma, and mucoepidermoid carcinoma (Ferreiro & Stylopoulos 1995). In addition, they characterize a much smaller range of neoplasms and tumour-like lesions, where oncocytic cells are the defining element. Diagnostic difficulties may arise especially if the cells lose their cytoplasmic eosinophilia, and give the appearance of clear cells. This may be due to either artefact or the accumulation of glycogen.

Apart from electron microscopy, the best method for demonstrating the mitochondria is phosphotungstic acid haematoxylin (PTAH) after 48 hour incubation (Brandwein & Huvos 1991), where they stain dark blue. In contrast, they are usually negative with PAS after diastase digestion. These staining reactions are the converse of those of the granules in acinic cell carcinoma. Oncocytic cells express cytokeratins but not S100 protein or α smooth muscle actin.

Non-neoplastic lesions characterized by oncocytes include focal oncocytosis, in which there is focal metaplasia of ducts and, to a lesser extent, acini. This change is not uncommonly seen with advancing age. In contrast, diffuse oncocytosis is very rare, and consists of complete metaplasia of all ductal and acinar cells in a parotid gland. It is thought to be due to an intracellular metabolic disorder of mitochondria.

Multifocal nodular oncocytic hyperplasia (MNOH) is often bilateral. It consists of large and small nodules of oncocytes, which often show clear cell

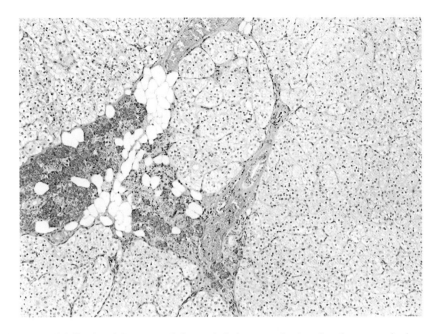

Fig 8.7. Multifocal nodular oncocytic hyperplasia is a metaplastic rather than a neoplastic process. It is often bilateral and composed of clear cells. H&E × 95.

change (Fig. 8.7). Sometimes, this takes the form of a single large lesion surrounded by much smaller satellite nodules in an otherwise normal gland.

At times a true encapsulated oncocytoma develops against the background of MNOH. The relation between the two has been compared to changes in thyroid adenomatous goitre versus adenoma, and is more obvious grossly than microscopically (Brandwein & Huvos 1991). In such cases, the tumour is generally composed of clear cells. Oncocytoma may occasionally have this appearance when it arises in an otherwise normal gland (Ellis 1988), but more often, it consists of cells with granular, light and dark, eosinophilic cytoplasm (Palmer et al 1990). The component cells, whether typically oncocytic or clear, are arranged in solid sheets or in nests and cords, which then form alveolar or organoid patterns. Some of these structures have small central lumina. A minor degree of cellular atypia with nuclear hyperchromatism and pleomorphism may be allowable (Goode 1991), but not to the extent seen in invasive oncocytic carcinoma. In addition, a mild chronic inflammatory cell infiltrate may be present. There is, therefore, a possible overlap with stroma-poor Warthin's tumour, where the lymphoid tissue is only patchy. The only value in making the distinction between the two is that Warthin's tumour is more likely to be multifocal or bilateral (Eveson 1992).

Other differential diagnoses of oncocytoma include pleomorphic adenoma with oncocytic change, which has a fibrous or myxochondroid stroma and, sometimes, psammoma bodies may be present (Palmer et al 1990). The differential diagnoses of the clear cell variant is summarized in Table 8.2.

Oncocytic carcinoma is a rare malignancy of the elderly and only a few dozen cases have been reported. The tumour is composed of oncocytes which show mitotic activity and nuclear pleomorphism, as well as invasion of surrounding tissues and blood vessels (Goode & Corio 1988). Perineural infiltration is also characteristic, but it has been described in non-metastasizing tumours – whether these were really benign or low grade malignancies was not apparent. However, it is likely that necrosis is a more reliable indicator of poor patient outcome (Brandwein & Huvos 1991). The literature is limited, but the consensus is that oncocytic carcinoma is an aggressive tumour with over half of reported patients either dying of disease or suffering recurrences (Scher et al 1991).

KEY POINTS FOR CLINICAL PRACTICE

1. Salivary gland tumours should be assessed using either the revised WHO or AFIP classifications.

2. The term 'monomorphic adenoma' is not a diagnostic category, as it includes various distinct entities, some of which are closely related to pleomorphic adenoma.

3. Adenocarcinoma includes several entities ranging from the relatively indolent polymorphous low grade adenocarcinoma to the usually fatal salivary duct carcinoma.

4. Many different salivary tumours are characterized by clear cells – most are malignant.

5. Malignancy develops in 3–4% of pleomorphic adenomas, the incidence increasing with time. Histological type and, especially, extent of invasion are important prognostic indicators.

REFERENCES

Adam P, Joubert M, Meyer-Seiler C et al 1994 Récidive aggressive d'une tumeur mixte des glandes salivaires accessoires à fort contingent myoépithélial. Rev Stomatol Chir Maxillofac 95: 427–430

Alós L L, Ribé A, Bombi J A et al 1995 Myoepithelial tumors of major and minor salivary glands. A clinicopathologic, immunohistochemical and flow cytometric study. Pathol Res Pract 191: 606 (abstract)

Barnes L, Appel B N, Perez H et al 1985 Myoepitheliomas of the head and neck: case report and review. J Surg Oncol 28: 21–28

Barnes L, Rao U, Krause J et al 1994 Salivary duct carcinoma: Part I. A clinicopathologic evaluation and DNA image analysis of 13 cases with review of the literature. Oral Surg Oral Med Oral Pathol 78: 64–73

Batsakis J G 1979 Tumors of the head and neck: clinical and pathological considerations. 2nd edn. Williams and Wilkins, Baltimore. p 9

Batsakis J G, El-Naggar A K 1991 Terminal duct adenocarcinoma of salivary tissues. Ann Otol Rhinol Laryngol 100: 251–253

Batsakis J G, Luna M A 1991 Basaloid salivary carcinoma. Ann Otol Rhinol Laryngol 100: 785–787

Batsakis J G, Luna M A, El-Naggar A K 1991 Basaloid monomorphic adenomas. Ann Otol Rhinol Laryngol 100: 687–690

Batsakis J G, El-Naggar A K, Luna M A 1992 Epithelial-myoepithelial carcinoma of salivary glands. Ann Otol Rhinol Laryngol 101: 540–542

Batsakis J G, Pinkston G R, Luna M A et al 1983 Adenocarcinomas of the oral cavity: a clinicopathologic study of terminal duct carcinomas. J Laryngol Otol 97: 825–835

Brandwein M S, Huvos A G 1991 Oncocytic tumors of major salivary glands: a study of 68 cases with follow-up of 44 patients. Am J Surg Pathol 15: 514–528

Brandwein M S, Jagirdar J, Patil J et al 1990 Salivary duct carcinoma (cribriform salivary carcinoma of excretory ducts): a clinicopathologic and immunohistochemical study of 12 cases. Cancer 65: 2307–2314

Brocheriou C, Auriol M, de Roquancourt A et al 1991 Carcinome épithélial-myoépithélial des glandes salivaires: étude de 15 observations et revue de la littérature. Ann Pathol (Paris) 11: 316–325

Cassidy M, Connolly C E 1994 Clear cell carcinoma arising in a pleomorphic adenoma of the submandibular gland. J Laryngol Otol 108: 529–532

Chen K T K 1983 Clear cell carcinoma of the salivary gland. Hum Pathol 13: 91–93

Colmenero C M, Patron M, Burgueño M et al 1992 Polymorphous low-grade adenocarcinoma of the oral cavity: a report of 14 cases. J Oral Maxillofac Surg 50: 595–600

Colmenero Ruiz C, Patrón Romero M, Martín Pérez 1993 Salivary duct carcinoma: a report of nine cases. J Oral Maxillofac Surg 51: 641–646

Corio R L 1991 Epithelial-myoepithelial carcinoma. In: Ellis G L, Auclair P L, Gnepp D R (eds) Surgical pathology of the salivary glands. Saunders, Philadelphia. pp 412–421

Corridan M 1956 Glycogen-rich clear-cell adenoma of the parotid gland. J Pathol Bacteriol 72: 623–626

Daley T D 1984 The canalicular adenoma: considerations on differential diagnosis and treatment. J Oral Maxillofac Surg 42: 728–730

Dardick I, van Nostrand A W P 1988 Polymorphous low-grade adenocarcinoma: a case report with ultrastructural findings. Oral Surg Oral Med Oral Pathol 66: 459–465

Dardick I, Thomas M J, van Nostrand A W P 1989 Myoepithelioma – new concepts of histology and classification: a light and electron microscopic study. Ultrastruct Pathol 13: 187–224

Deguchi H, Hamano H, Hayashi Y 1993 c-myc, ras p21 and p53 expression in pleomorphic adenoma and its malignant form of the human salivary glands. Acta Pathol Jpn 43: 413–422

Delgado R, Vuitch F, Albores-Saavedra J 1993 Salivary duct carcinoma. Cancer 72: 1503–1512

Di Palma S 1994 Epithelial-myoepithelial carcinoma with co-existing multifocal intercalated duct hyperplasia of the parotid gland. Histopathology 25: 494–496

Di Palma S, Guzzo M 1993 Malignant myoepithelioma of salivary glands: clinicopathological features of ten cases. Virchows Archiv A Pathol Anat 423: 389–396

Di Palma S, Guzzo M, Eveson J W 1993 Salivary duct carcinoma – a highly malignant tumour with close resemblance to breast ductal carcinoma. Pathol Res Pract 189: 681 (abstract)

Donath K, Seifert G, Schmitz R 1972 Zur Diagnose und Ultrastruktur des tubulären Speichelgangcarcinoms: Epithelial-myoepitheliales Schaltstückcarcinom. Virchows Archiv A Pathol Anat 356: 16–31

Ellis G L 1988 'Clear cell' oncocytoma of salivary gland. Hum Pathol 19: 862–867

Ellis G L, Auclair P L 1991 Classification of salivary gland neoplasms. In: Ellis G L, Auclair P L, Gnepp D R (eds) Surgical pathology of the salivary glands. Saunders, Philadelphia. pp 129–134

Ellis G L, Corio R L 1983 Acinic cell carcinoma: a clinicopathologic analysis of 294 cases. Cancer 52: 542–549

Ellis G L, Wiscovitch J G 1990 Basal cell adenocarcinomas of the major salivary glands. Oral Surg Oral Med Oral Pathol 69: 461–469

Evans R W, Cruickshank A H 1970 Epithelial tumours of the salivary glands. Saunders, Philadelphia. pp 19

Eveson J W 1992 Troublesome tumours 2: borderline tumours of salivary glands. J Clin Pathol 45: 369–377

Ferlito A, Gale N, Hvala H 1981 Laryngeal salivary duct carcinoma: a light and electron microscopic study. J Laryngol Otol 95: 731–738

Ferreiro J A, Stylopoulos N 1995 Oncocytic differentiation in salivary gland tumours. J Laryngol Otol 109: 569–571

Feyrter F 1963 Über das glykogenreiche retikulierte Adenom der Speicheldrüsen. Zeitschrift für Krebsforschung 65: 446–454

Fonseca I, Soares J 1993 Epithelial-myoepithelial carcinoma of the salivary glands. A study of 22 cases. Virchows Archiv A Pathol Anat 422: 389–396

Foote F W Jr, Frazell E L 1954 Atlas of tumor pathology. Section IV. Fascicle 11. Tumors of the major salivary glands. Armed Forces Institute of Pathology, Washington D.C. pp 8

Freedman P D, Lumerman H 1983 Lobular carcinoma of intraoral minor salivary gland origin: report of twelve cases. Oral Surg Oral Med Oral Pathol 56: 157–165

Gallimore A, Spraggs P, Allen J et al 1994 Basaloid carcinomas of salivary glands: a clinicopathological and immunohistochemical study. Histopathology 24: 139–144

Gnepp D R, Wenig B M 1991 Malignant mixed tumors. In: Ellis G L, Auclair P L, Gnepp D R (eds) Surgical pathology of the salivary glands. Saunders, Philadelphia. pp 350–368

Goode R K 1991 Oncocytoma. In: Ellis G L, Auclair P L, Gnepp D R (eds) Surgical pathology of the salivary glands. Saunders, Philadelphia. pp 225–237

Goode R K, Corio R L 1988 Oncocytic adenocarcinoma of salivary glands. Oral Surg Oral Med Oral Pathol 65: 61–66

Grenko R T, Gemryd P, Tytor M et al 1995 Salivary duct carcinoma. Histopathology 26: 261–266

Hamperl H 1931 Onkocyten und Geschwulste der Speicheldrusen. Virchows Archiv A Anat Pathol 282: 724–736

Hellquist H B, Karlsson M G, Nilsson C 1994 Salivary duct carcinoma – a highly aggressive salivary gland tumour with overexpression of c-erbB-2. J Pathol 172: 35–44

Hui K K, Batsakis J G, Luna M A et al 1986 Salivary duct adenocarcinoma: a high grade malignancy. J Laryngol Otol 100: 105–114

Jones H, Moshtael F, Simpson R H W 1992 Immunoreactivity of α smooth muscle actin in salivary gland tumours: a comparison with S 100 protein. J Clin Pathol 45: 938–940

Kemp B L, Batsakis J G, El-Naggar A K et al 1995 Terminal duct adenocarcinomas of the parotid gland. J Laryngol Otol 109: 466–468

Klijanienko J, Micheau C, Schwabb G et al 1989 Clear cell carcinoma arising in pleomorphic adenoma of the minor salivary gland. J Laryngol Otol 103: 789–791

Kratochvil F J 1991 Canalicular adenoma and basal cell adenoma. In: Ellis G L, Auclair P L, Gnepp D R (eds) Surgical pathology of the salivary glands. Saunders, Philadelphia. pp 202–224

Kumar R V, Kini L, Bhargava A K et al 1993 Salivary duct carcinoma. J Surg Oncol 54: 193–198

Littman C D, Alguacil-Garcia A 1987 Clear cell carcinoma arising in a pleomorphic adenoma of the salivary gland. Am J Clin Pathol 88: 239–243

Michal M, Skálová A, Simpson R H W et al 1996 Clear cell malignant myoepithelioma of the salivary glands. Histopathology 28: 309–315

Milchgrub S, Gnepp DR, Vuitch F et al 1994 Hyalinizing clear cell carcinoma of the salivary gland. Am J Surg Pathol 18: 74–82

Mills S E, Garland T A, Allen M S 1984 Low grade papillary adenocarcinoma of palatal salivary gland origin. Am J Surg Pathol 8: 367–374

Mohamed A H 1976 Ultrastructure of glycogen-rich clear cell carcinoma of the palate. J Oral Pathol 5: 103–121

Müller S, Vigneswaran N, Gansler T et al 1994 c-erbB-2 Oncoprotein expression and amplification in pleomorphic adenoma and carcinoma ex pleomorphic adenoma: relationship to prognosis. Modern Pathol 7: 628–632

Nagao K, Matsuzaki O, Saiga H et al 1981 Histopathologic studies on carcinoma in pleomorphic adenoma of the parotid gland. Cancer 48: 113–121

Ng W K, Ma L 1995 Pleomorphic adenoma with extensive lipometaplasia. Histopathology 27: 285–288

Nistal M, García-Viera M, Martínez-García C et al 1994 Epithelial-myoepithelial tumor of the bronchus. Am J Surg Pathol 18: 421–425

Ogawa I, Nikai H, Takata T et al 1991 Clear cell tumors of minor salivary gland origin: an immunohistochemical and ultrastuctural analysis. Oral Surg Oral Med Oral Pathol 72: 200–207

Ogawa I, Nikai H, Takata T et al 1992 Clear-cell variant of mucoepidermoid carcinoma: report of a case with immunohistochemical and ultrastructural observations. J Oral Maxillofac Surg 50: 906–910

Palmer T J, Gleeson M J, Eveson J W et al 1990 Oncocytic adenomas and oncocytic hyperplasia of salivary glands: a clinicopathological study of 26 cases. Histopathology 16: 487–493

Pesce C, Colacino R, Buffa P 1986 Duct carcinoma of the minor salivary glands: a case report. J Laryngol Otol 100: 611–613

Scher R L, Feldman P S, Lambert P R 1991 Oncocytic malignancy of the parotid gland. Otolaryngology – Head Neck Surg 105: 868–876

Sciubba J J, Brannon R B 1982 Myoepithelioma of salivary glands: report of 23 cases, Cancer 49: 562–572

Seifert G 1995 Differential diagnosis of clear cell and basal cell tumours of the salivary glands. Pathol Res Pract 191: 774 (abstract)

Seifert G, Sobin L H 1991 World Health Organization international histological classification of tumours: histological typing of salivary gland tumours. 2nd edn. Springer-Verlag, Berlin

Seifert G, Miehlke A, Haubrich J et al 1986 Diseases of the salivary glands: Pathology – Diagnosis – Treatment – Facial nerve surgery. Georg Thieme Verlag, Stuttgart. pp 171–285

Simpson R H W, Kitara-Okot P 1995 Clear cell salivary myoepithelioma. Pathol Res Pract 191: 780 (abstract)

Simpson R H W, Skálová A 1995 MIB 1 in polymorphous low grade adenocarcinoma and adenoid cystic carcinoma of the salivary glands. Pathol Res Pract 191: 779–780 (abstract)

Simpson R H W, Sarsfield P T L, Clarke T J et al 1990 Clear cell carcinoma of minor salivary glands. Histopathology 17: 433–438

Simpson R H W, Clarke T J, Sarsfield P T L et al 1991a Salivary duct adenocarcinoma. Histopathology 18: 229–235

Simpson R H W, Clarke T J, Sarsfield P T L et al 1991b Epithelial-myoepithelial carcinoma of salivary glands. J Clin Pathol 44: 419–423

Simpson R H W, Clarke T J, Sarsfield P T L et al 1991c Polymorphous low grade adenocarcinoma of the salivary glands: a clinicopathological comparison with adenoid cystic carcinoma. Histopathology 19: 121–129

Simpson R H W, Jones H, Beasley P 1995 Benign myoepithelioma of the salivary glands: a true entity? Histopathology 27: 1–9

Skálová A, Michal M 1990 Epimyoepithelial carcinoma of parotid gland. Zentralbl allg Pathol pathol Anat 136: 715–718

Skálová A, Leivo I, Michal M et al 1992 Analysis of collagen isotopes in crystalloid structures of salivary gland tumors. Hum Pathol 23: 748–754

Skorpil F 1937 K. Pathologické anatomii a histologii epithelovych nádoru slinnychzlaz. Prometheus, Praha

Skorpil F 1940 Über das Speicheldrüsenadenom. Virchows Archiv A Anat Pathol 306: 714–736

Slootweg P J 1993 Low-grade adenocarcinoma of the oral cavity: polymorphous or papillary? J Oral Pathol Med 22: 327–330

Szanto P A, Luna M A, Tortoledo M E et al 1984 Histologic grading of adenoid cystic carcinoma of the salivary glands. Cancer 54: 1062–1069

Takeda Y 1992 Malignant myoepithelioma of minor salivary gland origin. Acta Pathol Jpn 42: 518–522

Thackray A C, Sobin L H 1972 Histological typing of salivary gland tumours. World Health Organization, Geneva

Thackray A C, Lucas R B 1974 Tumors of the major salivary glands. Fascicle 10. 2nd series. Armed Forces Institute of Pathology, Washington D.C

Tortoledo M E, Luna M A, Batsakis J G 1984 Carcinomas ex pleomorphic adenoma and malignant mixed tumors: histomorphologic indexes. Arch Otolaryngol 110: 172–186

van Krieken J H J M 1993 Prostate marker immunoreactivity in salivary gland neoplasms: a rare pitfall in immunohistochemistry. Am J Surg Pathol 17: 410–414

Wenig B M, Gnepp D R 1991 Polymorphous low-grade adenocarcinoma of minor salivary glands. In: Ellis G L, Auclair P L, Gnepp D R (eds) Surgical pathology of the salivary glands. Saunders, Philadelphia. pp 390–411

Wenig B M, Hitchcock C L, Ellis G L et al 1992 Metastasizing mixed tumor of salivary glands: a clinicopathologic and flow cytometric analysis. Am J Surg Pathol 16: 845–858

9

Paediatric solid tumours

N. M. Smith, J. W. Keeling

The commonest solid tumours of early life are the embryonal tumours, so called because of their histological resemblance to stages of development of organs during embryonic and fetal life. The more frequent occurrence of embryonal tumours in individuals with certain syndromes and the familial occurrence of some of them promoted the concept of errors of development as important factors in their genesis. It was suggested that these observations were consistent with a two mutation model, where the initial error was a germ line mutation (Knudson & Strong 1972). It is now thought that many more stages are involved (Bolande 1995). More recently the demonstration of one or more chromosome abnormalities in either the host individual or the tumour has reinforced the view of a more complex chain of pre- and post-natal events.

These observations have practical importance, such as the need to organise long term protective medication or regular screening for individuals at risk. They also mean that biopsies from tumours in children should be handled according to a predetermined protocol so that essential investigations are not omitted.

Rapid and accurate diagnosis on tumours of children has become increasingly important as more specific (and toxic) chemotherapeutic regimes have evolved. The recognition of good or adverse prognostic features currently affects the choice of therapy of several tumours and it is likely that this will become more common. It is particularly important that in children, whose normal tissues are more sensitive to chemotherapy, a minimal yet adequate treatment is administered. Thus, the histopathologist's report influences therapy directly.

SPECIMEN HANDLING

Three important steps are necessary in order to make the best use of biopsy material from a child's tumour. The first is good liaison between clinician and histopathologist so that the laboratory is forewarned about the biopsy and accurate clinical information is available at the outset. The second is that the biopsy reaches the laboratory promptly and in a fresh, unfixed state. The third is that tumours are handled in the laboratory in a consistent fashion,

Table 9.1 Locations and types of cytogenetic abnormalities in childhood solid tumours

Neuroblastoma	1p- HSRs on chromosome 2 Double minutes	1p36 11	1pter-1p32 14q
PNET/Ewing's sarcoma	t(11q;22)(q24;q12) der (16)	t(11;22)(2,14,17,18) t(1;16)(q21;q13)	Trisomy 8 12q13-14
Desmoplastic small round cell tumour	t(11;22) (p13;q12)		
Nephroblastoma	del 11p13 11p15 16q	Partial trisomy 1q 12 7p	del 22 18
Extra-renal nephroblastoma	t(10;11) (q24;p15)		
Malignant rhabdoid tumour of kidney	22q 11		
Congenital mesoblastic nephroma	Trisomy 11	12q13-15	
Clear cell sarcoma of kidney	t(2;22) (q21;q11)	t(10;17)	
Hepatoblastoma	del 2q Trisomy 20 t(10;22)(q26;q11)	t(2;4) LOH at 11p15	Trisomy 2 del 17p
Rhabdomyosarcoma Embryonal	t(2;8) (q37;q13) 3p Trisomy 8 2q37	del 1p21-qter Trisomy 2 1q21 13q14	LOH at 11p15 Trisomy 20 2p25
Alveolar	t(2;13)(q35-37;q14)	t(1;13) (p36;q14)	
Alveolar soft part sarcoma	17q25		
Extra-renal rhabdoid tumour	t(11;22)(p15.5;q11.23)		
Pleuropulmonary blastoma	del 2q	Partial trisomy 2	
Malignant peripheral nerve sheath tumour	Monosomy 22		
Synovial sarcoma	t(X;18) (p11; q11.2)		

Non-Hodgkin's lymphoma
  Burkitt type
  Anaplastic large cell
  (Ki-1)
	t(8;14) (q24;q32)
	t(2;5) (p23;q35)
		t(8;22)(q24;q11)	t(2;8) (q13;q24)

Hodgkin's lymphoma	13p	14q32	t(2;5) (p23;q35)

LOH: Loss of heterozygosity   HSRs: Homogeneously staining regions

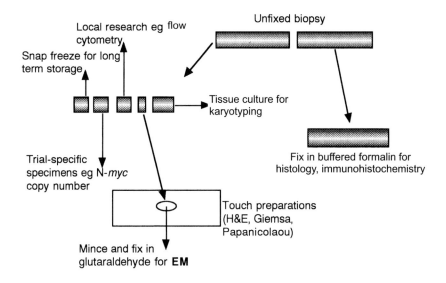

Fig. 9.1 Handling a paediatric tumour biopsy

according to a clearly drawn up and agreed protocol such as shown in Figure 9.1. Ideally, all of the procedures indicated should be carried out but biopsies are sometimes so small that it may be necessary to restrict these to the most appropriate. A well fixed sample for histology and immunohistochemistry and fresh tissue for culture and karyotyping are vital (Table 9.1).

Molecular techniques

The ability to relate phenotype to genotype has transformed the field of oncology and many laboratories and all paediatric pathologists require some level of understanding in this area (Demetrick 1994). Developments in fluorescent and immunologically detected in situ hybridization and increasing numbers of probes have realised the potential for examination of fresh and archival material for cytogenetic abnormalities. Aneuploidy is readily demonstrable (Poddighe et al 1992) and tumour-specific translocations such as t(11;22)(q24;q12) seen in the Ewing's sarcoma/PNET group of tumours are identifiable using such techniques on touch imprints (McManus et al 1995). Polymerase chain reaction (PCR) techniques are also available in the search for tumour-specific nucleic acid sequences, such as the EWS-FLI-I fusion transcript resulting from the t(11;22)(q24;q12) translocation (Downing et al 1993). The development of a related technique applicable to archival material will undoubtedly be highly informative (Williams & Williams 1995), and correlation of PCR with histological features (in situ PCR) may soon be feasible (Pan et al 1995). Comparative genomic hybridization (CGH) has been used to demonstrate amplification of N-myc in neuroblastomas and alveolar rhabdomyosarcomas (Bayani et al 1995).

Flow cytometry

DNA flow cytometry is used to quantify DNA content by assessing the ploidy status of a given tumour, and this may be predictive of tumour behaviour, response to therapy and prognosis (Brodeur et al 1992). Retrospective studies are enhanced by extension of this technique to formalin-fixed, paraffin embedded material (Dressler et al 1993).

Cytology

A well established technique in adult oncology, fine needle aspiration cytology (FNAC) is a relatively recent addition to paediatric practice and is still not used widely, possibly due to the lack of co-operation anticipated from younger patients. FNAC has been found to be useful in a wide variety of benign and malignant tumours (Buchino 1991). The diagnosis of primary and recurrent round 'blue' cell tumours of childhood is possible using ancillary tests such as immunohistochemistry, electron microscopy (McGahey et al 1992) and cytogenetics (Sreekantaiah et al 1992). Cytological examination of imprints and smears can be helpful when only a limited amount of tissue has been obtained at surgery and can conserve the sample for more useful studies (Wakely et al 1993). Peroperative diagnostic frozen section is difficult to justify in modern practice.

Autopsy

The importance of postmortem examination in the understanding of neoplasia at the molecular level has recently been emphasised (Kleiner et al 1995). In paediatric oncology the value of the autopsy has been shown by the discovery of findings which, if known in life, would have altered management. In up to a quarter of cases there may be an unsuspected infection by agents such as candida, aspergillus, *E coli* and pseudomonas, and pulmonary emboli and acute renal failure may also feature (Koszyca et al 1993). Changes in management of children with tumours mean that most now die at home and this is reducing an already low rate of autopsy in such cases. This low rate seems to be due to a combination of a low expectation of significant findings in an intensively investigated group and a reluctance to seek permission from bereaved families with whom clinical staff may have had a long and close relationship. The former is no more likely to be true in this group of patients than in other patients cared for in active academic units in whom postmortem examination has revealed significant numbers of unsuspected treatable conditions (Shanks et al 1990, Veress & Alafuzoff 1994).

Late effects of chemotherapy

As the efficacy of treatments for childhood cancer has improved over the last three decades, a significant number of patients have survived to early adulthood, almost 1 in 1000 of this age group. Two thirds of deaths are then due to recurrence of the primary tumour. Others die from second malignancy, ischaemic heart disease, chronic infection, and pneumonia or other respiratory problems (Nicholson et al 1994).

Much of the morbidity observed in these patients is related to tumour therapy, currently a combination of anti-cancer drugs, perhaps with the addition of radiotherapy. Some drugs are particularly associated with a risk of secondary leukaemia. VP16, VM26, cyclophosphamide, ifosfamide, chlorambucil, melphalan, busulphan, CCNU, BCNU, estramustine, thiotepa, nitrogen mustard, dacarbazine and procarbazine are noteworthy in this respect (Kissen & Wallace 1995). Although the overall risk is low, of the order of 1.2-1.3% over 10 years (Pui et al 1990), patients treated for non-Hodgkin lymphoma in the early 1980s are at higher risk, possibly because of the inclusion of radiotherapy in the treatment protocol at that time (Hawkins 1990). Tissues and organs within radiotherapy fields are at increased risk of malignant change (Scaradavou et al 1995); tumours of thyroid, breast, liver, intestines, bone and skin and soft tissue tumours have all been described. Non-neoplastic sequelae, such as deformity as a result of epiphyseal damage, are also recognised (Kissen & Wallace 1995). Cardiomyopathy is seen during and after anthracycline therapy; the extent of myocardial damage correlates with total drug dose (Pihkala et al 1994).

NEUROBLASTOMA

After leukaemias, CNS tumours and lymphomas, neuroblastoma is the next commonest childhood malignancy, affecting 1 in 100 000 children under 15 years of age and comprising 10% of tumours in this age group. Most of these tumours occur between birth and 5 years and neuroblastoma is an occasional cause of fetal hydrops when it arises during late fetal life. Amongst congenital tumours, 30-50% are neuroblastomas.

The classification of neuroblastoma is intimately related to grading and prognostic features (Beckwith & Martin, 1968, Shimada et al 1984). The study of Joshi et al (1992) revealed several histological features associated with better prognosis which included the presence of ganglion cells, tumour giant cells, a low (<10 per 10 high power fields) mitotic count, and focal calcification. A grading system has been proposed based on the low mitotic count as defined and the presence of calcification: Grade 1 – both features present; Grade 2 – one feature present; Grade 3 – neither feature present.

This grading system was shown to relate to prognosis better than the degree of differentiation or the age of the patient. Grade 1 and 2 tumours are more likely to be associated with good prognosis factors such as a serum lactate dehydrogenase level of less than 1500 iu/l, a single copy of N-myc, and hyper-diploid genome (Joshi et al 1993a).

Other biological factors shown to be of value in prognosis include the serum ferritin, and neuron specific enolase (NSE) levels (Brodeur et al 1993). Tumour expression of the *trk A* - encoded p140 receptor protein for nerve growth factor may be detected by immunohistochemistry and is also associated with a favourable outcome (Tanaka et al 1995).

Cytogenetics

Cytogenetic studies of neuroblastoma have concentrated on chromosome 1, as loss of material from the short arm of this chromosome has been observed in some cases. At least two tumour suppressor genes have been postulated at 1p36 and 1pter-1p32 and loss of the latter is associated with a poor prognosis (Takeda et al 1994). The 1p36 deletion has been reported as a constitutional finding in a child who developed neuroblastoma at 5 months of age and inheritance of this anomaly may mimic the apparently autosomal dominant pattern seen in a number of families (Biegel et al 1993). This deletion has been demonstrated in paraffin sections of neuroblastoma by in situ hybridization (Stock et al 1993). However, abnormalities of other chromosomes, including 14q and 11, have also been reported in neuroblastoma, suggesting that these loci may be involved in the pathogenesis of some cases (Srivatsan et al 1993).

Extensive studies of various gene products have been conducted in an attempt to relate these to outcome. The expression of protein gene product 9.5 (PGP9.5), p110 (Ramani & Dewchand 1995) and p53 (Wang et al 1995) have not yet demonstrated such a correlation. High levels of Ha-ras p21 have been shown to be associated with a favourable prognosis (Tanaka et al 1991), and conversely, there is a strong correlation between over-expression of N-myc and a poor outcome (Hiyama et al 1991). The over-expression of the apoptosis-suppressing protein bcl-2 has been shown to be an unfavourable factor in some studies (Castle et al 1993) but not others (Ramani & Lu 1994).

Abnormalities of apoptosis may explain the phenomenon of stage 4s disease, where spontaneous regression occurs in young infants (<1 yr) with neuroblastoma involving liver, bone marrow and subcutaneous tissues, but not cortical bone or lymph nodes (Pritchard & Hickman 1994). Relapse after apparent spontaneous regression of stage 4s disease indicates a possible overlap of stage 4s with stage 4 disease or a further mutation in susceptible cells (De Bernardi et al 1992, Pritchard & Hickman 1994).

Immunohistochemistry

In round 'blue' cell tumours of childhood, a panel of antibodies has become available for diagnosis and, to a limited degree, as an indicator of maturation. Those recommended include NSE, pan-neurofilament, chromogranins, vasoactive intestinal peptide (VIP), PGP9.5 and S100 protein (Wirnsberger et al

1992). A negative reaction for myogenic and leucocyte antigens must also be established.

Fine needle aspiration cytology

The cytological features of neuroblastoma correlate with its histological appearances, and cytological examination has been advocated as a primary diagnostic procedure and for the confirmation of metastatic disease (Joshi et al 1993b). There seems little chance of widespread acceptance of the technique, however, while tumour handling protocols require relatively large amounts of fresh, unfixed material for N-myc or other biological studies. The rapid development of molecular techniques is likely to reduce the need for large samples and lead to wider use of fine needle aspiration in this context, as the use of immunohistochemistry and EM is already established (Buchino 1991).

PRIMITIVE NEUROECTODERMAL TUMOUR (PNET)/EWING'S SARCOMA

Cytogenetic analysis of fresh tumour specimens has made a particular contribution to the understanding of the relationship between PNET and both soft tissue and skeletal Ewing's sarcoma. The finding of a common cytogenetic abnormality, t(11;22)(q24;q12), suggests that a phenotypic spectrum exists, from undifferentiated Ewing's sarcoma to PNET with neural morphological markers such as rosettes and positivity for 'neural' markers such as NSE, PGP9.5 and S100 (Carter et al 1990, Anon 1992, Dehner 1993). Tumours ultimately deemed PNET tend to have a worse prognosis (Anon 1992). The gene at 11q24 is referred to as FLI-1 and encodes a transcription factor. In the product of the translocated chromosome the DNA-binding domain of the FLI-1 protein is associated with the product of the EWS gene at 22q 12 which is an RNA binding protein (Zucman et al 1993). Antibodies to the abnormal protein product are becoming available (A McManus, personal communication), and demonstration of the chromosome lesion t(11;22)(q24;q12) by in situ hybridization is well established in some centres (Pinkerton et al 1994, McManus et al 1995).

Immunohistochemistry is more useful in the diagnosis of PNET/Ewing's sarcoma since antibodies were introduced against the product of the MIC2 gene present on the X and Y chromosomes, which is a cell surface glycoprotein (Perlman et al 1994, Weidner & Tjoe 1994). This protein is overexpressed in PNET/Ewing's sarcoma but positive staining must be interpreted as part of a panel of antibody reactions, as positivity has also been seen in normal tissues, rhabdomyosarcomas, ovarian granulosa cell tumours and T-lymphocytes (Ramani et al 1993, Chan et al 1995, Loo et al 1995). The involvement of the p53 protein in some of these tumours is suggested by the finding of amplification of the MDM2 gene at 12q13, which codes for a p53-binding protein in some cases (Ladanyi et al 1995).

Interestingly, aesthesioneuroblastoma, a locally aggressive round 'blue' cell tumour of the upper nasal passages and sinuses is negative for MIC2 by immunohistochemistry despite the reported presence of t(11;22) in derived cell lines (Nelson et al 1995).

INTRA-ABDOMINAL DESMOPLASTIC SMALL ROUND CELL TUMOUR

This tumour is also known as the intra-abdominal small round cell (or neu-roectodermal) tumour with divergent differentiation, and has a propensity for adolescent males (Gerald et al 1991, Variend et al 1991). The histological appearances are characteristic, with well defined islands of small round 'blue' cells separated by abundant fibroblastic stroma (Gerald et al 1991). A translocation involving the EWS gene on chromosome 22 has been observed in this tumour, t(11;22)(p13;q12) which, in this case, also involves the WTI gene at 11p13 (Sawyer et al 1992). The gene product is as yet unidentified but there is no over-expression of MIC2 which would enable the distinction from PNET/Ewing's sarcoma to be made (Resnick & Donovan 1995). The prognosis of desmoplastic small round cell tumour is poor.

RENAL TUMOURS

Primary renal tumours are the fourth commonest solid tumour of childhood (Stiller & Bunch 1990). They are also the subject of a significant therapeutic success with major improvements in 5 year survival (and cure) particularly for nephroblastoma. The relative proportions of tumour types are tabulated in Table 9.2.

Nephroblastoma

Many recent advances in our understanding of the significance of the pathol-ogy and biology of nephroblastoma are due to the work of the National

Table 9.2 Frequency of primary renal tumours of childhood. After Beckwith (1994)

Type of tumour	%
Nephroblastoma (Wilms' tumour)	85
Non-anaplastic	80
Anaplastic	5
Mesoblastic nephroma	5
Classical	1
Cellular	4
Clear cell sarcoma	4
Malignant rhabdoid tumour	2
Miscellaneous	4

Wilms' Tumour Study (NWTS). The classic histological pattern consists of an admixture of blastemal, stromal and epithelial elements, though biphasic and monomorphic tumours are not uncommon. Each component can exhibit a wide variety of histological patterns and differentiation which, in the absence of anaplasia, are of no prognostic significance. Blastemal cells are small, non-epithelial, non-stromal cells with little cytoplasm. They may manifest a diffuse, monomorphic pattern, a serpentine pattern with anastomosing cords separated by myxoid background, or a nodular pattern with rounded nests of blastema. Epithelial cells may exhibit tubular, glomeruloid, papillary, mucinous, squamous, neural and neuroendocrine patterns. Stromal cells include myxoid, fibroblastic, leiomyomatoid, rhabdomyoblastic, adipose, chondroid, osteoid or bone and neurogenic types.

Given the variety of cell types potentially present in nephroblastoma, current practice avoids terms such as 'fetal rhabdomyomatomous nephroblastoma' which are descriptive but do not provide prognostic information (Beckwith 1994).

Prognosis of nephroblastoma

Tumour staging is important in Wilms' tumour as there are major differences in chemotherapy regimes between stages. Pathological examination of tumour specimens is an important part of staging, but can be adequately performed only if these tumours are received fresh and intact. A systematic approach to tumour examination is important. The staging of nephroblastoma is defined in Table 9.3. Stage I tumours are confined to the kidney. Tumours that penetrate the renal capsule or extend beyond the hilar plane of the renal sinus are stage II. The presence of tumour in abdominal lymph nodes indicates stage III. It is important that potentially misleading lesions such as epithelial inclusions, squamous cells from metaplastic urothelium, mesothelial clusters, megakaryocytes, lympho-histiocytic aggregates and prominent post-capillary venules in lymph nodes are correctly interpreted (Weeks et al 1990).

The most important marker of poor prognosis in nephroblastoma is the presence of anaplastic nuclear changes. These are defined as the presence of *all* of the following: nuclear enlargement which is at least threefold compared to adjacent nuclei of the same cell type; hyperchromasia of the enlarged nuclei; and enlarged or multipolar mitoses (each limb of an X or Y-shaped figure should be as large as a normal metaphase) (Zuppan et al 1988, Beckwith 1994). Anaplastic nuclear change may be diffuse or focal. Because anaplastic nuclear changes identify chemo-resistant tumours, the significance of the observation depends on tumour stage. In stage I, after complete excision of the tumour, no further treatment is necessary and prognosis remains favourable. However, in stage IV, the presence of diffuse anaplastic nuclear changes indicates a rapidly fatal outcome, although focal changes are not so significant (Beckwith JB 1993, personal communication).

Table 9.3 Staging of pediatric renal tumours according to the National Wilms' Tumour Study

Stage I	Tumour is limited to kidney and is completely resected Renal capsule is intact, not penetrated by tumour Sinus infiltration does not extend beyond hilus There is no extrarenal spread
Stage II	Tumour extends beyond kidney but is completely resected Tumour penetrates through renal capsule Sinus infiltration is beyond hilar plane Tumour is in renal vein Biopsy has been performed or local spillage has occurred but is confined to ipsilateral flank There is no residual tumour, and specimen margins are uninvolved
Stage III	Residual non-hematogenous tumour that is confined to abdomen Any abdominal nodes are involved There is diffuse peritoneal contamination by tumour There are peritoneal implants Tumour extends beyond specimen margins
Stage IV	Hematogenous metastases
Stage V	Bilateral renal tumours

Other factors indicative of good prognosis in stage I nephroblastoma are age less than 2 years at diagnosis and tumour specimen weight (combined weight of tumour and residual normal renal tissue removed at nephrectomy) of less than 550g (Green et al 1994).

In stage 2 or 3 tumours with favourable histology (i.e. non-anaplastic), the presence of tumour at the resection margin predicts the likelihood of abdominal recurrence and death (Breslow et al 1991) and aneuploidy also confers a poor prognosis (Gururangan et al 1992). Mutation of p53 has been observed in both favourable and unfavourable histology nephroblastoma, limiting its use in prognosis (Lemoine et al 1992, Bardeesy et al 1994).

In many centres chemotherapy is administered prior to nephrectomy, resulting in widespread necrosis of undifferentiated, proliferating elements and sparing of mature cell types such as rhabdomyoblasts and epithelia. Anaplastic nuclear changes are unchanged by treatment and retain their significance for prognosis (Brisigotti et al 1992). The assessment of proliferative activity by silver staining of nucleolar organising regions (Ag NORs) and immunostaining of proliferating cell nuclear antigen (PCNA) has been shown to relate to prognosis in post-chemotherapy nephroblastoma (Delahunt et al 1994).

Risk factors and precursors of nephroblastoma

Epidemiological studies have shown that parental environmental exposures might be associated with nephroblastoma. Olshan et al (1993) found no such

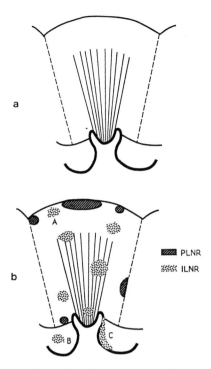

a

b

PLNR
ILNR

Fig. 9.2 (**a**) Diagram of renal lobe with adjoining calyx and intervening sinus. (**b**) Distribution of perilobar (PLNR) and intralobar (ILNR) nephrogenic rests. (After Beckwith JB et al 1990 Pediatr Pathol 10:1–36, with permission.)

links with maternal factors including smoking, coffee or tea consumption, hypertension, hormone exposure, hair dye use, infection during pregnancy, or high birthweight. It was suggested, however, that paternal factors such as occupation before conception were more important. Molecular and genetic studies of conditions predisposing to nephroblastoma, such as Wilms'-Aniridia-Genitourinary abnormalities-related mental Retardation (WAGR), Beckwith-Wiedemann, Denys-Drash and Bloom syndromes have implicated three genes, WT1, WT2 and WT3. The gene WT1 is located on chromosome 11p13 and encodes a DNA-binding protein which regulates events during nephrogenesis (Bard 1992); it has been shown to be partly deleted in WAGR with resultant homozygosity (Gessler et al 1993) and to contain mis-sense mutations in Denys-Drash syndrome. The occurrence of WT1 mutations in tumours of the gonads in Denys-Drash syndrome and acute myeloid leukaemia in a survivor of nephroblastoma suggests a wider role for this gene (Pritchard Jones et al 1994). However, abnormalities of WT1 are seen in a small number of sporadic childhood nephroblastomas. A WT2 locus at 11p15 close to the gene for Beckwith-Wiedemann syndrome is suggested, as is WT3, which is not on chromosome 11 and is yet to be identified (Hodgson & Maher 1993). Other chromosomes important in the pathogenesis of some cases of nephroblastoma include 7p, 12, 16q and 18 (Sawyer et al 1994, Brown et al 1993). The genes H-ras, K-ras, N-ras, p53 and RB are not implicated in Wilms' tumour (Waber et al 1993).

The expression of insulin-like growth factor binding protein II (IGFBP2) by the blastema of nephroblastoma has led to the suggestion that WT1 may exert an effect via regulation of this protein, for instance by altering expression of other growth factors and their receptors (Vincent et al 1994). The modes of action of the other WT genes have not yet been delineated, but abnormalities of insulin-like growth factor II have been reported in Beckwith-Wiedemann syndrome (Schneid et al 1993).

Nephrogenic rests and their significance

The biology and significance of persistent embryonal remnants in the kidney, nephrogenic rests, have been examined in depth in recent years (Beckwith et al 1990, Beckwith 1993, Bove et al 1995). Beckwith (1993) emphasised the biological differences between perilobar (PLNR) and intralobar (ILNR) nephrogenic rests (Fig. 9.2) and defined them in terms which imply a level of activity – regressing, sclerosing, obsolescent, hyperplastic, neoplastic and nephroblastomosis. Relationships between the different types are illustrated in Figure 9.3. Bove et al (1995) attempted to measure the activity of nephrogenic rests using the number of AgNORs and PCNA activity, the size of rests and nuclear morphology and cytoplasmic filament expression as an index of cell differentiation. This led to a better definition between dormancy or hyperplasia in nephrogenic rests and demonstrated differences between hyperplastic and neoplastic rests.

Both intralobar and perilobar nephrogenic rests are associated with bilateral nephroblastomas which tend to be synchronous in perilobar and metachronous

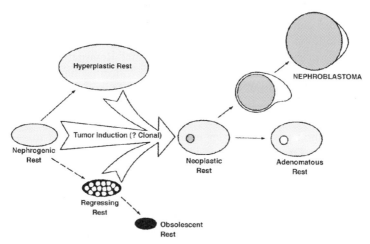

Fig. 9.3 Diagrammatic representation of rest fates. (After Beckwith JB et al 1990 Pediatr Pathol 10: 1–36, with permission)

in intralobar types. Nephrogenic rests are not the only precursors of nephroblastoma, as evidenced by familial cases of nephroblastoma where no such rests could be found. Nephroblastoma arising in association with intralobar rests presents significantly earlier than that associated with perilobar rests.

Extrarenal Wilms' tumours

Some of these tumours arise as the predominant component of teratoma (which must be excluded by wide sampling) and some are assumed to have developed in embryonic remnants or rests, such as ectopic metanephrogenic blastema (Sarode et al 1992), or in small renal duplications (Beckwith JB 1994, personal communication). This tumour most frequently arises in the retroperitoneum and presents as a mass or causes abdominal distension (Coppes et al 1991). It is identical in appearance to the Wilms' tumour in the kidney, exclusion of which is integral to the diagnosis, and seems to respond to similar, stage dependent chemotherapeutic regimes (Fahner et al 1993). The authors have seen a case that had a karyotype including t(10;11)(q24;p15), which is interesting given the association of renal Wilms' tumours with abnormalities of chromosome 11p (Heim & Mitelman 1992).

Multicystic renal tumours

Cystic renal tumours exhibit a range of appearances which relates to biological activity. At the histologically mature end of the spectrum are the benign cystic nephroma and the cystic partially differentiated nephroblastoma for which complete excision is curative. At the other end is the cystic variant of otherwise typical nephroblastoma. Benign cystic nephroma is a multiloculated cystic lesion with cysts lined by flattened epithelium and a stromal component which is entirely mature. It usually presents as a painless mass in the flank, but occasionally haematuria may be the presenting symptom. It is unlikely to be confused with partial or segmental renal dysplasia, being clearly demarcated from the adjacent normal kidney and lacking immature collecting ducts surrounded by concentric layers of mesenchyme. When the stroma includes immature, embryonal cell types such as islands of blastema or immature tubular or glomerular structures, the term cystic partially differentiated nephroblastoma is appropriate. Where the stromal component is indistinguishable from that of typical nephroblastoma, the tumour is categorised as a cystic nephroblastoma. (Domizio & Risdon 1991, Beckwith 1994).

Other renal tumours

Nephrogenic adenofibroma

This is a rare tumour of young people (mean age 13.3 years, range 3.5–23 years) characterised by a benign mesenchymal stroma surrounding tubulo-papillary blastema disposed in nodules (Hennigar & Beckwith 1992). It may be distinguished from nephroblastoma by a lack of encapsulation and an irregular margin which interdigitates with adjacent renal parenchyma. Derivation from multiple nephrogenic rests is postulated (Hennigar & Beckwith 1992). Although nephrectomy is curative, concurrent collecting duct carcinoma has been seen in association with nephrogenic adenofibroma. The distinction between nephrogenic adenofibroma and metanephric adenoma can be difficult; some cases appear to fulfil the criteria of more than one entity (Davis et al 1995).

Renin-secreting juxtaglomerular cell tumour

This is an unusual cause of hypertension in paediatric practice. The lesion is typically up to 5 cm in greatest dimension, encapsulated, and composed of cells with uniform round nuclei and abundant pale cytoplasm, which are arranged in sheets or nests separated by vascular septa. Renin content may be confirmed by immunohistochemical or electron microscopic examination (Abbi et al 1993) or by in situ hybridisation (Kodet et al 1994). The tumour may exhibit extra-capsular extension but behaves in a benign fashion (Kodet et al 1994).

Ossifying renal tumour of infancy

This tumour usually presents with haematuria. Most patients have been males and the tumours were solitary and left sided. The lesions appear to originate in the renal papillae and comprise varying proportions of an osteoid 'core' with osteoblasts and fusiform or epithelioid spindle cells. The tumour grows into the pelvicalyceal system and may superficially resemble a staghorn calculus. Origin from intralobular nephrogenic rests is postulated (Sotelo-Avila et al 1995).

Malignant rhabdoid tumour of kidney

This highly aggressive tumour occurs in a distinctly younger age group than nephroblastoma, with a median age of 13 months, and is rare over 5 years (Beckwith 1994). Despite intensive chemotherapy 1 year mortality is 75% and death occurs from widespread metastatic disease. The tumour is associated with hypercalcaemia and PNET of the posterior fossa. Histologically, a monomorphous, diffuse, invasive tumour is seen, composed of cells which ideally satisfy three criteria, namely abundant, variably eosinophilic cytoplasm, large vesicular nuclei with prominent central nucleoli, and a hyaline inclusion adjacent to the nucleus. Immunohistochemistry is positive for vimentin, cytokeratin and epithelial membrane antigen. Different areas in a tumour may show a variety of appearances, including spindle and epithelioid cells, a vascular or sclerosing stroma, but the classic pattern is usually also present (Beckwith 1994).

It is now apparent that rhabdoid-like or 'pseudo rhabdoid' cells may be seen in congenital mesoblastic nephroma, renal lymphoma, nephroblastoma, rhabdomyosarcoma and other tumours (Weeks et al 1991). Thus, a wide variety of tumours may mimic the appearance of malignant rhabdoid tumour, particularly in an extra-renal location.

Cytogenetic studies have shown that karyotypic changes are detectable in less than half of cases (Douglas et al 1990). Changes in chromosome 22 in the renal lesion and associated brain tumours are described (Fort et al 1994, Shashi et al 1994). Cell lines seem to express c-myc, rather than the N-myc expressed by nephroblastomas (Gansler et al 1991, Ota et al 1993).

Congenital mesoblastic nephroma

This is the commonest kidney tumour in the first year of life and presents during the first month in 70% of cases. Some achieve large size in fetal life and may cause hydrops. Of the two main types described, the classical is less common than the cellular (or atypical). Classical cases tend to arise as single central masses, have an indistinct margin, and exhibit early extension into hilar structures; this can render assessment of completeness of excision difficult. Microscopically this tumour shows a uniform, fibromatosis-like spindle cell appearance and it entraps islands of renal tissue which may undergo dysplastic changes (Beckwith 1994). In contrast, the cellular variant may be multifocal and arise within the classical form, has a sharp, distinct, pushing margin, and microscopically appears as a spindle 'blue' cell or plump cell tumour with higher cell density and mitotic count than the classical form. Both types may recur locally within a year if incompletely excised. Additionally, the cellular variant may metastasize commonly to lung, and invasion of the heart has also been described (Vujanic et al 1993).

The finding of concurrent perilobar nephrogenic rests in one case indicates a relationship between this tumour and nephroblastoma. It is suggested that the type of tumour which arises is determined by the stage of development at which the mutational event occurs (Vujanic et al 1995), before metanephric differentiation in the case of congenital mesoblastic nephroma and after this stage in nephroblastoma. This theory is supported by the lack of N-myc or WT1 expression in congenital mesoblastic nephroma, both factors expressed in the epithelium of the developing kidney and in nephroblastomas (Tomlinson et al 1992). The cytogenetics are more akin to leiomyoma than nephroblastoma, with trisomy 11 and breakpoints at 12q13-15, as described in leiomyoma (Carpenter et al 1993).

LIVER TUMOURS

Hepatoblastoma

Hepatoblastoma is the commonest malignant liver tumour in children in Europe and North America with an incidence of 1 in 100 000 (about eight new cases each year in the UK). Because this tumour is uncommon, significant numbers of cases can be reviewed only within collaborative projects. The amount of material from individual cases and the histological appearances of most tumours are variable hence attempts at classification have proved difficult. This probably explains the failure to confirm prognostic features between studies (Variend 1993). Classifications based on epithelial type only (Haas et al 1989) or on epithelial and mesenchymal components (Conran et al 1992) are both in current use. There is some evidence for a better prognosis in pure fetal type tumours (Weinberg & Finegold 1983, Haas et al 1989) whilst macrotrabecular and anaplastic tumours do worse (Haas et al 1989). Tumours which are completely resectable are most frequently of pure fetal type and resectability appears to be the most useful prognostic feature (Conran et al 1992).

Only a small number of cases have been subjected to DNA analysis. In the series of Conran et al (1992) this was of no prognostic value. Schmidt et al (1993) found that diploid tumours behaved more favourably but the difference did not reach statistical significance. Abnormalities of chromosomes 2, 17 and 20 have been reported in hepatoblastoma (Tonk et al 1994) as has loss of heterozygosity at 11p15.5 (Simms et al 1995). A single case report documents t(10;22)(q26;q11) in an undifferentiated hepatoblastoma (Hansen et al 1992). P53 protein expression has been described in small cell, embryonal and macrotrabecular hepatoblastoma (Ruck et al 1994, Chen et al 1995), and a possible prognostic link is postulated (Ruck et al 1994).

Undifferentiated (embryonal) sarcoma

Undifferentiated, or embryonal sarcoma of the liver is seen in older children. It has a distinctive histological appearance, with a thick pseudo-capsule and non-neoplastic bile duct remnants at the periphery of the tumour, which is composed of spindle cells, some with bizarre nuclear and cytoplasmic morphology (Leuschner et al 1990). Immunohistochemistry of this tumour reveals a diverse pattern of differentiation, with mesenchymal, muscle, epithelial and neural marker positivity (Variend 1993). The prognosis is poor, but cure is possible in those few cases where complete resection and chemotherapy are combined, and one third of patients will survive beyond 3 years (Leuschner et al 1990).

RHABDOMYOSARCOMA

Rhabdomyosarcoma is the commonest sarcoma in children. Classic sites are the head and neck and urogenital triangle. It can also arise in the limbs but less commonly. Table 9.4 shows the conventional classification of rhabdomyosarcoma as well as the recently devised scheme relating subtypes to prognosis.

Two recently defined subtypes are the *spindle cell/leiomyomatoid embryonal tumour* and the *solid alveolar* type. The former comprises approximately 5%

Table 9.4 Classifications of rhabdomyosarcoma (RMS)

Conventional classification (Enzinger & Weiss 1995) is:	
Embryonal RMS	botryoid
	spindle cell/leiomyomatoid
	conventional
Alveolar RMS	classic
	solid
Pleomorphic	
Classification relating histology to prognosis (Newton et al 1995)	
1. Superior prognosis	botryoid
	spindle cell/leiomyomatoid
2. Intermediate prognosis	embryonal
3. Poor prognosis	alveolar
	undifferentiated sarcoma
4. Prognosis not evaluable	rhabdoid features

of all cases (Wijnaendts et al 1994) but 27% of paratesticular rhabdomyosarcomas (Leuschner et al 1993). At this site it may be confused with
a fibrosarcoma. It is composed of spindle cells arranged in a storiform or
whorled arrangement. In most cases, individual cells show ovoid nuclei with
large nucleoli. In a minority, cytoplasmic eosinophilia and bundling of cells
produces a leiomyosarcomatoid pattern. Spindle cell/leiomyomatoid tumours
express vimentin and myoglobin more frequently than other varieties of rhabdomyosarcomas (Leuschner et al 1993). Paratesticular spindle cell/leio-
myomatoid tumour has a relatively favourable course, but in other sites this
histology confers a worse prognosis (Leuschner et al 1993). Solid alveolar
rhabdomyosarcoma has been defined on the basis of the cytological similarity
to the classic alveolar variety, both entities showing cells with large, round,
coarse, irregular nuclei and several prominent nucleoli in a solid compact con-
figuration. Solid alveolar tumours lack the discohesive areas seen in classic
alveolar rhabdomyosarcoma, and are composed of densely packed round cells
traversed and surrounded by dense fibrous tissue (Tsokos et al 1992). Small
numbers of multinucleated myoblastic or strap cells with cross-striation in the
cytoplasm may be present, as in the classic type. In the past, solid alveolar
rhabdomyosarcoma was probably placed in the embryonal subgroup on the
basis of the lack of an alveolar pattern. Correct designation of this tumour is
important, however, as it confers the same poor prognosis as the classic type
(Tsokos et al 1992).

The pleomorphic variant comprises about 3% of childhood rhabdomyosarcomas (Kodet et al 1993), predominantly as an anaplastic variant of the
embryonal type. Anaplasia, defined as 'the presence of cells with large lobated
nuclei at least three times larger than the common tumour cell population in
rhabdomyosarcoma', is an indicator of unfavourable prognosis (Kodet et al
1993). Grading is based on differentiation (assessed by the presence of rhabdomyoblasts), maturation (degree and pattern), proliferation (based on
mitotic activity and necrosis), and architecture (characterised by the presence

Table 9.5 Cytogenetic abnormalities in rhabdomyosarcoma

Embryonal:	Loss of heterozygosity at 11p15	(Scrable et al 1989)
	Trisomy 8	(Dietrich et al 1993)
	Trisomy 2	(Wang-Wuu et al 1988)
	1q21,2p25,2q37,13q14	(Whang-Peng et al 1992)
Alveolar:	t(2;13)(q35;q14)	(Biegel et al 1995)
	t(1;13)(p36;q14)	(Davis et al 1994)
	N-myc amplification	(Driman et al 1993)

of myxoid areas and fibrous septa), and it correlates well with clinical course (Wijnaendts et al 1994). In this study, the three features which correlated with a favourable outcome in all types of rhabdomyosarcomas were a high degree of maturation (the surface area of the cytoplasm exceeding that of the nucleus in the most mature rhabdomyoblasts), absence of tumour necrosis, and no fibrous septa.

Cytogenetic analysis of rhabdomyosarcoma has revealed differences between the various subtypes (Table 9.5). The t(2;13) is the most consistently detected abnormality, and is present in classic and solid alveolar tumours (Parham et al 1994a). This translocation brings part of the transcription factor gene PAX3 on chromosome 2 into proximity with a disrupted transcription factor gene on chromosome 13 termed FKHR (fork head in rhabdomyosarcoma); the resulting PAX3-FKHR transcript may promote tumour growth (Galili et al 1993). Changes seen in embryonal rhabdomyosarcoma are less characteristic. This may reflect difficulties in diagnosis with the inclusion of other primitive tumours in this group. This may be avoided in future by the use of monoclonal antibodies against the protein product of the MyoD1 gene, which encodes a nuclear phosphoprotein in skeletal muscle (Wesche et al 1995).

ALVEOLAR SOFT PART SARCOMA

Alveolar soft part sarcoma arising in childhood tends to affect the head and neck, particularly the orbit and tongue. The alveolar pattern caused by central detachment of cells in nests is sometimes less prominent in children than in adults but other typical features, e.g. PAS positive cytoplasmic crystals, are present. The immunohistochemical localisation of myosin and desmin (Sciot et al 1993), and the expression of nuclear phosphoprotein MyoD1 (Rosai et al 1991) strongly suggest skeletal muscle differentiation. Rearrangement of chromosome 17q has been described (Sciot et al 1993).

EXTRARENAL RHABDOID TUMOUR

Unlike the extrarenal Wilms' tumour, which is thought to arise from true ectopic renal elements, extrarenal rhabdoid tumours are a phenotypically similar but heterogeneous group (Parham et al 1994b). They have been reported in a variety of sites including brain, liver, soft tissue, skin, vulva, nasopharynx, tongue, orbit, heart, thymus, bladder, prostate and pelvis (Berry & Vujanic 1992). Diagnosis is based on the resemblance of the tumour cells to those of renal rhabdoid tumour, minimal criteria being large nucleoli, abundant cytoplasm and eosinophilic filamentous cytoplasmic inclusions. These 'rhabdoid' cells are, however, also seen as a component of a wide variety of other tumours including small cell tumours of childhood, malignant nerve sheath tumours, melanoma, hepatoblastoma and rhabdomyosarcoma (Parham et al 1994b). The characteristic immunohisto-chemical profile is positivity for vimentin, keratin and epithelial membrane antigen (Kodet et al 1991). Recently, scepticism has been expressed as to extrarenal rhabdoid tumour being an entity, as careful and exhaustive immunohistochemistry and electron microscopy may reveal features of dif-ferentiation indicating a more conventional diagnosis (Parham et al 1994b). A possible relationship with PNET/Ewing's sarcoma has been suggested on the basis of a t(11;22)(p15.5;q11.23) in one cell line (Karnes et al 1991). There remain, however, a group of tumours of this phenotype which defy all efforts to arrive at a more definitive diagnosis and it seems useful to refer to them by the terms 'primitive malignant tumour with rhabdoid features' (Berry & Vujanic 1992) or 'poorly differentiated neoplasm with rhabdoid fea-tures' (Parham et al 1994b).

UNUSUAL SARCOMAS

Infantile rhabdomyofibrosarcoma has recently been separated from infantile fibrosarcoma. This new entity has the fascicular spindle cell appearance of infantile fibrosarcoma, but shows metastatic potential, positivity for sarcom-ere-specific actin and desmin, and exhibits electron microscopic evidence of sarcomere-like structures. The cytogenetic abnormalities reported in infan-tile fibrosarcoma or rhabdomyosarcoma are not seen, but changes involving chromosomes 19 and 22 have been identified in infantile rhabdomyofibrosar-coma (Lundgren et al 1993).

PLEUROPULMONARY BLASTOMA

Pulmonary blastoma is a rare malignancy of lung which occurs most com-monly in adults. It is characterised by a mixture of malignant epithelial and blastemal-mesenchymal elements resembling fetal lung at 10-16 weeks of ges-tation. The childhood form of the tumour, pleuropulmonary blastoma, differs in several ways from the adult tumour. It can occur in extrapulmonary sites such as mediastinum and pleural cavity, it may be cystic (Hachitanda et al 1993), and the epithelial elements are not malignant. The mesenchymal-blastemal component may exhibit rhabdomyosarcomatous, chondrosarcomatous, osteosarcomatous, lipoblastic or anaplastic features (Sciot et al 1994) and is the sole component of any metastasis. Pleuropulmonary blastoma may arise in association with cystic adenomatoid malformation of the lung (Cohen et al 1991). A cytogenetic abnormality, partial trisomy of chromosome 2, is described. Similar karyotypic abnormalities have been seen in hepatoblastoma and embryonal rhabdomyosarcoma (Sciot et al 1994).

TUMOURS OF SKIN

Malignant melanoma and Spitz naevus

Malignant melanoma does occur in children but is extremely rare at about 6 per 850 000 biopsies (Mehregan & Mehregan 1993). Risk factors include transplacental spread of maternal melanoma, neurocutaneous melanosis, giant congenital naevus, multiple dysplastic naevi and xeroderma pigmentosum but primary nodular malignant melanoma can also occur (Mchregan & Mehregan 1993). The main differential diagnosis is Spitz naevus, and in some cases it may be impossible to distinguish between the two lesions. The occurrence of cutaneous lesions of Spitz type which metastasise to a single ipsilateral lymph node and do not disseminate further is also described (Smith et al 1989, Barnhill et al 1995). Such local spread must be distinguished from benign but atypical naevus cell aggregates in the capsule, perisinusoidal tissue, trabeculae and lymphatics, as seen, for example, in nodes draining congenital naevi (Hara 1993).

The features which favour a diagnosis of malignancy are the presence of atypical mitoses, mitoses at the margins, a high mitotic rate, ulceration, prominent pigment granules, areas of clear cell differentiation, a pushing and crowded lower margin (Busam & Barnhill 1995, Gray & Smith 1995), and the presence of large numbers of plasma cells in any inflammatory infiltrate (Smith et al 1989). The presence of nuclear pseudo-inclusions does not permit discrimination between benign and malignant lesions (Rose 1995). Pagetoid spread is seen in both benign and malignant melanocytic lesions and may be the predominant growth pattern in either case (Busam & Barnhill 1995). A lack of cytological atypia in the intra-epidermal component favours a benign process (Haupt & Stern 1995). Aneuploidy suggests a malignant process (De Wit et al 1994).

Merkel cell carcinoma

Merkel cell carcinoma is usually a lesion of the elderly but has been described in girls of 7, 13 and 14 years. The tumours had typical electron microscopic and immunohistochemical features, with perinuclear intermediate filaments, neurosecretory granules and perinuclear positivity for cytokeratin and neurofilaments (Schmid et al 1992).

LYMPHOMA

Classification

The most recent proposal attempts to reconcile the differences between North American and European diagnostic terms, in the form of the Revised European-American Lymphoma (REAL) classification (Chan et al 1994). This system has three main categories, Hodgkin's disease, B-cell neoplasms and T-cell and postulated natural killer cell neoplasms. In paediatric practice, virtually all non-Hodgkin's lymphomas are high grade and most are extranodal and non-follicular.

Anaplastic large cell lymphoma

Immunophenotyping has led to the virtual abandonment of the term 'malignant histiocytosis', as most have been shown to be of T-cell origin (Wilson et al 1990) and in the anaplastic group. Most are positive for the Ki-1 antigen (CD30) and a chromosomal abnormality, t(2;5)(p23;q35) is consistently found (Smith et al 1993). This translocation produces a fusion product of a kinase gene termed alk, related to insulin receptor genes known to regulate cellular growth, and a nuclear phosphoprotein nucleophosmin termed npm. The protein encoded has tyrosine kinase activity (Orscheschek et al 1995). The t(2;5)(p23;q35) abnormality has also been found in Hodgkin's disease (Orscheschek et al 1995) but this finding has been questioned by others (Chan et al 1995, Downing et al 1995, Poppema 1995).

Hodgkin's disease

Hodgkin's disease is a heterogeneous condition associated in up to 50% of cases with infection by the Epstein-Barr virus (EBV) (Delabie et al 1995, Morris et al 1995). Clonal abnormalities of 14q and 13p have been described (Poppema 1995), as has t(2;5)(p23;q35), as noted above (Orscheschek et al 1995). The major differential uncertainities may be resolved by the use of a broad pool of antibodies allowing distinction between Hodgkin's disease, anaplastic large cell lymphoma (many of which were previously assigned to lymphocyte-depleted Hodgkin's disease), T-cell rich B-cell lymphoma (previously probably called diffuse lymphocyte predominant Hodgkin's disease), and nodular lymphocyte predominant Hodgkin's disease, which is now known to be a B-cell lymphoma Indeed, some authorities feel that the term Hodgkin's disease should only be used for the nodular sclerosing and mixed cellularity subtypes, which are likely to represent different entities (Wright 1995).

REFERENCES

Abbi RK, McVicar M, Teichberg S et al 1993 Pathologic characterization of a renin-secreting juxtaglomerular cell tumor in a child and review of the pediatric literature. Pediatr Pathol

13: 443–451

Anonymous 1992 Ewing's sarcoma and its congeners: an interim appraisal. Lancet 339: 99–100

Bard J 1992 The molecular basis of nephrogenesis and congenital kidney disease. Arch Dis Child 67: 983–984

Bardeesy N, Falkoff D, Petruzzi MJ et al 1994 Anaplastic Wilms' tumour, a subtype displaying poor prognosis, harbours p53 gene mutations. Nat Genet 7: 91–97

Barnhill RL, Flotte TJ, Fleischli M et al 1995 Cutaneous melanoma and atypical Spitz tumors in childhood. Cancer 76: 1833–1845

Bayani J, Thorner P, Zielenska M et al 1995 Application of a simplified comparative genomic hybridization technique to screen for gene amplification in pediatric solid tumors. Pediatr Pathol Lab Med 15: 831–844

Beckwith JB 1993 Precursor lesions of Wilms' tumor: Clinical and biological implications. Med Ped Oncol 21: 158–168

Beckwith JB 1994 Renal neoplasms of childhood. In: Sternberg SS (ed) Diagnostic surgical pathology, 2nd ed, Raven Press, New York pp 1741–1766

Beckwith JB, Martin RF 1968 Observations on the histopathology of neuroblastomas. J Ped Surg 3: 106–110

Beckwith JB, Kiviat NB, Bonadio JF 1990 Embryology and development. Nephrogenic rests, nephroblastomatosis, and the pathogenesis of Wilms' tumor. Pediatr Pathol 10: 1–36

Berry PJ, Vujanic GM 1992 Malignant rhabdoid tumour. Histopathology 20: 189–193

Biegel JA, White PS, Marshall HN et al 1993 Constitutional 1p36 deletion in a child with neuroblastoma. Am J Hum Genet 52: 176–182

Biegel JA, Nycum LM, Valentine V et al 1995 Detection of the t(2;13)(q35;q14) and PAX3–FKHR fusion in alveolar rhabdomyosarcoma by fluorescence in situ hybridization. Genes Chromosom Cancer 12: 186–192

Bolande RP 1995 The prenatal origins of cancer. In Reed GB, Claireaux AE, Cockburn F (eds) Diseases of the fetus and newborn, 2nd ed, Chapman and Hall Medical, London pp 67–82

Bove KE, Lewis C, Kiser Debrosse B 1995 Proliferation and maturation indices in nephrogenic rests and Wilms' tumor; the emergence of heterogeneity from dormant nodular renal blastema. Pediatr Pathol Lab Med 15: 223–244

Breslow N, Sharples K, Beckwith JB et al 1991 Prognostic factors in non metastatic, favorable histology Wilms' tumor. Results of the third National Wilms' Tumor Study. Cancer 68: 2345–2353

Brisigotti M, Cozzutto C, Fabbretti G et al 1992 Wilms' tumor after treatment. Pediatr Pathol 12: 397–406

Brodeur GM, Azar C, Brother M et al 1992 Neuroblastoma. Effect of genetic factors on prognosis and treatment. Cancer 70: 1685–1694

Brodeur GM, Pritchard J, Berthold F et al 1993 Revisions of the international criteria for neuroblastoma diagnosis, staging and response to treatment. J Clin Oncol 11: 1466–1477

Brown KW, Wilmore HP, Watson JE et al 1993 Low frequency of mutations in the WT1 coding region in Wilms' tumor. Genes Chromosom Cancer 8: 74–79

Buchino JJ 1991 Cytopathology in pediatrics. In: Wield GL (ed) Monographs in Clinical Cytology Vol 13 Karger, Basel pp 34–118

Busam KJ, Barnhill, RL 1995 Pagetoid Spitz nevus. Intraepidermal Spitz nevus with prominent pagetoid spread. Am J Surg Pathol 19: 1061–1067

Carpenter PM, Mascarello JT, Krous HF et al 1993 Congenital mesoblastic nephroma. Cytogenetic comparison to leiomyoma. Pediatr Pathol 13: 435–441

Carter RL, Al-Sam SZ, Corbett RP et al 1990 A comparative study of immunohistochemical staining for neuron-specific enolase, protein gene product 9.5 and S-100 protein in neuroblastoma, Ewing's sarcoma and other round cell tumours in children. Histopathology 16: 461–467

Castle VP, Heidelberger KP, Bromberg J et al 1993 Expression of the apoptosis-suppressing protein bcl-2 in neuroblastoma is associated with unfavourable histology and N-myc amplification. Am J Pathol 143: 1543–1550

Chan JKC, Banks PM, Cleary ML et al 1994 A proposal for classification of lymphoid neoplasms (by the International Lymphoma Study Group). Histopathology 25: 517–536

Chan JKC, Tsang WYW, Seneviratne S et al 1995 The MIC2 antibody 013. Practical application for the study of thymic epithelial tumors. Am J Surg Pathol 19: 1115–1123

Chan WC, Elmberger G, Lozano MD et al 1995 Large-cell anaplastic lymphoma-specific translocation in Hodgkin's disease. Lancet 345: 921

Chen TC, Hsieh LL, Kuo TT 1995 Absence of p53 gene mutation and infrequent overexpression of p53 protein in hepatoblastoma. J Pathol 176: 243–247

Cohen M, Emms M, Kaschula ROC 1991 Childhood pulmonary blastoma: a pleuropulmonary variant of the adult-type pulmonary blastoma. Pediatr Pathol 11: 737–749

Conran RM, Hitchcock CL, Waclawiw MA et al 1992 Hepatoblastoma: the prognostic significance of histologic type. Pediatr Pathol 12: 167–183

Coppes MJ, Wilson PCG, Wietzman S 1991 Extrarenal Wilms' tumor: staging treatment and prognosis. J Clin Oncol 9: 167–174

Davis CJ, Barton JH, Sesterhenn IA et al 1995 Metanephric adenoma. Clinicopathological study of fifty patients. Am J Surg Pathol 19: 1101–1114

Davis RJ, D'Cruz CM, Lovell MA et al 1994 Fusion of PAX7 to FKHR by the variant t(1;13)(p36;q14) translocation in alveolar rhabdomyosarcoma. Cancer Res 54: 2869–2872

De Bernardi B, Pianca C, Boni L et al 1992 Disseminated neuroblastoma (Stage IV and IV-s) in the first year of life. Outcome related to age and stage. Cancer 70: 1625–1633

Dehner LP 1993 Primitive neuroectodermal tumor and Ewing's sarcoma. Am J Surg Pathol 17: 1–13

Delabie J, Weisenburger DD, Chan WC 1995 Hodgkin's disease: a monoclonal lymphoproliferative disorder? Histopathology 27: 93–96

Delahunt B, Farrant GJ, Bethwaite PB et al 1994 Assessment of proliferative activity in Wilms' tumour. Anal Cell Pathol 7: 127–138

Demetrick DJ 1994 Molecular biology primer for the pediatric pathologist. Pediatr Pathol 14: 339–367

De Wit PEJ, Kerstens HMJ, Poddighe PJ et al 1994 DNA in situ hybridization as a diagnostic tool in the discrimination of melanoma and Spitz naevus. J Pathol 173: 227–233

Dietrich CU, Jacobsen BB, Starklint H et al 1993 Clonal karyotypic evolution in an embryonal rhabdomyosarcoma with trisomy 8 as the primary chromosomal abnormality. Genes Chromosom Cancer 7: 240–244

Domizio P, Risdon, RA 1991 Cystic renal neoplasms of infancy and childhood: a light microscopical, lectin histochemical and immunohistochemical study. Histopathology 19: 199–209

Douglass EC, Valentine M, Rowe ST et al 1990 Malignant rhabdoid tumor: a highly malignant childhood tumor with minimal karyotypic changes. Genes Chromosom Cancer 2: 210–216

Downing JR, Head DR, Parham DM et al 1993 Detection of the (11;22)(q24;q12) translocation of Ewing's sarcoma and peripheral neuroectodermal tumour by reverse transcription polymerase chain reaction. Am J Pathol 143: 1294–1300

Downing JR, Ladanyi M, Raffeld M et al 1995 Large-cell anaplastic lymphoma-specific translocation in Hodgkin's disease. Lancet 345: 918–919

Dressler LG, Duncan MH, Varsa EE et al 1993 DNA content measurement can be obtained using archival material for DNA flow cytometry. A comparison with cytogenetic analysis in 56 pediatric solid tumours. Cancer 72: 2033–2041

Driman D, Thorner PS, Greenberg ML et al 1994 MYCN gene amplification in rhabdomyosarcoma. Cancer 73: 2231–2237

Enzinger FM, Weiss SW 1995 Soft tissue tumours. 3rd ed, Mosby, St Louis pp 539–577

Fahner JB, Switzer R, Freyer DR et al 1993 Extrarenal Wilms' tumor: unusual presentation in the lumbosacral region. Am J Pediatr Hematol Oncol 15: 117–119

Fort DW, Tonk VS, Tomlinson GE et al 1994 Rhabdoid tumor of the kidney with primitive neuroectodermal tumor of the central nervous system: associated tumors with different histologic, cytogenetic and molecular findings. Genes Chromosom Cancer 11: 146–152

Galili N, Davis RJ, Fredericks WJ et al 1993 Fusion of a fork head domain gene to PAX3 in the solid tumour alveolar rhabdomyosarcoma. Nature Gen 5: 230–235

Gansler T, Gerald W, Anderson G et al 1991 Characterization of a cell line derived from rhabdoid tumor of kidney. Hum Pathol 22: 259–266

Gerald WL, Miller HK, Battifora H et al 1991 Intra-abdominal desmoplastic small round-cell tumor. Report of 19 cases of a distinctive type of high-grade polyphenotypic malignancy affecting young individuals. Am J Surg Pathol 15: 499–513

Gessler M, Konig A, Moore J et al 1993 Homozygous inactivation of WT1 in a Wilms' tumor associated with the WAGR syndrome. Genes Chromosom Cancer 7: 131–136

Gray ES, Smith N 1995 Paediatric surgical pathology. An illustrated handbook of the paediatric biopsy. Churchill Livingstone, Edinburgh, pp 167–189

Green DM, Beckwith JB, Weeks DA et al 1994 The relationship between microsubstaging variables, age at diagnosis, and tumor weight of children with stage 1/favorable histology Wilms' tumor: a report from the National Wilms' Tumor Study. Cancer 74: 1817–1820

Gururangan S, Dorman A, Ball R et al 1992 DNA quantitation of Wilms' tumour (nephroblastoma) using flow cytometry and image analysis. J Clin Pathol 45: 498–501

Haas JE, Muczynski KA, Krailo M et al 1989 Histopathology and prognosis in childhood hepatoblastoma and hepatocarcinoma. Cancer 64: 1082–1095

Hachitanda Y, Aoyama C, Sato JK et al 1993 Pleuropulmonary blastoma in childhood. A tumor of divergent differentiation. Am J Surg Pathol 17: 382–391

Hansen K, Bagtas J, Mark HF et al 1992 Undifferentiated small cell hepatoblastoma with a unique chromosomal translocation: a case report. Pediatr Pathol 12: 457–462

Hara K 1993 Melanocytic lesions in lymph nodes associated with congenital naevus. Histopathology 23: 445–451

Haupt HM, Stern JB 1995 Pagetoid melanocytosis. Histologic features in benign and malignant lesions. Am J Surg Pathol 19: 792–797

Hawkins MM 1990 Risks of myeloid leukaemia in children treated for solid tumours. Lancet 336: 887

Heim S, Mitelman F 1992 Cytogenetics of solid tumours. In: Anthony PP, MacSween RNM (eds) Recent advances in histopathology Vol 15, Churchill Livingstone, Edinburgh pp 37–66

Hennigar RA, Beckwith JB 1992 Nephrogenic adenofibroma – a novel kidney tumor of young people. Am J Surg Pathol 16: 325–334

Hiyama E, Hiyama K, Yokoyama T et al 1991 Immunohistochemical analysis of N-myc protein expression in neuroblastoma: correlation with prognosis of patients. J Ped Surg 26: 838–843

Hodgson SV, Maher ER 1993 A practical guide to human cancer genetics. University Press, Cambridge pp 72–74

Joshi VV, Cantor AB, Altshuler G et al 1992 Age-linked prognostic categorization based on a new histologic grading system of neuroblastomas – a clinicopathologic study of 211 cases from the pediatric oncology group. Cancer 69: 2197–2211

Joshi VV, Cantor AB, Brodeur GM et al 1993a Correlation between morphologic and other prognostic markers of neuroblastoma. A study of histologic grade, DNA index, N-myc gene copy number, and lactic dehydrogenase in patients in the pediatric oncology group. Cancer 71: 3173–3181

Joshi VV, Silverman JF, Altshuler G et al 1993b Systematization of primary histopathologic and fine needle aspiration cytologic features and description of unusual histopathologic features of neuroblastic tumours: A report from the pediatric oncology group. Hum Pathol 24: 493–504

Karnes PS, Tran TN, Cui MY et al 1991 Establishment of a rhabdoid tumour cell line with a specific chromosomal abnormality, 46,XY t(11;22)(p15.5;q11.23). Cancer Genet Cytogenet 56: 31–38

Kissen GDN, Wallace WHB 1995 Long term follow up therapy based guidelines. The United Kingdom Children's Cancer Study Group Late Effects Group. Pharmacia, Milton Keynes

Kleiner DE, Emmert-Buck MR, Liotta LA 1995 Necropsy as a research method in the age of molecular pathology. Lancet 346: 945–948

Knudson AG, Strong LC 1972 Mutation and cancer: a model for Wilms' tumor of the kidney. J Nat Cancer Inst 48: 313–324

Kodet R, Newton WA, Sachs N et al 1991 Rhabdoid tumors of soft tissues: A clinicopathologic study of 26 cases enrolled in the intergroup rhabdomyosarcoma study. Hum Pathol 22: 674–684

Kodet R, Newton WA, Hamoudi AB 1993 Childhood rhabdomyosarcoma with anaplastic (pleomorphic) features. Am J Surg Pathol 17: 443–453

Kodet R, Taylor M, Vachalova H et al 1994 Juxtaglomerular cell tumor. An immunohistochemical, electron-microscopic, and in situ hybridization study. Am J Surg Pathol 18: 837–842

Koszyca B, Moore L, Toogood I et al 1993 Is postmortem examination useful in pediatric oncology? Pediatr Pathol 13: 709–715

Ladanyi M, Lewis R, Jhanwar SC et al 1995 MDM2 and CDK4 gene amplification in Ewing's sarcoma. J Pathol 175: 211–217

Lemoine NR, Hughes CM, Cowell JK 1992 Aberrant expression of the tumour suppressor gene p53 is very frequent in Wilms' tumours. J Pathol 168: 237–242

Leuschner I, Schmidt D, Harms D 1990 Undifferentiated sarcoma of the liver in childhood: morphology, flow cytometry and literature review. Hum Pathol 21: 68–76

Leuschner I, Newton WA, Schmidt D et al 1993 Spindle cell variants of embryonal rhabdomyosarcoma in the paratesticular region. Am J Surg Pathol 17: 221–230

Loo KT, Leung AKF, Chan JKC 1995 Immunohistochemical staining of ovarian granulosa cell tumours with MIC2 antibody. Histopathology 27: 388–390

Lundgren L, Angervall L, Stenman G et al 1993 Infantile rhabdomyofibrosarcoma: a high-grade sarcoma distinguishable from infantile fibrosarcoma and rhabdomyosarcoma. Hum Pathol 24: 785–795

McGahey BE, Moriarty AT, Nelson WA et al 1992 Fine-needle aspiration biopsy of small round blue cell tumors of childhood. Cancer 69: 1067–1073

McManus A, Gusterson BA, Pinkerton CR et al 1995 Diagnosis of Ewing's sarcoma and related tumours by detection of chromosome 22q12 translocations using fluorescence in situ hybridization on tumour touch imprints. J Pathol 176: 137–142

Mehregan AH, Mehregan DA 1993 Malignant melanoma in childhood. Cancer 71: 4096–4103

Morris JDH, Eddleston ALWF, Crook T 1995 Viral infection and cancer. Lancet 346: 754–758

Nelson RJ, Perlman EJ, Askin FB 1995 Is esthesioneuroblastoma a peripheral neuroectodermal tumor? Hum Pathol 26: 639–641

Newton WA, Gehan EA, Webber BL et al 1995 Classification of rhabdomyosarcomas and related sarcomas. Pathological aspects and proposal for a new classification – an Intergroup Rhabdomyosarcoma Study. Cancer 76: 1073–1085

Nicholson HS, Fears TR, Byrne J 1994 Death during adulthood in survivors of childhood and adolescent cancer. Cancer 73: 3094–3102

Olshan AF, Breslow NE, Falletta JM et al 1993 Risk factors for Wilms' tumor: report from the National Wilms' Tumor Study. Cancer 72: 938–944

Orscheschek K, Merz H, Hell J et al 1995 Large-cell anaplastic lymphoma-specific translocation (t[2;5] [p23;q35]) in Hodgkin's disease: indication of a common pathogenesis? Lancet 345: 87–90

Ota S, Crabbe DCG, Tran TN et al 1993 Malignant rhabdoid tumor: a study with two established cell lines. Cancer 71: 2862–2872

Pan LX, Diss TC, Isaacson PG 1995 The polymerase chain reaction in histopathology. Histopathology 26: 201–217

Parham DM, Shapiro DN, Downing JR et al 1994a Solid alveolar rhabdomyosarcomas with the t(2;13). Report of two cases with diagnostic implications. Am J Surg Pathol 18: 474–478

Parham DM, Weeks DA, Beckwith JB 1994b The clinicopathologic spectrum of putative extrarenal rhabdoid tumors: an analysis of 42 cases studied with immunohistochemistry or electron microscopy. Am J Surg Pathol 18: 1010–1029

Perlman EJ, Dickman PS, Askin FB et al 1994 Ewing's sarcoma – routine diagnostic utilization of MIC2 analysis: a pediatric oncology group/children's cancer group intergroup study. Hum Pathol 25: 304–307

Pihkala J, Sariola H, Saarinen UM 1994 Myocardial function and postmortem myocardial histology in children given anthracycline therapy for cancer. Pediatr Hematol Oncol 11: 259–269

Pinkerton CR, Pritchard-Jones K, McManus A et al 1994 Small round cell tumours of childhood. Lancet 344: 725–729

Poddighe PJ, Ramaekers FCS, Hopman AHN 1992 Interphase cytogenetics of tumours. J Pathol 166: 215–224

Poppema S 1995 Large-cell anaplastic lymphoma-specific translocation in Hodgkin's disease. Lancet 345: 919

Pritchard J, Hickman JA 1994 Why does stage 4s neuroblastoma regress spontaneously? Lancet 344: 869–870

Pritchard-Jones K, Renshaw J, King-Underwood L 1994 The Wilms' tumor (WT1) gene is mutated in a secondary leukaemia in a WAGR patient. Hum Mol Genet 3: 1633–1637

Pui CH, Hancock ML, Raimondi SC et al 1990 Myeloid neoplasia in children treated for solid tumours. Lancet 336: 417–421

Ramani P, Lu QL 1994 Expression of bcl-2 gene product in neuroblastoma. J Pathol 172: 273–278

Ramani P, Dewchand H 1995 Expression of mdr1/p-glycoprotein and p110 in neuroblastoma. J Pathol 175: 13–22

Ramani P, Rampling D, Link M 1993 Immunocytochemical study of 12E7 in small round-cell tumours of childhood: an assessment of its sensitivity and specificity. Histopathology 23: 557–561

Resnick MB, Donovan M 1995 Intra-abdominal desmoplastic small round cell tumor with extensive extra-abdominal involvement. Pediatr Pathol Lab Med 15: 797–803

Rosai J, Dias P, Parham DM et al 1991 Myo D1 protein expression in alveolar soft part sarcoma as confirmatory evidence of its skeletal muscle nature. Am J Surg Pathol 15: 974–981

Rose DSC 1995 Nuclear pseudoinclusions in melanocytic naevi and melanomas. J Clin Pathol 48: 676–677

Ruck P, Xiao JC, Kaiserling E 1994 P53 protein expression in hepatoblastoma: an immunohistochemical investigation. Pediatr Pathol 14: 79–85

Sarode VR, Savitri K, Banerjee CK et al 1992 Primary extrarenal Wilms' tumour: identification of a putative precursor lesion. Histopathology 21: 76–78

Sawyer JR, Tryka AF, Lewis JM 1992 A novel reciprocal chromosome translocation t(11;22)(p13;q12) in an intra-abdominal desmoplastic small round-cell tumor. Am J Surg Pathol 16: 411–416

Sawyer JR, Goosen LS, Stine KC et al 1994 Telomere fusion as a mechanism for the progressive loss of the short arm of chromosome 11 in an anaplastic Wilms' tumor. Cancer 74: 767–773

Saxena R, Leake JL, Shafford EA et al 1993 Chemotherapy effects on hepatoblastoma: a histological study. Am J Surg Pathol 17: 1266–1271

Scaradavou A, Heller G, Sklar CA et al 1995 Second malignant neoplasms in long-term survivors of childhood rhabdomyosarcoma. Cancer 76: 1860–1867

Schmid CH, Beham A, Feichtinger J et al 1992 Recurrent and subsequently metastasizing Merkel cell carcinoma in a 7 year old girl. Histopathology 20: 437–439

Schmidt D, Wischmeyer P, Leuschner I et al 1993 DNA analysis in hepatoblastoma by flow and image cytometry. Cancer 72: 2914–2919

Schneid H, Seurin D, Vazquez MP et al 1993 Parental allele specific methylation of the human insulin-like growth factor II gene and Beckwith-Wiedemann syndrome. J Med Genet 30: 353–362

Sciot R, Dal Cin P, De Vos R et al 1993 Alveolar soft-part sarcoma: evidence for its myogenic origin and for the involvement of 17q25. Histopathology 23: 439–444

Sciot R, Dal Cin P, Brock P et al 1994 Pleuropulmonary blastoma (pulmonary blastoma of childhood): genetic link with other embryonal malignancies? Histopathology 24: 559–563

Scrable H, Witte D, Shimada H et al 1989 Molecular differential pathology of rhabdomyosarcoma. Genes Chromosom Cancer 1: 23–35

Shanks JH, McCluggage G, Anderson NH et al 1990 Value of the necropsy in perioperative deaths. J Clin Pathol 43: 193–195

Shashi V, Lovell MA, von Kap-herr C et al 1994 Malignant rhabdoid tumor of the kidney: involvement of chromosome 22. Genes Chromosom Cancer 10: 49–54

Shimada H, Chatten J, Newton WA et al 1984 Histopathologic prognostic factors in neuroblastic tumors: definition of subtypes of ganglioneuroblastoma and an age-linked classification of neuroblastomas. JNCI 73: 405–416

Simms LA, Reeve AE, Smith PJ 1995 Genetic mosaicism at the insulin locus in liver associated with childhood hepatoblastoma. Genes Chromosom Cancer 13: 72–73

Smith KJ, Barrett TL, Skelton HG et al 1989 Spindle cell and epithelioid cell nevi with atypia and metastasis (malignant Spitz nevus) . Am J Surg Pathol 13: 931–939

Smith NM, Byard RW, Vasiliou M et al 1993 Pediatric anaplastic large cell (CD30+) lymphomas associated with the t(2;5)(p23:q35) chromosomal abnormality. Int J Surg Pathol 1: 43–50

Sotelo-Avila C, Beckwith JB, Johnson JE 1995 Ossifying renal tumor of infancy: a clinicopathologic study of nine cases. Pediatr Pathol Lab Med 15: 745–762

Sreekantaiah C, Appaji L, Hazarika D 1992 Cytogenetic characterisation of small round cell tumours using fine needle aspiration. J Clin Pathol 45: 728–730

Srivatsan ES, Ying KL, Seeger RC 1993 Deletion of chromosome 11 and of 14q sequences in neuroblastoma. Genes Chromosom Cancer 7: 32–37

Stiller CA, Bunch KJ 1990 Trends in survival for childhood cancer in Britain diagnosed 1971-85. Br J Cancer 62: 806–815

Stock C, Ambros IM, Mann G et al 1993 Detection of 1p36 deletions in paraffin sections of neuroblastoma tissues. Genes Chromosom Cancer 6: 1–9

Takeda O, Homma C, Maseki N et al 1994 There may be two tumor suppressor genes on chromosome arm 1p closely associated with biologically distinct subtypes of neuroblastoma. Genes Chromosom Cancer 10: 30–39

Tanaka T, Slamon DJ, Shimada H et al 1991 A significant association of Ha-ras p21 in neuroblastoma cells with patient prognosis. Cancer 68: 1296–1302

Tanaka T, Hiyama E, Sugimoto T et al 1995 trk A gene expression in neuroblastoma. Cancer 76: 1086–1095

Tomlinson GE, Argyle JC, Velasco S et al 1992 Molecular characterization of congenital mesoblastic nephroma and its distinction from Wilms' tumor. Cancer 70: 2358–2361

Tonk VS, Wilson KS, Timmons CF et al 1994 Trisomy 2, trisomy 20, and del(17p) as sole chromosomal abnormalities in three cases of hepatoblastoma. Genes Chromosom Cancer 11: 199–202

Tsokos M, Webber BL, Parham DM et al 1992 Rhabdomyosarcoma – a new classification scheme related to prognosis. Arch Pathol Lab Med 116: 847–855

Variend S, Gerrard M, Norris PD et al 1991 Intra-abdominal neuroectodermal tumour of childhood with divergent differentiation. Histopathology 18: 45–51

Variend S 1993 Paediatric neoplasia. Kluwer, Dordrecht

Veress B, Alafuzoff I 1994 A retrospective analysis of clinical diagnoses and autopsy findings in 3042 cases during two different time periods. Hum Pathol 25: 140–145

Vincent TS, Garvin AJ, Gramling TS et al 1994 Expression of insulin-like growth factor binding protein 2 (IGFBP-2) in Wilms' tumors. Pediatr Pathol 14: 723–730

Vujanic GM, Delemarre JFM, Moeslichan S et al 1993 Mesoblastic nephroma metastatic to the lungs and heart – another face of this peculiar lesion. Pediatr Pathol 13: 143–153

Vujanic GM, Sandstedt B, Dijoud F et al 1995 Nephrogenic rest associated with a mesoblastic nephroma – what does it tell us? Pediatr Pathol Lab Med 15: 469–475

Waber PG, Chen J, Nisen PD 1993 Infrequency of ras, p53, WT1, or RB gene alterations in Wilms' tumors. Cancer 72: 3732–3738

Wakely PE, Sprague RI, Kornstein MJ 1989 Extrarenal Wilms' tumor: an analysis of four cases. Hum Pathol 20: 691–695

Wakely PE, Frable WJ, Kornstein MJ 1993 Role of intraoperative cytopathology in pediatric surgical pathology. Hum Pathol 24: 311–315

Wang DG, Johnston CF, Anderson N et al 1995 Overexpression of the tumour suppressor gene p53 is not implicated in neuroendocrine tumour carcinogenesis. J Pathol 175: 397–401

Wang-Wuu S, Soukup S, Ballard E et al 1988 Chromosomal analysis of sixteen human rhabdomyosarcomas. Cancer Res 48: 983–987

Weeks DA, Beckwith JB, Mierau GW 1990 Benign nodal lesions mimicking metastases from pediatric renal neoplasms: A report of the National Wilms' Tumor Study pathology center. Hum Pathol 21: 1239–1244

Weeks DA, Beckwith BJ, Mierau GW et al 1991 Renal neoplasms mimicking rhabdoid tumor of kidney: A report from the National Wilms' Tumor Study pathology center. Am J Surg Pathol 15: 1042–1054

Weidner N, Tjoe J 1994 Immunohistochemical profile of monoclonal antibody 013: antibody that recognizes glycoprotein p30/32[MIC2] and is useful in diagnosing Ewing's sarcoma and peripheral neuroepithelioma. Am J Surg Pathol 18: 486–494

Weinberg AG, Finegold MJ 1983 Primary hepatic tumors of childhood. Hum Pathol 14: 512–537

Wesche WA, Fletcher CDM, Dias P et al 1995 Immunohistochemistry of MyoD1 in adult pleomorphic soft tissue sarcomas. Am J Surg Pathol 19: 261–269

Whang-Peng J, Knutsen T, Theil K et al 1992 Cytogenetic studies in subgroups of rhabdomyosarcoma. Genes Chromosom Cancer 5: 299–310

Wijnaendts LCD, Van der Linden JC, Van Unnik AJM et al 1994 Histopathological features and grading in rhabdomyosarcomas of childhood. Histopathology 24: 303–309

Williams GH, Williams ED 1995 Identification of tumour-specific translocations in archival material. J Pathol 175: 279–281

Wilson MS, Weiss LM, Gatter KC et al 1990 Malignant histiocytosis – a reassessment of cases previously reported in 1975 based on paraffin section immunophenotyping studies. Cancer 66: 530–536

Wirnsberger GH, Becker H, Ziervogel K et al 1992 Diagnostic immunohistochemistry of neuroblastic tumours. Am J Surg Pathol 16: 49–57

Wright DH 1995 Out of the Hodgkin's maze? J Pathol 177: 331–333

Zucman J, Melot T, Desmaze C et al 1993 Combinatorial generation of variable fusion proteins in the Ewing family of tumours. EMBO J 12: 4481–4487

Zuppan CW, Beckwith JB, Luckey DW 1988 Anaplasia in unilateral Wilms' tumor: a report from the National Wilms' Tumor Study pathology center. Hum Pathol 19: 1199–1209

10

Interstitial nephritis

A. J. Howie

Inflammation of interstitial tissues of the kidney has several controversial aspects. Even the name commonly applied to it, tubulo-interstitial nephritis, can be criticized. This name is misleading because it implies equal involvement of tubules and interstitial tissues in the process and an equal contribution to whatever changes occur. Although interstitial inflammation may damage tubules, tubules may be normal when there is interstitial inflammation, and may be damaged by something else even when there is interstitial inflammation. A more useful approach is to consider tubules and interstitial tissues separately.

Importance of interstitial changes in renal function

Renal interstitial inflammation, if it has a significant clinical effect, is associated with a reduction of renal excretory function. This means a reduction in glomerular filtration rate, shown by such changes as a rise in serum creatinine concentration and a fall in creatinine clearance. The information that is usually given on request forms accompanying renal biopsy specimens is that there is acute or chronic renal failure or renal impairment.

There is a paradox. Renal excretory function is expressed as a measure of glomerular function, namely, glomerular filtration rate, and yet interstitial changes can cause impairment of renal function, which they must do by having an effect on glomeruli. To emphasize the paradox, morphological changes in glomeruli themselves are known to have little correlation with glomerular filtration rate (Risdon et al 1968, Newbold & Howie 1990).

Observations are not in dispute that a correlation can be shown between measures of interstitial changes including inflammation and measures of glomerular filtration rate (Schainuck et al 1970, Bohle et al 1987, Howie et al 1990). This evidence has been taken by some to show that, although the explanation is not obvious, the prime determinant of glomerular filtration rate is the state of interstitial tissues.

The hypothesis is made that interstitial events such as inflammation and fibrosis destroy the capillaries around tubules. These capillaries are derived from the efferent arterioles leaving glomeruli. Loss of capillaries causes ischaemia of tubules, which will eventually atrophy. Loss of peritubular capillaries also causes a rise in glomerular capillary pressure, which leads either to reduced glomerular perfusion or glomerular enlargement. Large glomeruli are at risk of global sclerosis and as the number of glomeruli declines, so does the glomerular filtration rate (Fine et al 1993, Bohle et al 1994).

A few other observations contradict this and suggest that glomerular filtration rate does not depend upon interstitial tissues, and that the correlations commonly found are indirect and due to another factor. It has been reported that in patients with IgA nephropathy, although there was a correlation between renal interstitial volume and creatinine clearance at the time of their first renal biopsy, there was no correlation between change in interstitial volume in repeat renal biopsy specimens and change in creatinine clearance (Bennett et al 1982). There was no difference in interstitial inflammation and interstitial oedema between those in oliguric acute renal failure and others who had recently recovered from acute renal failure (Solez et al 1979).

Another factor that has a better correlation with renal function than the state of interstitial tissues is the state of tubules (Solez et al 1979, Howie 1994). Renal failure has different mechanisms in different diseases and even at different times in the same disease (Solez 1992a, Bonventre 1993). An important factor is reduced perfusion of the cortex (Trueta et al 1947). This causes reduced glomerular filtration rate directly and it damages tubules, especially the proximal tubule and the thick limb of the loop of Henle, both of which are sensitive to ischaemia (Howie et al 1990, Howie 1994). Tubules can also be damaged by toxins and immunological mediators. Tubular damage itself can contribute to renal failure by allowing glomerular filtrate to leak into interstitial tissues, by activation of the tubulo-glomerular feedback mechanism so that an increased sodium load at the macula densa, due to decreased tubular reabsorption, leads to reduced glomerular filtration, and possibly by obstruction of tubules, although it is not clear how obstruction could ever be overcome and allow recovery, if it is indeed a significant mechanism (Bohle et al 1990, Solez 1992a).

Implications of this are that interstitial inflammation can cause tubular damage which may be associated with clinical renal impairment, but that interstitial changes themselves, including inflammation, while they are often seen in renal impairment and can be correlated with it, are not directly responsible.

Interstitial nephritis is usually divided into acute and chronic forms, and this is useful in clinical practice. This is because acute tubular damage is potentially reversible as long as viable cells remain but chronic tubular damage, that is, atrophy, is irreversible.

ACUTE INTERSTITIAL NEPHRITIS

This morphological change is relatively straightforward. The kidneys are normal in size or may be enlarged. There is expansion of interstitial tissues of the kidneys by oedema and inflammatory cells which is more obvious in

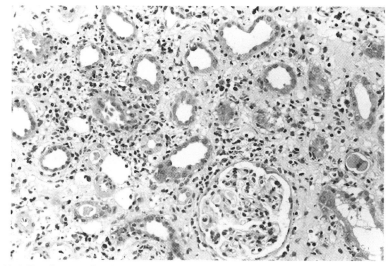

Fig. 10.1 Renal cortex showing acute interstitial nephritis, in this case due to a non-steroidal anti-inflammatory drug. Tubules are acutely damaged. There is interstitial oedema with an inflammatory cell infiltrate. H & E × 250.

the cortex than in the medulla. Although this condition is called acute, neutrophil polymorphs are absent or few, and if they are seen in greater numbers, there is a likelihood of other conditions, especially ascending infection and pyaemic abscesses. These conditions should not be called acute interstitial nephritis, but are often included in that diagnosis. The infiltrating cells are usu-

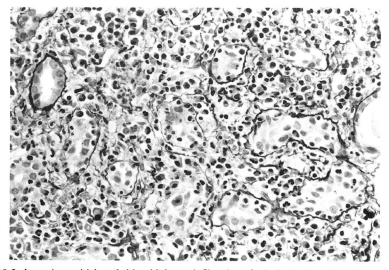

Fig. 10.2 Acute interstitial nephritis with heavy infiltration of tubules by chronic inflammatory cells, in this case associated with vasculitis in the Churg-Strauss syndrome. Periodic acid – methenamine silver. × 400.

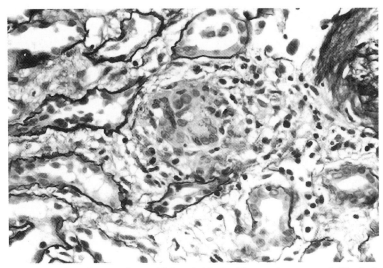

Fig. 10.3 A granuloma in acute interstitial nephritis, in this case due to a penicillin derivative. Periodic acid-methenamine silver. × 500.

ally lymphocytes with various numbers of macrophages, plasma cells and eosinophils (Fig. 10.1). Eosinophils are helpful to the histopathologist as they indicate a functionally significant infiltrate but they are not always seen. Another helpful sign, although again it is not always found, is the presence of lymphocytes within tubular epithelium (Fig. 10.2). This feature is sometimes called tubulitis, especially in cellular rejection of renal transplants, which can be regarded as an example of acute interstitial nephritis (Solez et al 1993).

Tubular cells are acutely damaged. This means that the number of tubules appears roughly normal and they are not shrunken or markedly dilated, but the epithelium shows various changes, such as loss of brush border, irregularity, flattening and vacuolation. Frank necrosis of epithelium and bare areas of basement membrane are hardly ever seen, but the fact that mitoses can often be found and that proliferation markers are strongly expressed in damaged tubules indicate that there must be loss of cells (Howie et al 1995). Apoptosis may be the mechanism of such cell loss (Bonventre 1993, Wolf & Neilson 1995).

Sometimes, macrophages and other cells aggregate into small granulomas, usually with ill-defined edges (Fig. 10.3). These are different from granulomas in sarcoidosis in which they are more clearly outlined and are associated with chronic damage to the kidney (Fig. 10.4).

Causes and associations of acute interstitial nephritis

This change can either be the only disease in the kidney or may be found with other abnormalities such as disorders of glomeruli and blood vessels. Acute

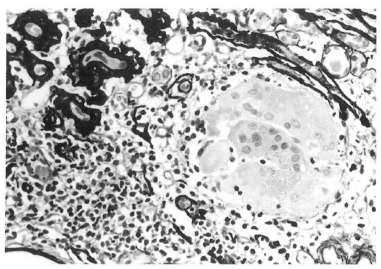

Fig. 10.4 A granuloma in the kidney with chronic damage to tubules in sarcoid. Periodic acid – methenamine silver. × 400.

interstitial nephritis is often found in active lupus nephritis and acute post-infective glomerulonephritis. Acute interstitial nephritis is also almost universal in active renal vasculitis (Fig. 10.2) but granulomas are not a feature, even in Wegener's granulomatosis (Adu & Howie 1995).

Acute interstitial nephritis as the only change in the kidney is seen as a reaction to drugs, in infections and in association with disease outside the kidney. In practice in some cases no cause or association are ever identified. The disease may also be superimposed on another renal disorder such as diabetic glomerulonephropathy and can be responsible for an acute deterioration in renal function.

The drugs most often associated with acute interstitial nephritis are non-steroidal anti-inflammatory drugs and antibiotics, especially penicillins and cephalosporins (Figs 10.1, 10.3) but many others have been reported (Colvin & Fang 1989, Solez 1992b).

Among the infections associated with acute interstitial nephritis are leptospirosis and those caused by the various hantaviruses causing haemorrhagic fever with renal syndrome (Papadimitriou 1995). In the past, many other infective causes were reported, such as diphtheria and scarlet fever. Whether the infections or treatments for them or complications including other infections caused the acute interstitial nephritis is now difficult to say.

The association of acute interstitial nephritis with uveitis is given the acronym TINU, meaning tubulo-interstitial nephritis with uveitis. This is usually a disease of women who have acute renal impairment and proteinuria, sometimes with arthralgia. Uveitis may be the reason for presentation initially or may become apparent after acute interstitial nephritis is diagnosed.

The cause is not known and the connection between the uveal tract and renal tubules is not explained (Heptinstall 1992).

Notes on the diagnosis of acute interstitial nephritis

Acute interstitial nephritis as the only change in the kidney is rare. Among 3700 non-transplant renal biopsy specimens seen by the author from 1980 to 1995 inclusive, the diagnosis was made in 55, that is, 1.5% of the total, excluding the many examples of acute interstitial nephritis in lupus nephropathy, acute post-infective glomerulonephritis and vasculitis, but including a few examples of the disease superimposed on other diseases. Of these 55, 15 were attributed to non-steroidal anti-inflammatory drugs, seven to antibiotics, two to both simultaneously, and six to six other drugs. One was thought to be due to leptospirosis on serological evidence although no leptospires were detectable in the biopsy specimen, and one to another undiagnosed infective agent guessed to be a virus. Three were associated with uveitis. In 20, no cause was found. In every case with a known aetiology, renal failure improved after appropriate treatment.

The rarity of the disease means that much of the literature is based on single case reports. Clinical clues are usually necessary to indicate probable causes or associations of acute interstitial nephritis found in a renal biopsy specimen. Immunohistological and electron microscopical investigations are rarely useful in diagnosis but are important in research.

Pathogenesis of acute interstitial nephritis

All examples of acute interstitial nephritis, as defined here, are probably due to an immune response to tubular antigens (Neilson 1989). Drugs may bind to tubular structures and make them immunogenic. Infective agents may mimic endogenous antigens and provoke an autoimmune response, or may invade tubular cells directly and be the target for an immune response (Papadimitriou 1995). The immune response is usually initiated by T lymphocytes, and most lymphocytes in acute interstitial nephritis are T cells. There is usually a mixture of CD4-positive and CD8-positive T cells in various proportions and the assessment of the relative numbers of these is of little practical value in diagnosis (Neilson 1989, Strutz & Neilson 1994).

Rarely, antibodies to tubular basement membranes occur, sometimes associated with antibodies to glomerular basement membrane as in Goodpasture's syndrome (Heptinstall, 1992). Apparent deposition of antigen-antibody complexes in tubular basement membrane may also occur, most often in systemic lupus erythematosus (Cameron 1992, Heptinstall 1992). Most examples of acute interstitial nephritis have no linear or granular deposition of immunoproteins in tubular basement membranes and tubular damage in these is unlikely to be related to antibody-dependent complement activation.

CHRONIC INTERSTITIAL NEPHRITIS

This term and its synonym, chronic tubulo-interstitial nephritis, are widely used but are unsatisfactory and almost meaningless. They give the impression of a specific diagnosis but in practice are of little help. The terms are now used so frequently and uncritically that the literature on them is virtually the same as that on renal disease as a whole. The impression is given that, unlike acute interstitial nephritis, chronic interstitial or tubulo-interstitial nephritis is one of the commonest disorders of the kidney.

The problem is that these terms are applied to late changes in the kidney of many different causes, often but not always associated with two symmetrically shrunken kidneys. They refer to the combination of tubular atrophy, interstitial fibrosis and a lymphocytic infiltrate in the kidney, usually with intimal thickening in arteries (Fig. 10.5). Glomeruli may give clues to the underlying disease or may show secondary changes including global sclerosis of some and compensatory enlargement of others, with development of overload-type segmental lesions. There are areas of sclerosis and hyalinosis in large glomeruli, usually next to the arterioles at the glomerular hilum, apparently due to excessive glomerular filtration (Newbold & Howie 1990, Howie et al 1993). These may be thought to indicate a primary glomerular disorder.

Chronic interstitial nephritis is analogous to the term cirrhosis of the liver, a morphological description of late changes of many different causes. Indeed, there is justification for the term cirrhosis of the kidney (Cameron 1992). This would at least avoid the implications that in every case interstitial inflammation is continuing and is the main reason for the renal damage, and that all authors who use the term chronic interstitial or tubulo-interstitial

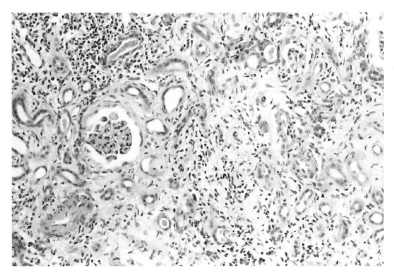

Fig. 10.5 Renal cortex showing tubular atrophy, interstitial fibrosis and a lymphocytic infiltrate, often described as chronic interstitial or tubulo-interstitial nephritis, in this case several months after an episode of acute renal failure due to rhabdomyolysis. H & E × 200.

nephritis are describing the same disease. The confusion arises because the mechanisms of chronic damage are similar in virtually all progressive renal diseases.

Pathogenesis of interstitial fibrosis

Some regard interstitial fibrosis as the more important event in chronic renal damage, with tubular atrophy as an incidental and minor feature. Probably a more accurate view is that tubular damage progressing to atrophy is the crucial event and that interstitial fibrosis accompanies this. The importance of this is that efforts to prevent or reverse fibrosis are likely to have no effect on renal function if tubules have already atrophied.

Damage to tubular cells can be caused by many things such as ischaemia, immunological attack and toxins filtered by glomeruli. Proteins that normally are not filtered by glomeruli may be damaging to tubular cells, as shown by an increased proliferation rate in tubules in the nephrotic syndrome (Howie et al 1995). This may explain the clinical observations that renal impairment can occur in the nephrotic syndrome even when there is no conventionally accepted cause such as fluid depletion, and that the amount of proteinuria correlates with progression of glomerular disorders. Other endogenous substances when filtered in abnormal amounts by glomeruli may also be toxic, such as light chains and haemoglobin (Fine et al 1993).

If some nephrons are lost from any cause, those surviving have an increased demand for oxygen. This may be accompanied by increased production of reactive oxygen species, namely, superoxide anion, hydrogen peroxide and hydroxyl radical. Ammonia production is also increased in surviving nephrons. These and other chemicals in abnormal kidneys may have toxic effects on tubular or interstitial cells and provoke inflammation (Bonventre 1993, Nath et al 1994).

Damaged tubular cells, and tubular cells stimulated by cytokines such as gamma-interferon from inflammatory cells, may express antigens not normally found on them such as histocompatibility antigens, including class 2. These allow them to act as antigen-presenting cells and lead to more damage by activation of T lymphocytes (Cameron 1992). Glomerular basement membrane material is one substance postulated to be an antigen that can be presented by tubular cells (Bohle et al 1994).

Adhesion molecules such as intercellular adhesion molecule 1 may also have increased expression by damaged tubular cells and allow inflammatory cells to localize around tubules (Cameron 1992).

Damaged tubular cells can secrete many substances. These include cytokines such as interleukin 6 and tumour necrosis factor alpha that attract inflammatory cells and fibroblasts, collagens, not only of basement membrane types but of interstitial types, and growth factors such as platelet-derived growth factor that stimulate interstitial fibroblasts to make interstitial collagens and other extracellular substances (Fine et al 1993).

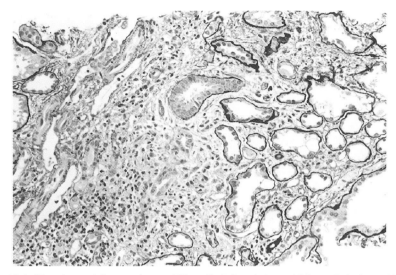

Fig. 10.6 Chronic renal damage that could be called chronic interstitial or tubulo-interstitial nephritis. Several tubular cells contain a single large vacuole characteristic of hypokalaemia, in this case due to chronic diarrhoea. Periodic acid – methenamine silver. × 250.

Inflammatory infiltrates in chronically damaged kidneys could be attracted by new antigens in abnormal tubules or by cytokines released from them, and are not necessarily evidence that the damage was initially due to the infiltrates (Fine et al 1993). Interstitial fibrosis is likely to be a consequence of tubular damage, rather than a cause of it (Dodd 1995).

Causes and associations of so-called chronic interstitial nephritis

If possible, the histopathologist should try to determine the cause of chronic renal damage, although this can be difficult in a nephrectomy specimen or autopsy kidney, and even more difficult in a renal biopsy. Lists of causes and associations of chronic interstitial or tubulo-interstitial nephritis are arbitrary in what is included and excluded, but the following are among such causes and associations.

Persistence of acute interstitial nephritis with progression to chronic renal damage

This is difficult to verify. To be sure of the diagnosis, there would have to be a renal biopsy specimen showing acute interstitial nephritis, without recovery from acute renal failure, which itself would raise doubts about the diagnosis of acute interstitial nephritis. Although many people in the armed forces in the Korean war had a hantavirus infection and went on to renal failure, there was a possibility that they initially had a complication such as haemolytic-uraemic syndrome rather than acute interstitial nephritis (Papadimitriou 1995). True progression of acute interstitial nephritis to chronic interstitial

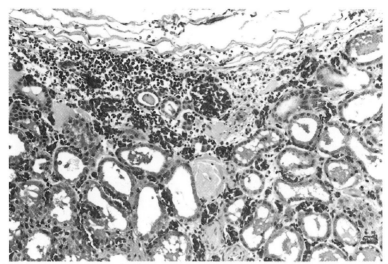

Fig. 10.7 Renal cortex just under the capsule in a nephrectomy specimen, showing a small wedge-shaped area of ischaemic damage, with changes that could be called chronic interstitial or tubulo-interstitial nephritis. H & E x 200.

nephritis is possible but can only be established by rigorous exclusion of the many other so-called causes, and this is hardly ever achieved.

Exogenous toxins causing chronic tubular damage

All chronic tubular damage is accompanied by interstitial fibrosis and a variable amount of chronic inflammatory cells. In the past, lead was a common environmental toxin, and one of its effects was to poison renal tubules. One of the most prominent figures in the American revolution, John Paul Jones, died in France in 1792 aged 45. His body was examined in 1905. The kidneys were small and were said to show chronic interstitial nephritis (Dale 1952). This was guessed to be due to lead (Neilson 1989). Cadmium, mercury and lithium are also tubular toxins. Balkan endemic nephropathy occurs in well-defined areas, seems likely to have a toxic cause and is included in lists of chronic interstitial nephritis (Hall & Batuman 1991). Environmental toxins even today may be important causes of chronic renal failure (Nuyts et al 1995). A history of exposure to a toxin will suggest the diagnosis.

Disorders of urinary drainage and of the renal medulla

Reflux nephropathy alias chronic pyelonephritis, urinary tract obstruction, renal papillary necrosis including that due to analgesic nephropathy, malako-plakia and sickle cell disease are said to be causes of chronic interstitial nephritis. A sensible approach is to give the specific diagnosis, which should be suggested by appropriate clinical and pathological features.

Various hereditary and metabolic disorders

These cause chronic tubular damage either by obstructive effects, such as gout, cystinuria and uraemic medullary cystic disease (juvenile nephronophthisis), or by toxic effects such as hypercalcaemia, cystinosis and hypokalaemia (Fig. 10.6). Occasionally myeloma and amyloid are causes of chronic interstitial nephritis. Most of these diagnoses should be straightforward.

Chronic ischaemic damage

Tubules are sensitive to ischaemia and will atrophy if it is prolonged. Histopathologists are familiar with the little depressed areas on the capsular surface of kidneys of virtually all elderly people at autopsy, and these show changes typical of so-called chronic interstitial nephritis (Fig. 10.7). Renal artery stenosis has a more severe effect. Many histopathologists accept that systemic hypertension of the so-called benign type produces similar damage, although there is a view that such hypertension never causes clinically significant renal impairment (Kincaid-Smith 1982). Renal ischaemia can also be produced by drugs such as cyclosporin (McNally & Feehally 1992). There seems little point in using the label chronic interstitial nephritis for ischaemic damage.

Sarcoidosis and tuberculosis

Sarcoidosis can have a few effects on the kidney including hypercalcaemic damage. Granulomas can be found in the kidney in both sarcoidosis and in tuberculosis, and are usually associated with chronic damage (Fig. 10.4).

Miscellaneous

Late glomerular disorders are accompanied by tubular atrophy and other features of so-called chronic interstitial nephritis. Sometimes glomerular diseases such as Alport's hereditary nephropathy are listed as causes of chronic interstitial nephritis. There are many possible explanations for chronic interstitial nephritis in the nephropathy of human immunodeficiency virus infection, and one is the frequent finding of a segmental sclerosing glomerulopathy (D'Agati et al 1989). Irradiation of the kidney and Sjögren's syndrome are among the other causes or associations of chronic interstitial nephritis that are frequently listed.

KEY POINTS FOR CLINICAL PRACTICE

1. Interstitial nephritis is conventionally divided into acute and chronic. This has practical value.

2. Acute interstitial nephritis is a clinically useful diagnosis if confined to morphological changes of an interstitial inflammatory infiltrate of lymphocytes and eosinophils, with acute tubular damage.

3. Acute interstitial nephritis can be associated with reactions to drugs such as non-steroidal anti-inflammatory drugs, infections such as leptospirosis, and systemic diseases such as vasculitis.

4. Chronic interstitial nephritis and chronic tubulo-interstitial nephritis are non-specific terms applied to virtually all late renal diseases and have therefore little use as diagnoses or as guides to nephrologists in management. This is because the mechanisms of chronic damage are similar in many different renal diseases.

5. If possible, the histopathologist should try to determine the specific disease underlying the largely non-specific morphological features of so-called chronic interstitial or tubulo-interstitial nephritis.

REFERENCES

Adu D, Howie A J 1995 Vasculitis in the kidney. Curr Diagn Pathol 2: 73–77

Bennett W M, Walker R G, Kincaid-Smith P 1982 Renal cortical interstitial volume in mesangial IgA nephropathy: dissociation from creatinine clearance in serially biopsied patients. Lab Invest 47: 330–335

Bohle A, Mackensen-Haen S, Gise H 1987 Significance of tubulointerstitial changes in the renal cortex for the excretory function and concentration ability of the kidney: a morphometric contribution. Am J Nephrol 7: 421–433

Bohle A, Christensen J, Kokot F et al 1990 Acute renal failure in man: new aspects concerning pathogenesis. Am J Nephrol 10: 374–388

Bohle A, Wehrmann M, Mackensen-Haen S et al 1994 Pathogenesis of chronic renal failure in primary glomerulopathies. Nephrol Dial Transplant (Suppl 3): 4–12

Bonventre J V 1993 Mechanisms of ischemic acute renal failure. Kidney Int 43: 1160–1178

Cameron J S 1992 Tubular and interstitial factors in the progression of glomerulonephritis. Pediatr Nephrol 6: 292–303

Colvin R B, Fang L S T 1989 Interstitial nephritis. In: Tisher CC, Brenner BM (eds) Renal pathology with clinical and functional correlations. Lippincott, Philadelphia: pp 728–776

D'Agati V, Suh J, Carbone L et al 1989 Pathology of HIV-associated nephropathy: a detailed morphologic and comparative study. Kidney Int 35: 1358–1370

Dale P M 1952 Medical biographies: the ailments of thirty-three famous persons. University of Oklahoma, Norman: pp 127–135

Dodd S M 1995 The pathogenesis of tubulointerstitial disease and mechanisms of fibrosis. Curr Top Pathol 88: 51–67

Fine L G, Ong A C M, Norman J T 1993 Mechanisms of tubulo-interstitial injury in progressive renal diseases. Eur J Clin Invest 23: 259–265

Hall P W, Batuman V 1991 Introduction: Balkan endemic nephropathy. Kidney Int 40 (Suppl 34): 1–3

Heptinstall R H 1992 Pathology of the kidney. 4th edn. Little, Brown, Boston: pp 1315–1368

Howie A J 1994 Morphometric studies of acute renal failure using anti-brush-border and other antisera. Nephrol Dial Transplant 9 (Suppl 4): 37–39

Howie A J, Gunson B K, Sparke J 1990 Morphometric correlates of renal excretory function. J Pathol 160: 245–253

Howie A J, Lee S J, Green N J et al 1993 Different clinico-pathological types of segmental sclerosing glomerular lesions in adults. Nephrol Dial Transplant 8: 590–599

Howie A J, Rowlands D C, Reynolds G M et al 1995 Measurement of proliferation in renal biopsy specimens: evidence of subclinical tubular damage in the nephrotic syndrome. Nephrol Dial Transplant 10: 2212–2218

Kincaid-Smith P S 1982 Renal hypertension. In: Kincaid-Smith PS, Whitworth JA (eds) Hypertension - mechanisms and management. ADIS Health Science, New York, pp 94–101

McNally P G, Feehally J 1992 Pathophysiology of cyclosporin A nephrotoxicity: experimental and clinical observations. Nephrol Dial Transplant 7: 791–804

Nath K A, Fischereder M, Hostetter T H 1994 The role of oxidants in progressive renal injury. Kidney Int 45 (Suppl 45): 111–115

Neilson E G 1989 Pathogenesis and therapy of interstitial nephritis. Kidney Int 35: 1257–1270

Newbold K M, Howie A J 1990 Determinants of glomerular cross-sectional area. J Pathol 162: 329–332

Nuyts G D, Van Vlem E, Thys J et al 1995 New occupational risk factors for chronic renal failure. Lancet 346: 7–11

Papadimitriou M 1995 Hantavirus nephropathy. Kidney Int 48: 887–902

Risdon R A, Sloper J C, De Wardener H E 1968 Relationship between renal function and histological changes found in renal biopsy specimens from patients with persistent glomerular nephritis. Lancet 2: 363–366

Schainuck LI, Striker GE, Cutler RE et al 1970 Structural-functional correlations in renal disease. Part 2: the correlations. Hum Pathol 1: 631–641

Solez K 1992a Acute renal failure (acute tubular necrosis, infarction, and cortical necrosis). In: Heptinstall RH Pathology of the kidney. 4th edn. Little, Brown, Boston: pp1235–1314

Solez K 1992b Renal complications of therapeutic and diagnostic agents, analgesic abuse, and addiction to narcotics. In: Heptinstall RH Pathology of the kidney. 4th edn. Little, Brown, Boston: pp1369–1431

Solez K, Morel–Maroger L, Sraer J 1979 The morphology of 'acute tubular necrosis' in man: analysis of 57 renal biopsies and a comparison with the glycerol model. Medicine 58: 362–376

Solez K, Axelsen R A, Benediktsson H et al 1993 International standardization of criteria for the histologic diagnosis of renal allograft rejection: the Banff working classification of kidney transplant pathology. Kidney Int 44: 411–422

Strutz F, Neilson E G 1994 The role of lymphocytes in the progression of interstitial disease. Kidney Int 45 (Suppl 45): 106–110

Trueta J, Barclay A E, Daniel P M et al 1947 Studies of the renal circulation. Blackwell, Oxford

Wolf G, Neilson E G 1995 Cellular biology of tubulointerstial growth. Curr Top Pathol 88: 69–97

11

The histopathologist and the law

B. H. Knight

Since I last wrote a chapter on this subject in 1987 for the 13th edition of 'Recent Advances', a number of significant developments have occurred which affect the legal aspects of laboratory practice in the United Kingdom. The introduction of so-called 'Crown Indemnity', the advent of National Health Service (NHS) Trusts, and an increase in private pathology practice have all affected matters such as medical negligence and vicarious liability.

Although, compared to ward based clinical disciplines laboratory medicine is still not in the 'front-line' for allegations of malpractice, such problems have steadily increased, especially as some aspects of 'pathology' in the broadest sense have moved nearer the patient and become more interventionist. Haematology in particular throws up an increasing number of problems, and recent errors in cytology and surgical biopsy reporting have led to prominent media interest.

The Medical Protection Society received 206 enquiries from members engaged in laboratory medicine during the four years between 1991–1995. Although many of these were merely requests for information, a number related to allegations of negligence, or concerned a wide spectrum of other problems experienced by doctors in the various branches of pathology.

In addition to purely legal matters, there have been a number of guidelines issued by the Royal College of Pathologists on various matters (usually published in the College Bulletin), as well as dictats from the Department of Health (DOH) and the General Medical Council, some of which have a direct bearing on laboratory practice. Only those with direct relevance to histopathology will be discussed in the following pages.

RETENTION OF REPORTS AND SPECIMENS

A working party of the Royal College of Pathologists reported on this matter in 1995. It pointed out that the DOH has guidance on the preservation, retention and destruction of records (HC89/20) which the Chief Medical Officer has indicated applies also to the preservation of pathological material and other biological samples. The Public Records Act 1959–67 also affect pathology records in that any records more than 60 years old (which may well exist in large hospitals and university departments) cannot be destroyed before the Local Records Office is consulted.

Although the subject is complex and the DOH and College documents should be studied whenever there is any doubt, the following are the minimum recommended times for retention, though in many cases these should be exceeded and permanent retention considered for anything with particular medical or historic interest:

- Request forms – 1 month after the final report has been issued.

- Day books and specimen receipt books – 2 years.

- Protocols of standard procedures– permanent or until procedures are discontinued.

- Laboratory file cards or bench records – 2 years.

- Surgical (histopathology) reports – hard copy lodged in patient's notes. Bound copies kept permanently in the laboratory.

- Post mortem reports – reports lodged in patient's records (but note caution later for Coroners' autopsies). Bound copies of autopsy reports kept permanently.

- Body fluids (eg for cytology) – 48 hours after final report has been issued.

- Wet formalin-fixed tissue – 4 weeks after final report.

- Frozen sections – four weeks after final report.

- Paraffin wax and EM blocks – estimated lifetime of patient or permanently.

- Histology sections – 10 years or permanently if possible.

- Cytology slides – 10 years if abnormal, otherwise five years.

It is not practicable to retain indefinitely all human tissues removed at operation and it is often impossible to foresee which tissues may be needed at a later date for clinical or medico-legal purposes. It is reasonable to keep all tissues for that length of time which allows the clinician in charge of the case to comment on the histological report and permits further samples to be taken if additional clinical problems come to light as a result of that report.

This time period should also enable the clinician to inform the histopathologist of any possible medico-legal complication. When these are foreseen, it is suggested that the unprocessed tissue be kept for a minimum of one year and much longer if possible. If relevant and practicable, a photographic record of the macroscopic appearances should be retained for a minimum of 10 years. Normally a four week period is the minimum time for retention of surgical specimens after the date of issue of the report.

Currently the statutory limit for the initiation of legal actions (usually limited to six years) is often extended, but the great majority of legal actions are initiated within 10 years. It is therefore suggested that blocks and slides should be kept for a minimum of 10 years. Because a significant number of patients return for several biopsies over a much longer period, the current practice of retaining slides for 30 years or even longer is commended.

POSTAL DESPATCH OF PATHOLOGY SPECIMENS

There are strict rules about the transit of pathological samples by post, but in histopathology these are rarely likely to be potentially infective and would consist mostly of paraffin wax blocks, glass slides, and occasionally formalin-fixed wet tissue. Full details were given in the Bulletin of the Royal College of Pathologists in April 1992. Unless the conditions of the 1986 'Post Office Guide' concerning prohibited or restricted articles is adhered to, specimens will be destroyed by the postal authorities. Only First Class or Datapost may be used, not parcel post. Where any potentially leaking liquid is involved which includes formalin, then the container must not exceed 50 ml, which would exclude most larger specimens. The container must be hermetically sealed, such as a heat-sealed plastic bag or a screw-top container. There must be sufficient absorbent material around the primary package to absorb all the fluid contained in the package. The whole must then be placed in a container specified by the regulations.

There are no particular regulations for sending slides and blocks, apart from the common-sense necessity to avoid damage to the specimens.

CONSENT FOR AUTOPSY

The majority of autopsies are now conducted at the direction of the Coroner or Procurator Fiscal, where consent is not required. In the remaining clinical 'consent' autopsies, the legal situation concerning such autopsies must be fully appreciated. Permission is derived from the Human Tissue Act (1961) which also governs the donation of tissues for therapeutic, research and teaching purposes. This Act provides that the person lawfully in possession of the body (usually the hospital authority in the shape of the NHS Trust, District Health Authority or the managers of a private institution) may give consent for an autopsy to be carried out, if having made such reasonable enquiries as may be practicable, is satisfied that:

1. The deceased person had not indicated during life that he or she had objected to a post mortem examination.

2. The surviving spouse or any relative does not object to a post mortem examination.

In practice, these provisions are satisfied by obtaining positive consent from the next-of-kin or a near relative, who signs a printed form to confirm the absence of objection. This form is witnessed by a member of the hospital staff. These forms are not statutory but usually conform to a format devised by the DOH.

There is a sub-section on the form (which can be deleted by the relative if they so desire) which allows the retention of tissues for the purposes of treatment, research and teaching. It should be appreciated that if the section consenting to removal of tissues is deleted, the pathologist cannot retain material other than that related to the investigation of the cause of death or other disease processes found in the body, such as histology, microbiology, virology etc.

Occasionally other clinicians, especially surgeons, wish to practice new operative techniques or otherwise investigate anatomical structures. As no tissue is being removed, the Human Tissue Act is not operative but it would be both unethical and unwise to allow this to be done without the consent of the relatives. Such consent, as with the removal of tissues, must be obtained with sufficient information for the relatives to understand what is proposed to be done. Any transgression of this doctrine of 'informed consent' runs the risk of complaint from the relatives and although there is no legal property in a dead body, the public concern and especially the unwelcome attention of the media (who have a morbid delight in exposing anything to do with mortuaries or dead bodies) makes it very unwise to transgress any ethical boundaries. The Human Tissue Act is somewhat vague in that it does not define 'reasonable enquiries' nor 'relative' but it is interpreted as meaning that there is no need to seek every relative throughout the world and that the signature of a spouse, other next of kin, or executor is satisfactory.

Sometimes, the absence of the next of kin may lead to another relative giving consent and occasionally there is dispute between relatives about the granting of consent. This should be a matter for the hospital administration, not the histopathologist. Some histopathologists have been reluctant to accept doubtful consent though it is unlikely that they could ever suffer any legal consequences, as the permission granted is derived from the Health Authority or Trust, via the Human Tissue Act and not directly to the histopathologist from the relative. The histopathologist cannot be legally responsible as long as a properly signed and witnessed consent form is presented to him or her – though acrimony and adverse publicity might be most unwelcome consequences. With the increased ethnic mix in the UK, notice should be taken of the desires of various religions, though where consent autopsies are concerned, consent is usually withheld by those who object – a different situation from the Coroners' autopsy.

In respect of medico-legal autopsies, the Coroner or Procurator Fiscal directs a histopathologist to carry out an autopsy on his behalf and no consent is involved. The Coroner cannot command a histopathologist to perform an autopsy if the latter does not wish to, though this would be a rare event except where he or she feels that a different type of expert would be more suitable, such as in highly specialized fields, in suspicious or criminal cases or where the professional skill of a clinical colleague in the same hospital has been complained about. Theoretically, the Coroner can order any registered medical practitioner who was in attendance on the deceased before death to carry out an autopsy, but this is an anachronism from former years, as now the Coroners' Rules (1981) indicate that only a histopathologist with proper laboratory facilities should undertake medico-legal autopsies.

Where the death is due to criminal action or is suspicious, or in certain circumstances such as causing death by dangerous driving, the Coroner is advised by his Rules to seek the advice of the Chief Officer of Police as to the most appropriate choice of who should carry out the autopsy. This is almost invariably a Home Office histopathologist of whom there are about 48 in England and Wales, but this is an advisory, not a mandatory provision.

In Scotland, the Procurator Fiscal must seek the authority of the Sheriff if he or she desires an autopsy, but it is the former who actually directs the individual to proceed. If the Procurator Fiscal decides that an autopsy is not required, permission may be requested for a 'consent' examination. In England and Wales, the Coroner cannot object to a consent examination once he or she has declined to accept jurisdiction over a death reported to him or her.

The situation sometimes arises where a clinician requests an autopsy on a patient and obtains a signed consent from relatives, but the histopathologist considers that the case should have been reported to the Coroner or Procurator Fiscal. The histopathologist should try to persuade the clinician to contact the Coroner, but if this advice is not followed, he or she must decide whether to decline the performance of the autopsy or to report it directly. The decision depends upon the facts of the case, but if the cause of death is unknown or totally speculative, or if trauma or some unnatural event may have been a factor in a death, the histopathologist or the clinician should report the death for medico-legal investigation as otherwise an unacceptable death certificate may be rejected by the Registrar and further delay imposed on the bereaved relatives.

REPORTS ON CORONER'S AND PROCURATOR FISCAL AUTOPSIES

In an earlier section about retention of reports, it was indicated that autopsy reports should be filed in the clinical notes of the deceased patient. This is certainly recommended in clinical 'consent' autopsies, but care must be taken with medico-legal autopsies as the report was commissioned by the Coroner or Procurator Fiscal and is their property: the information contained in the report is privy to them.

In sudden natural deaths, there is usually no problem about sending copies of the report to the attending physician or GP and placing a copy in the clinical records, though it is as well to get general agreement from the Coroner or Procurator Fiscal to this routine. If there is to be an inquest or fatal accident enquiry, then the autopsy report should not be placed in the notes or given to the clinician before the court hearing, except with the specific consent of the Coroner or Procurator Fiscal. Some Coroners become extremely irate if, unbeknown to them, doctors, relatives or lawyers appear at the inquest with a copy of the report, as the usual civil and criminal court procedure of disclosure and exchange of documents do not apply to the Coroner's inquest.

RETENTION OF MATERIAL FROM AUTOPSIES

In England and Wales, when a death is reported to the Coroner and that law officer orders an autopsy, the retention of relevant material is not only sanctioned but is mandatory. The Coroner's Rules (1984) state:

A person making a post-mortem examination shall make provision, so far as possible, for the preservation of material which in his opinion bears upon the cause of death, for such period as the Coroner thinks fit.

In most cases, the specific direction of the Coroner to retain such tissues in each case is not necessary and the length of time for which they are to be retained is usually determined by the particular circumstances.

The statutory duty to retain organs and tissues from a Coroner's autopsy strictly applies only to those tissues where further examination is relevant to the cause of death or to an interpretation of the nature of the associated injuries or conditions. It is also intended to preserve relevant material for later examination by another histopathologist acting on behalf of a third party, such as any person accused of causing the death. This duty does not cover incidental lesions unrelated to the nature of the death, though in most instances it can be legitimately argued that all abnormalities must be investigated to determine their relevance.

The retention of material for teaching and research purposes is not covered by the Coroner's permission and indeed, the Coroner cannot grant such permission as it is not within his power to do so. He can forbid the use of tissues for such purposes, but positive permission can be obtained only under the terms of the Human Tissue Act (1961).

Until some years ago the most common example of confusion over such permission was the collection of pituitary glands for the extraction of growth hormone, now made obsolete by synthetic production. In spite of frequent claims to the contrary, the Coroner has no authority to grant permission for the removal of pituitaries or for organs for transplantation – he or she can offer only an absence of objection.

Similarly, there is no power to sanction the use of material for research or teaching purposes. As a significant proportion of the contents of pathology museums come from Coroner's autopsies, these are in the strict terms of the law illegally obtained, as the seeking of consent from the relatives of the subjects of medico-legal autopsies is most uncommon.

Where non-Coroner's autopsies (the so-called 'hospital' cases) are concerned, the retention of tissues is governed by the Human Tissue Act referred to above. This also regulates the obtaining of permission for the autopsy itself and for tissues for transplantation. The procedure has been described in the preceding section and it will be recalled that the standard permission form signed by the next-of-kin has a clause giving additional consent for the removal of limited amounts of tissue for therapeutic use, teaching and research.

If this clause is struck out by the signatory, then obviously no tissue can be removed. However, though it has never been tested in the courts, it would seem reasonable to retain the minute amounts of tissue needed for the preparation of histological sections; this must surely be accepted as part of the general autopsy for which permission has been granted. Nevertheless, cases have occurred in the United States where relatives have insisted that even histological blocks and sections be returned to the body before burial. Retention of whole brains for neuropathological examination may also prove to be a problem in the future as it has happened in Australia in recent years.

PRE-AUTOPSY TESTING FOR HIV AND HEPATITIS

In 1995, some confusion arose over the ethical right to conduct pre-autopsy testing for antibodies to Hepatitis B and C and to HIV virus. This confusion has not yet been totally resolved as the direction published by the General Medical Council (1995) has not been universally accepted. The problem arose because of the increasing incidence of hepatitis and HIV infection, especially in relation to Coroner's and Procurator Fiscal cases from the community. Many histopathologists feel that when the history suggests the possibility of infectivity, this should be made known before the autopsy so that a decision can be made whether or not to proceed, whether to increase the precautions in the autopsy room and to limit access of observers such as police, photographers etc. and perhaps also to modify the choice of anatomical pathology technician (APT) involved in the dissection.

An alternative school of thought holds that all autopsies should be conducted with maximum health and safety procedures as recommended by the Health Services Advisory Committee (1991–92), so that it does not matter whether the cadaver is infected or not. This idealistic view may be difficult to carry out in practice, especially where there is a heavy load of medico-legal autopsies, with a number of tables working in one autopsy room. It also does not solve the problem of choosing the most appropriate APT with experience and of limiting the access to police, scenes of crime officers, photographers etc.

The General Medical Council indicated in their direction that testing for HIV and hepatitis was legitimate if it assisted in determining the cause of death but this is rarely a valid reason, as the mere fact of serological positivity is usually irrelevant in determining the cause of death, especially in most Coroner's and police cases. The advice was also ambiguous in indicating whether pre-autopsy HIV testing was permissible for screening **all** cadavers or whether it should be confined to high-risk groups such as intravenous drug users and homosexuals.

The Royal College of Pathologists issued a report of a working party on 'HIV and the Practice of Pathology' in July 1995 which contains the following advice:

'Pre-autopsy HIV Testing'

Histopathologists are concerned about the likelihood of unknown HIV-positive cadavers being presented for autopsy, either through a hospital request or via the Coroner or Procurator Fiscal. For medico-legal autopsies, the Coroner can grant permission for HIV serology to be done as a test intended to provide information which may assist the histopathologist in making a diagnosis. In hospital autopsies, where permission for autopsy is given by the possessor of the body, a histopathologist can test likewise, since a major role of the autopsy is to establish a diagnosis. Legal opinion obtained by the Royal College of Pathologists and the statements of the General Medical Council are unanimous on this point. Prior consent of relatives is not required when HIV infection is suspected in a cadaver. Discussions are in progress between the GMC and DOH whether histopathologists are justified in testing all cadavers for HIV prior to autopsy. In practice, outside certain risk groups (e.g. known intravenous drug users) there appears to be little epidemiological or economic justification to do this at present.

If the previous unknown HIV-seropositive state of a patient is discovered through testing at autopsy, the duty of care and confidentiality does not cease with the patient's death. If there is a surviving spouse or sexual partner, then a breach of confidentiality is justified by the need to advise him or her of exposure to infection.

In practice such a responsibility usually devolves through the histopathologist to the patient's clinicians.

LIABILITY FOR LABORATORY STAFF

The situation has altered somewhat since 1990 when State Indemnity (sometimes called 'Crown Indemnity') was introduced. A general principle of law is that the master is responsible for the errors of his servants and this applies to the relationship between a hospital authority or Trust and the employed doctors. However, historically in about 1953, soon after the advent of the National Health Service, there was an agreement between the then Ministry of Health and the medical profession that doctors in hospital employ would assume financial responsibility for their own errors in return for clinical freedom. This responsibility was then indemnified by membership of a medical protection or defence organisation.

In 1990, due to the rising costs of indemnity, which were largely subsidised by the NHS, the latter reverted to the usual master-servant relationship, together with the financial implications. This applied only to medical staff of NHS hospitals whilst they were carrying out their contractual functions in the hospital. All other professional activities were excluded, such as general practice, locum work, emergency and 'Good Samaritan' episodes. Also the responsibility of the hospital authority was strictly confined to professional negligence during contractual work and did not extend to professional misconduct, Coroner's enquiries, courts-martial, disputes with employers, etc., for which membership of a protection organisation was still almost mandatory.

In respect of laboratory medicine, this means that all staff, from consultant to cleaner, are directly the responsibility of the hospital Trust or whatever management structure is in place. Though the employer in NHS hospitals now assumes the financial responsibility for malpractice, the plaintiff-patient can sue whom they wish and the doctor or any other member of staff can be joined with the employer as co-defendants.

Though the employer will no longer look to the doctor for a financial contribution, there is still the same responsibility on the head of a laboratory to take all measures to avoid negligent actions by himself or herself and the rest of the staff. Though the consultant is now unlikely to be sued directly, the Trust or other employing agency may well hold him responsible and internal enquiries may be arduous and inimical – and in these days of fixed-term contracts, may well have career consequences. It is therefore imperative that a histopathologist in charge of a department takes the same care to avoid mishaps as when he could be sued directly. The consultant histopathologist's responsibility for the safe working of his department depends upon his having established a satisfactory working regime.

The histopathologist should sanction the appointment only of suitably qualified and experienced staff. Furthermore, a safe and reliable system of working, which would be approved by a substantial body of peers, must be devised and implemented. Not only that, but the histopathologist must ensure that all members of his staff are fully aware of this system of working and that a written code of procedures be provided and measures taken to ensure that every member of staff is fully conversant with such a written code.

This is similar to the requirements for health and safety procedures in laboratory and mortuary, for which the head of department has direct legal responsibility, being liable for criminal penalties of fines and theoretically, even imprisonment, if these are breached and a prosecution results.

In the negligence sphere, the Trust or other employing authority will delegate responsibility to the consultant histopathologist to see that all the staff abide by a written code of procedures in order to minimise the risk of negligent action.

If a consultant has abided by the above measures, then he or she no longer has vicarious liability for errors. As an example, a claim which came to the Medical Protection Society involved a MLSO who erroneously reported a blood type on a pregnant woman. He recorded the Rhesus factor as being positive, though the patient herself knew from a previous pregnancy that she was

Rh negative. She told the consultant obstetrician of the earlier result, but he preferred the evidence of the laboratory report. She later developed antibodies and sued the obstetrician and haematologist. The latter could successfully deny any liability on the grounds that the fully-trained MLSO had not followed the written standing orders for the laboratory.

Sometimes, medical staff will attempt to avoid liability by claiming that shortage of resources was responsible for the error. This might be shortage of suitably qualified staff or specialised equipment, but liability cannot be evaded retrospectively by complaining about the lack of resources after the mishap has occurred. If any doctors feel that lack of resources may lead to a potentially dangerous situation, they must indicate this in full detail and in writing to the employing authority in advance, so that if the expected error occurs they can point to a previous warning. It is emphasised that this cannot be done in retrospect, as not uncommonly has been attempted.

Generally, a histopathologist will be personally responsible for any report which bears his or her signature. For this reason, it is now uncommon for a consultant to sign multiple reports on serial or automated analyses in the specialties other than histopathology. Consultants have a responsibility for doing all they can to ensure that the staff, equipment and methodology are completely satisfactory, but they obviously cannot personally guarantee that every test gives a correct result. It is quite different when they provide an opinion, such as that on a histological section, which they themselves write or dictate and sign.

THE PATHOLOGIST IN PRIVATE PRACTICE

The legal position of pathologists in private practice varies according to their contractual relationships. If they work entirely for themselves, then obviously they will be personally liable in law for everything they and staff employed by them do in a professional capacity. If they are associated with a private hospital or laboratory, the position will vary according to whether they act as salaried employees – when the employers will be liable for negligence – or as contractors, when they will carry their own risks. If there is a mutual association with other doctors, then the laws of partnership will apply and each partner will be jointly and severally liable for the misdeeds of each other. In these circumstances, it is usual for a deed of indemnity to be drawn up between the partners, as in general practice, so that the innocent members can recover from the guilty one any financial loss in the way of damages awarded against the partnership. Naturally, it is imperative to maintain current membership of a medical protection society.

In relation to laboratory staff, the liability of pathologists in private practice depends on their contractual status. If they all are in the employ of a private hospital, then the situation is as stated above for NHS hospitals. If the pathologists run a private laboratory and employ their own staff, then they are undoubtedly vicariously responsible for all their acts and misdeeds, though possibly they could try to recover a contribution from the erring employee in a separate 'third party action', which is hardly likely to succeed if the employee has little wealth and no indemnity.

Outside the NHS, the pathologist has no obligation to belong to a medical protection organisation. However, just as a general practitioner – who is an independent contractor, and not an employee of, the Health Service – would be foolhardy not to obtain complete indemnity, so the pathologist in private practice would be taking a devastating risk by not seeking the cover of a medical protection society or some other form of insurance.

CONSENT FOR DIAGNOSTIC PROCEDURES

In the past, the pathologist tended to be laboratory-bound, the passive recipient of material supplied by clinicians. In haematology, this era has long passed and even the histopathologist now ventures into the wards and clinics to obtain his own diagnostic samples. Though his surgical colleagues still provide most biopsy material, techniques such as needle aspiration, bone marrow biopsy and the removal of lymph nodes may be carried out by the histopathologist.

Any procedure, even the taking of a venous blood sample, must be subsequent to the obtaining of a valid consent from the patient. In clinical practice, most diagnostic measures are carried out on the basis of implied consent. This means that the very fact of a patient presenting in the hospital, clinic or surgery gives tacit permission for the doctor to proceed. However, this implication extends only to preliminary acts such as palpation, percussion and auscultation. Where more complex or intimate procedures are required, the patient must give express consent, ie specific consent for that particular procedure. Often, such permission is gained merely through the courtesies of speech – such as the request, 'Do you mind rolling up your sleeve, as I want to take a sample of blood from your arm?'.

Oral consent is as equally valid as written consent but is much harder to prove if a dispute occurs at a later date. For complex procedures – such as surgical operations and always when a general anaesthetic is to be given – written, witnessed consent must be obtained, though this will rarely concern the pathologist. To be valid, consent must be obtained in the light of a reasonable explanation of what is to be done and a realistic account of substantial risks arising from the procedure – in other words, to be valid, consent must be 'informed'. Again, the magnitude of the minor procedures usually undertaken by pathologists make this aspect much less important than it is to surgeons, but cases have occurred where mishaps in taking blood or during percutaneous biopsy have led to legal proceedings. Examples are untoward reactions, sometimes fatal, from local anaesthetic agents or associated adrenaline; damaged nerve plexuses during removal of lymph nodes; and arterial injury during venepuncture.

The patient should always be told what is to be performed and the reasons for the procedure. It is unrealistic to enumerate the slight risks before proceeding to a venepuncture, for instance puncture of the brachial artery, but patients have sued on the grounds that they were not warned of this risk! Damage to the brachial plexus during the biopsy of a supraclavicular lymph node also gave rise to a negligence action.

Without valid consent, the patient can sue for assault and battery or for negligence in not explaining the risks. Every possible risk does not have to be enumerated and peer review would be used to discover what risks other doctors would have disclosed to their patients in the same circumstances.

MEDICO-LEGAL REPORTS AND STATEMENTS: CONFIDENTIALITY

Most requests made of histopathologists for reports of a medico-legal nature concern autopsies, but depending upon the field of interest of the individual, other matters may require written opinions. Examples include tissue diagnoses in occupational diseases or reports following trauma of many kinds. Whatever the subject of the report, certain guidelines must be followed. The most important relates to medical confidentiality, which persists whether or not the patient is still alive.

When an autopsy is performed for the Coroner or Procurator Fiscal, then the report is at their behest and is privy to them. However, unless criminal proceedings are pending, it is standard practice to give a copy of the report to the medical attendant with the proviso discussed above that reports should not be provided prior to an inquest without the express permission of the Coroner. The relatives or their representative are entitled to a copy, but this should not be provided by the histopathologist: they should apply directly to the Coroner.

In a 'consent' autopsy where the Coroner or Procurator Fiscal is not involved, the autopsy report belongs to the Trust or Health Authority. Whilst every effort should be made to explain and interpret the results to any close relative who desires to know, the actual report should not be handed over. If some legal action against the hospital or a doctor is brought, then there are proper procedures which the family's lawyers can follow. This is no concern to the histopathologist, who should refer any requests for documents to the Trust or Health Authority legal department.

Where a request for a further opinion on an autopsy is received from a solicitor, the histopathologist is entitled to give such opinion if it is obvious that the solicitor has already obtained a copy of the autopsy report from the Coroner or hospital. However, if the letter does not clearly state that the lawyer is acting on behalf of the family of the deceased – he may be acting for the 'opposition' – then no opinion must be given until an affirmative reply is received to a request for confirmation that they indeed represent the next-of-kin.

Similar safeguards must be employed in matters other than autopsy reports, such as further opinions on biopsy reports. Even if another histopathologist requests the loan of sections or blocks, the reasons for his wishing to see them must be established. A number of doctors have recently been admonished by the General Medical Council for carelessly giving reports to solicitors without ensuring that the patient had consented.

If a request is received for an opinion on an autopsy, biopsy or other pathological report which was not originally carried out by the recipient of the request, then no question of confidentiality arises, as the original report will have been supplied by the applicant. However, where such a report comes from a colleague in the same vicinity, it may be a matter of common sense, tact and ethics (rather than strict law) for the second histopathologist to decline to offer a strongly contrary opinion, suggesting to the applicants that they should go further afield to seek another view of the matter.

In the records of the Medical Protection Society there are a number of cases which illustrate the problems relating to confidentiality over histology reports. For instance, a patient complained that notification of her diagnosis of cancer was passed by a pathologist working in a private laboratory to a tumour registry without her consent, from where details appeared in a research publication. Other cases refer to the disclosure of information to overseas lawyers and the undesirability of sending copies of diagnoses of non-notifiable venereal disease to consultants other than the one requesting the investigation.

Once the matter of consent is settled, the form of the report must be considered. Usually, the factual matters set out in an original autopsy report need amplification and interpretation for a lay, legal or police reader. An opinion expressed on the basis of a pathological finding makes the writer an 'expert witness', with a commensurate increase in the fee for the report and for any subsequent attendance at a court hearing. For example, the fact that pulmonary emboli and deep vein thrombosis were present will be converted into an 'expert opinion' if an elaboration is provided about the predisposing factors, such as trauma and immobility.

The pathologist should beware of trespassing too far into clinical opinions, but he is entitled to comment on general medical matters that his past training and experience warrant. The form of the report naturally depends on the nature of the opinion. Where histological matters are concerned, a diagnosis coupled with an opinion about aetiology especially in traumatic and occupational lesions and prognosis might well be offered. In autopsy matters, the field is much broader. Unless the letter of request makes it obvious, it may be advisable to seek more specific instructions as to the points that require clarification.

ALLEGATIONS OF NEGLIGENCE

Patients, their surviving relatives, or their lawyers often make allegations of negligence against doctors, but the proportion of complaints which succeed is relatively small. For such an allegation to be substantiated, the plaintiff (the patient) must show that the defendant (the doctor):

1. Had a duty of care towards the patient;

2. was in breach of that duty;

3. and that the patient suffered damage as a result.

Although these criteria apply just as much to a histopathologist as to a ward clinician, the laboratory-based doctor is in a rather different and usually safer position than his colleagues on the wards. However, in the increasingly common situation of direct contact for the purpose of taking tissue samples and in the area of incorrect diagnosis, the histopathologist may be vulnerable. If a clinician asks a histopathologist to carry out a diagnostic test and the latter negligently gives an erroneous answer then, if the patient suffers damage in the broadest sense through inappropriate actions due to an incorrect laboratory result, it is the pathologist who is liable.

These events are more frequent in the quantitative results generated by haematology and biochemistry departments than in the more descriptive opinions of histopathology and microbiology, but no specialty is exempt. In histopathology, errors of diagnosis – especially in exfoliative cytology – form the largest group of problems. It must be noted that an error of diagnosis in a biopsy is by no means necessarily negligent. There may be a wide range of differing opinion upon a given section, but where the defendant is at variance with a majority of opinion amongst his peers, then his position is weak. However, it must be noted that it is not necessary that unanimous agreement be obtained – it is sufficient to have a substantial number of fellow pathologists who would support the diagnosis, as all such opinions are subjective and are based on experience rather than on absolute criteria. Peer review is the essence of the criterion of negligence: the fact that an expert specialising in some exotic tumour could have named the condition correctly does not make the general histopathologist in a district general hospital negligent because he failed to recognise it – though in certain circumstances, he may be held negligent in not seeking further advice.

By way of illustration, a few examples of allegations of negligence against histopathologists are summarised below. These are cases from the files of the Medical Protection Society.

A histopathologist examined sections from a lump in the breast and an axillary lymph node. The latter showed carcinomatous deposits and, as a result, the patient underwent courses of chemotherapy with distressing side effects. At another hospital, a pelvic mass was removed, which appeared benign. During the investigation of this mass, the previous breast histology was obtained from the first hospital and no malignancy was observed. The original pathologist reviewed the sections and discovered that the lymph node had been cut from a paraffin block of another case and the slide had been mislabelled by the technical staff. Liability had to be admitted, but as the pathologist had instituted a secure system of working which had not been adhered to by the medical laboratory scientific officer, the hospital authorities paid the substantial damages.

In another breast case where the patient took legal action, a histopathologist reported a needle biopsy of a breast mass as an invasive adenocarcinoma. The patient underwent an excision and an axillary clearance, but subsequent examination of the biopsy by another pathologist revealed plasma-cell mastitis related to duct ectasia. Liability had to be accepted by the medical protection organisation on behalf of the first pathologist.

In the case of a woman diagnosed as having a serous cystadenocarcinoma of the ovary, no report was made to the surgeons on an omental biopsy and peritoneal washings taken at operation and the laboratory was blamed for loss of the specimens. Because peritoneal metastatic spread could not be confirmed nor excluded, prophylactic radiotherapy was undertaken, with adverse side effects including loss of hair. However, the system of recording the receipt and disposal of specimens in the laboratory was proved by the histopathologist to be totally reliable and it was accepted that the specimens could never have arrived from the operating theatre.

Cervical cytology provides a number of complaints by patients. In one, taken during pregnancy because of an erosion, the smear was reported as 'slightly atypical' and a repeat recommended after parturition. No communication was made of this to either the patient or her general practitioner. A further smear was taken later due to bleeding, when the cervix looked 'suspicious'. This was reported as being 'badly fixed' but negative for abnormal cells. Later a cervical wart was found but was not biopsied. It was two years from the date of the first smear that malignant cells were finally reported. Such a history is unfortunate but negligence would be hard to prove given the limitations of cervical cytology.

Over the years, the records of the protection and defence organisations reveal a small but significant number of errors over biopsies and cytology, the latter providing more legal problems than the former. As in many other medical mishaps, human errors over the identification of specimens, labelling and transposition and the failure to deliver reports are more frequent than professional incompetence.

However, an action for negligence was brought against a histopathologist recently by a senior medical laboratory scientific officer who had contracted pulmonary tuberculosis after assisting at an autopsy on a deceased patient suffering from the disease. The grounds for the action was that no special precautions against infection were observed, though the patient had had liver biopsies taken several days before death. The histopathologist had taken no steps to ascertain whether these biopsies revealed the presence of infection, which in the event turned out to be a particularly fulminating variety of tuberculosis. The histopathologist considered that the liver biopsies showed histiocytosis and not tuberculosis and he did not institute strict safety measures during the autopsy. The claim eventually lapsed, so no conclusion was reached as to liability.

As indicated at the beginning of this chapter, the medical protection and defence organisations receive many approaches each year from doctors involved in laboratory medicine. These cover a wide spectrum of issues and most do not concern allegations of negligence; however, such allegations are by no means infrequent, including a number involving histopathology. It is of interest to examine the most recent four-year period from the records of the Medical Protection Society, which has over 140 000 members in many parts of the world.

Between March 1991 and March 1995, there were 206 requests from doctors in laboratory medicine, of which 43 concerned errors in surgical histology and cytology and 15 involved autopsies and Coroner's work. As this period was after the introduction of 'State Indemnity', these numbers probably excluded most from British NHS hospitals and thus the true number of problems in the UK is almost certainly far greater. The allegations of errors in biopsies followed a pattern similar to an analysis of previous years. The 36 cases involved misdiagnosis of:

Melanomas and naevi	13
Hodgkin's and other lymphomas	5
Carcinoma of breast	4
Carcinoma of uterus	2
Carcinoma of stomach	2
Miscellaneous	10

The 'miscellaneous' cases included a chondrosarcoma, a trophoblastic neoplasm, a pelvic tumour, a prostatitis misdiagnosed as cancer, and several unspecified errors, including two allegations of incompetence by colleagues. In seven complaints about cytology, four were false-negative screening errors and several involved delegated responsibility to MLSOs, as well as three recall system faults, one resulting in death due to delayed diagnosis.

In relation to autopsies many diverse concerns were recorded, from Buddhist complaints about mortuary procedures to delays in providing reports to Coroners. Relatives complained about autopsy consent and several Coroners developed bad relationships with their histopathologists. There was even one allegation of assault upon a histopathologist by a Coroner's officer. Many contacts with the Medical Protection Society from laboratory doctors concerned administrative matters such as Category II work, problems with delegation of duties to MLSOs, sexual harassment, and a number involved problems with confidentiality of reports – several concerning the fax transmission of reports. Several defamation allegations occurred between colleagues, and there was a host of terms of service queries which made it obvious that in spite of the advent of State Indemnity, continued membership of a protection or defence organisation is as essential as ever.

KEY POINTS FOR CLINICAL PRACTICE

1. Adhere closely to guidelines for retention of specimens, slides, blocks and reports.

2. In equivocal biopsies, obtain a range of opinions from other histopathologists.

3. Never delegate duties unless you are confident that the delegatee has sufficient experience and ability.

4. Have written protocols for all technical procedures and ensure that your staff confirms to you that they are aware of them.

5. Never begin an autopsy until you have confirmed the identity of the deceased and that either written consent has been obtained or that the Coroner or Procurator Fiscal has authorised the examination.

6. If you consider that a shortfall in resource allocation gives rise to a potentially unsafe or unsatisfactory system of working, notify the Trust or other employing authority in writing in advance of any untoward event occurring.

REFERENCES

Royal College of Pathologists, Marks and Spencer Publications Unit 1995. The retention and storage of pathological records and Archives. Royal College of Pathologists, London.
Department of Health, Health Circular HC89/20 1989
Preservation, retention and destruction of records, responsibilities of health authorities under the Public Records Acts. Department of Health, London
Public Records Acts 1959–67. HMSO, London
Searle S J 1992 Pathological specimens in the post; articles sent for medical examination or analysis. Bull Roy Coll Pathol 78: 16–17
Human Tissue Act 1961. HMSO, London or in Cadaveric organs for transplantation – a code of practice including the diagnosis of brain death. 1983, Department of Health, London. pp. 30–33
Coroner's Rules 1984. HMSO, London
General Medical Council 1995: Testing deceased patients for communicable diseases before post-mortem. Bull Roy Coll Pathol 89: 4–5
Health Services Advisory Committee: safe working and the preparation of infection in the mortuary and post-mortem room. FM6 – 1991–92. Health and Safety Commission, London
Royal College of Pathologists, Marks and Spencer Publications Unit, 1995. HIV and the practice of pathology – report of the Working Party of the Royal College of Pathologists, London

Index